D0713604

PROCEDURES MANUAL
to Accompany

DENTAL HYGIENE
Theory and Practice

PROCEDURES MANUAL
to Accompany

DENTAL HYGIENE
Theory and Practice

Michele Leonardi Darby, BSDH, MS
Eminent Scholar, University Professor, Graduate Program Director
Gene W. Hirschfeld School of Dental Hygiene
College of Health Sciences
Old Dominion University
Norfolk, Virginia

Margaret M. Walsh, RDH, MS, MA, EdD
Professor
Department of Preventive and Restorative Dental Sciences
School of Dentistry
University of California–San Francisco
San Francisco, California

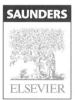

SAUNDERS

ELSEVIER

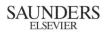

11830 Westline Industrial Drive
St. Louis, Missouri 63146

PROCEDURES MANUAL TO ACCOMPANY DENTAL HYGIENE: THEORY AND PRACTICE   ISBN: 978-1-4160-6100-7

Copyright © 2010 by Saunders, an imprint of Elsevier Inc.

All rights reserved. No part of this publication may be reproduced or transmitted in any form or by any means, electronic or mechanical, including photocopy, recording, or any information storage and retrieval system, without permission in writing from the publisher.

Permission is hereby granted to reproduce the *procedures and client education handouts* in this publication in complete pages, with the copyright notice, for instructional use and not for resale.

Although for mechanical reasons all pages of this publication are perforated, only those pages imprinted with an Elsevier Inc. copyright notice are intended for removal.

Permissions may be sought directly from Elsevier's Rights Department: phone: (+1) 215 239 3804 (US) or (+44) 1865 843830 (UK); fax: (+44) 1865 853333; e-mail: healthpermissions@elsevier.com. You may also complete your request on-line via the Elsevier website at http://www.elsevier.com/permissions.

Notice

Knowledge and best practice in this field are constantly changing. As new research and experience broaden our knowledge, changes in practice, treatment and drug therapy may become necessary or appropriate. Readers are advised to check the most current information provided (i) on procedures featured or (ii) by the manufacturer of each product to be administered, to verify the recommended dose or formula, the method and duration of administration, and contraindications. It is the responsibility of the practitioner, relying on their own experience and knowledge of the patient, to make diagnoses, to determine dosages and the best treatment for each individual patient, and to take all appropriate safety precautions. To the fullest extent of the law, neither the Publisher nor the Authors assume any liability for any injury and/or damage to persons or property arising out of or related to any use of the material contained in this book.

The Publisher

ISBN: 978-1-4160-6100-7

Vice President and Publisher: Linda Duncan
Senior Editor: John J. Dolan
Managing Editor: Kristin Hebberd
Developmental Editor: Brian S. Loehr
Publishing Services Manager: Patricia Tannian
Senior Project Manager: Kristine Feeherty
Design Direction: Maggie Reid

Working together to grow
libraries in developing countries

www.elsevier.com | www.bookaid.org | www.sabre.org

ELSEVIER   BOOK AID International   Sabre Foundation

Printed in the United States of America

Last digit is the print number: 9 8 7 6 5 4 3 2 1

PREFACE

The dental hygienist must master core clinical procedures to achieve clinical competence. These procedures are often complex and multifaceted, and they require significant study and practice to master. The purpose of this manual is to place the essential information and tools dental hygienists need for chairside practice into an organized and handy reference manual that holds a vital place within the clinical environment. Both dental hygiene students and practitioners can quickly and easily glean valuable instruction and client education information, making this book a must-have for any practitioner.

AUDIENCE

This manual is designed to assist all levels of dental hygienist—from students gaining experience in the clinical realm to expert practitioners who have been working with clients for years. Users can consult this book within the healthcare environment for a refresher on procedures; for information, advice, and tips on specific oral health issues (including the effects of certain diseases and conditions, communication, care and prevention, and documentation); and for handy client education materials, the latter of which are easily reproducible.

ORGANIZATION

The manual has three discrete parts, as follows:
- Part I: Dental Hygiene Procedures
- Part II: Client Education Handouts
- Part III: Assessment, Evaluation, and Client Care Resources

In addition, the parts are preceded by two documents foundational to the practice of dental hygiene:
1. *Standards for Clinical Dental Hygiene Practice*
2. *American Dental Hygienists' Association Code of Ethics for Dental Hygienists*

CONTENT

- *Detailed Procedures:* Approximately 85 procedures contain step-by-step descriptions with information about the steps, material, and equipment necessary to master them. Rationales are included to ensure that the dental hygienist comprehends the science underlying each step, as are all associated illustrations and tables to ensure that the reader has quick access to all the information.
- *Client Education Handouts:* Approximately 40 educational materials cover a wide variety of common and specialty issues about which dental hygienists must educate clients with whom they work. Three main divisions—(1) general dentistry, (2) pediatric dentistry, and (3) periodontics—tackle topics such as missing teeth, oral malodor, a child's first visit to the dentist, and periodontal disease. Certain handouts contain associated artwork to help clients visualize many dental procedures and diseases.
- *Assessment, Evaluation, and Client Care Resources:* This section contains a variety of useful summary tables and boxes from the text, organized into 10 subsections that address communication, documentation, care and prevention, and the special needs of certain clients, among others. Many of the materials within this section can also be used as educational resources.
- *Foundational Documents:* The American Dental Hygienists' Association *Code of Ethics for Dental Hygienists* forms a framework around which the dental hygienist makes everyday decisions, whereas the *Standards of Clinical Dental Hygiene Practice* is the basis for clinical excellence and managing legal risks. These two documents are foundational to the profession and as part of the manual.

FEATURES

- Procedures include step-by-step detail with simple, clear illustrations and rationales.
- Client education handouts and physical assessment, communication, and oral care management resources provide tips and advice—targeted resources for the educator and advocacy roles of the dental hygienist in the prevention of oral diseases.
- Spiral binding and perforated pages make this a portable and easy-to-use manual for chairside reference.

Michele Leonardi Darby
Margaret M. Walsh

To my parents, for their unwavering focus on what really matters in life.
To my husband, Dennis, and our children, Devan and Blake, for making everything worthwhile.
MLD

To the memory of my parents, who gave me so much love and support over the years,
and to Jerry and T.J., for their love and encouragement.
MMW

This work is dedicated to the next generation of dental hygiene students and
practitioners who will improve the health of all people worldwide.

CONTENTS

Standards for Clinical Dental Hygiene Practice

INTRODUCTION

One hallmark of a true profession is its willingness to assume responsibility for the quality of care that its members provide. In 1985, the American Dental Hygienists' Association (ADHA) took a major step toward fulfillment of that responsibility with the development of *Applied Standards of Clinical Dental Hygiene Practice.*[1] This document builds on those Standards and promotes dental hygiene practice based on current and relevant scientific evidence.

The *Standards for Clinical Dental Hygiene Practice* outlined in this document guide the individual dental hygienist's practice, whereas the *Accreditation Standards for Dental Hygiene Education Programs*[2] are chiefly concerned with the structure and conduct of dental hygiene education programs. Dental hygienists remain individually accountable to the standards set by the discipline and by applicable federal, state, and local statutes and regulations that define and guide professional practice.[3,4] These *Standards* should not be considered as a substitute for professional clinical judgment.

In the context of an evolving healthcare system for the twenty-first century, dental hygienists are valued members of the healthcare workforce. Dental hygienists have the knowledge, skills, and professional responsibility to provide oral health promotion and health protection strategies for individuals as well as groups. These updated *Standards* for clinical dental hygiene practice outline the expectations of the professional role within which dental hygienists should practice. These *Standards* promote the knowledge, attitudes, beliefs, practices, and behaviors that support and enhance oral health with the ultimate goal of improving overall health.

The primary purpose of the *Standards for Clinical Dental Hygiene Practice* is to assist dental hygiene clinicians in the provider-patient relationship. In addition, dental hygienists employed in other professional roles such as educator, researcher, advocate, and administrator/manager can use these *Standards* to facilitate the implementation of collaborative, patient-centered care in multidisciplinary teams of health professionals. This collaboration can occur in a variety of practice settings including community and public health centers, hospitals, school-based programs, long-term care facilities, outreach, and home care programs. The secondary purpose of these *Standards* is to educate other healthcare providers, policy makers, and the public about the clinical practice of dental hygiene.

The purpose of medical and dental science is to enhance the health of individuals as well as populations. Dental hygienists use scientific evidence in the oral healthcare decision-making process impacting their patient care. The dental hygienist is expected to respect the diverse values, beliefs, and cultures present in individuals and groups or communities served. In working with patients, dental hygienists must support the right of the individual to have access to the necessary information and provide opportunities for dialogue to allow the individual patient to make informed care decisions without coercion. Facilitating effective communication may require an interpreter and/or translator based on the patient and practitioner's need to communicate. Dental hygienists must realize and establish their professional privileges in accordance with the rights of individuals and groups. In addition, when participating in activities where decisions are made that have an impact on health, dental hygienists are obligated to assure that ethical and legal issues are addressed as part of the decision-making process. Dental hygienists are bound by the ethical provisions of the American Dental Hygienists' Association.[3]

The *Standards for Clinical Dental Hygiene Practice* provide a framework for clinical practice that focuses on the provision of patient-centered comprehensive care. The *Standards* describe a competent level of dental hygiene care[2,5-7] as demonstrated by the critical thinking model known as the process of care. As noted in various dental hygiene textbooks,[6,7] the five components of the dental hygiene process of care include assessment, dental hygiene diagnosis, planning, implementation, and evaluation. The dental hygiene process encompasses all significant actions taken by dental hygienists and forms the foundation of clinical decision making. This document expands the process to include a sixth component, documentation.

DEFINITION OF DENTAL HYGIENE PRACTICE

Dental hygiene is the science and practice of the recognition, treatment, and prevention of oral diseases.[6] The dental hygienist is a preventive oral health professional who has graduated from an accredited dental hygiene program in an institution of higher education, licensed in dental hygiene, who provides educational, clinical, research, administrative, and therapeutic services supporting total health through the promotion of optimal oral health.[7] In practice, dental hygienists integrate the roles of clinician, educator, advocate, manager, and researcher to prevent oral diseases and promote health.

Dental hygienists work in partnership with dentists. Dentists and dental hygienists practice together as colleagues, each offering professional expertise for the goal of providing optimum oral healthcare to the public. The distinct roles of the dental hygienist and dentist complement and augment the effectiveness of each professional and contributes to a cotherapist environment. Dental hygienists are viewed as experts in their field, are consulted about appropriate dental hygiene interventions, are expected to make clinical dental hygiene decisions, and are expected to plan, implement, and evaluate the dental hygiene component of the overall care plan.[8] The dental hygienist establishes the dental hygiene diagnosis, which is an integral component of the comprehensive dental diagnosis established by the dentist.

Reprinted from American Dental Hygienists' Association: *Standards for clinical dental hygiene practice,* Chicago, 2008 (March 10), Author.

Each state has defined its own specific regulations for dental hygiene licensure. Depending on the state regulations, dental hygienists:

- Perform oral healthcare and risk assessments that include the review of patients' health history, taking and recording blood pressure, dental and periodontal charting, oral cancer screening, and evaluation of oral disease/health;
- Evaluate a patient's current health status including all medications;
- Perform an extraoral and intraoral examination and oral cancer screening;
- Complete a comprehensive dental and periodontal charting that includes a detailed description and evaluation of the gingiva and periodontium;
- Develop a dental hygiene diagnosis[2, 5-10] (as a component of the dental diagnosis) based on the oral health findings;
- Expose, process, and interpret dental radiographs (x-rays);
- Remove biofilm plaque and calculus (soft and hard deposits) from teeth both coronal and apical to (above and below) the gingival margin (gumline) using dental instruments;
- Apply caries-preventive agents such as fluorides and sealants to the teeth;
- Discuss the progress being made toward isolating evidence that notes the potential association between systemic and oral health and disease;
- Administer local controlled and sustained release antimicrobial agents;
- Administer pain control agents such as local anesthetic and /or nitrous oxide analgesia;
- Provide patient education on biofilm plaque control and home care protocol by incorporating techniques and products that will become part of an individualized self-care oral hygiene program;
- Counsel and coordinate tobacco cessation programs; and
- Educate patients on the importance of good nutrition for maintaining optimal oral health.[11]

EDUCATIONAL PREPARATION

The registered dental hygienist (RDH) or licensed dental hygienist (LDH) is educationally prepared for practice upon graduation from an accredited dental hygiene program (certificate, associate, or baccalaureate) within an institution of higher education and qualified by successful completion of a national written board examination and state or regional clinical examination for licensure. In 1986, the ADHA declared its intent to establish the baccalaureate degree as the minimum entry level for dental hygiene practice.[11,12]

PRACTICE SETTING

Dental hygienists can apply their professional knowledge and skills in a variety of public and private work settings as clinicians, educators, researchers, administrators, managers, health advocates, and consultants. Clinical dental hygienists

Reprinted from American Dental Hygienists' Association: *Standards for clinical dental hygiene practice,* Chicago, 2008 (March 10), Author.

may be employed in a variety of healthcare settings including private dental offices, schools, public health clinics, hospitals, managed care organizations, correctional institutions, or nursing homes.[6,7]

PROFESSIONAL RESPONSIBILITIES AND CONSIDERATIONS

Dental hygienists are responsible and accountable for their dental hygiene practice, conduct, and decision making. Throughout their professional career in any practice setting a dental hygienist is expected to:

- Understand and adhere to the ADHA Code of Ethics.
- Maintain a current license to practice including certifications as appropriate.
- Demonstrate respect for the knowledge, expertise, and contributions of dentists, dental hygienists, dental assistants, dental office staff, and other healthcare professionals.
- Articulate the roles and responsibilities of the dental hygienist to the patient, interdisciplinary team members, referring providers, and others.
- Apply problem-solving processes in decision-making and evaluate these processes.
- Demonstrate a professional image and demeanor.
- Maintain compliance with established infection control standards following the most current guidelines to reduce the risks of healthcare-associated infections in patients, and illnesses and injuries in healthcare personnel.
- Recognize diversity. Incorporate cultural and religious sensitivity in all professional interactions.
- Access and use current, valid, and reliable evidence in clinical decision making through analyzing and interpreting the literature and other resources.
- Maintain awareness of changing trends in dental hygiene, health, and society that impact dental hygiene care.
- Support the dental hygiene profession through ADHA membership.
- Interact with peers and colleagues to create an environment that supports collegiality and teamwork.
- Take action to prevent situations where patient safety and well-being could potentially be compromised.
- Contribute to a safe, supportive, and professional work environment.
- Participate in activities to enhance and maintain continued competence, and address professional issues as determined by appropriate self-assessment.
- Commit to lifelong learning to maintain competence in an evolving healthcare system.

DENTAL HYGIENE PROCESS OF CARE

The purpose of the dental hygiene process of care is to provide a framework where the individualized needs of the patient can be met, and to identify the causative or influencing factors of a condition that can be reduced, eliminated, or prevented by the dental hygienist.[6,7] There are five components to the dental hygiene process of care (assessment, dental hygiene diagnosis, planning, implementation, and evaluation). This document expands the process to include a sixth component, documentation.

The dental hygiene diagnosis is a key component of the process and involves assessment of the data collected, consultation with the dentist and other healthcare providers, and informed decision making. The dental hygiene diagnosis and care plan are incorporated into the comprehensive plan that includes restorative, cosmetic, and oral health needs that the patient values. The dental hygienist is a licensed professional who is responsible for making informed, evidence-based decisions and is accountable for his/her actions.[8] All components of the process of care are interrelated and depend upon ongoing assessments and evaluation of treatment outcomes to determine the need for change in the care plan. These *Standards* follow the dental hygiene process of care to provide a structure for clinical practice that focuses on the provision of patient-centered comprehensive care.

STANDARDS OF PRACTICE

Standard 1: Assessment

Assessment is the systematic collection, analysis, and documentation of the oral and general health status and patient needs. The dental hygienist conducts a thorough, individualized assessment of the person with or at risk for oral disease or complications. The assessment process requires ongoing collection and interpretation of relevant data. A variety of methods may be used including radiographs, diagnostic tools, and instruments.

I. Patient History

a. Record personal profile information such as demographics, values and beliefs, cultural influences, knowledge, skills, and attitudes.
b. Record current and past dental and dental hygiene oral health practices.
c. Collection of health history data includes the patient's:
  1. current and past health status
  2. diversity and cultural considerations (e.g., age, gender, religion, race, ethnicity)
  3. pharmacologic considerations (e.g., prescription, recreational, over the counter [OTC], herbal)
  4. additional considerations (e.g., mental health, learning disabilities, phobias, economic status)
  5. record vital signs and compare with previous readings
  6. consultation with appropriate healthcare provider(s) as indicated

II. Perform a Comprehensive Clinical Evaluation, which Includes

a. A thorough examination of the head and neck and oral cavity including an oral cancer screening, evaluation of trauma, and a temporomandibular joint (TMJ) assessment
b. Evaluation for further diagnostics including radiographs
c. A comprehensive periodontal evaluation that includes the documentation of:
  1. Full mouth periodontal charting
    - Probing depths
    - Bleeding points
      - Suppuration
      - Mucogingival relationships/defects
      - Recession
      - Attachment level/attachment loss
  2. Presence, degree, and distribution of plaque and calculus
  3. Gingival health/disease
  4. Bone height/bone loss
  5. Mobility and fremitus
  6. Presence, location, and extent of furcation involvement
d. A comprehensive hard tissue evaluation that includes the charting of existing conditions and oral habits
  1. demineralization
  2. caries
  3. defects
  4. sealants
  5. existing restorations and potential needs
  6. anomalies
  7. occlusion
  8. fixed and removable prostheses
  9. missing teeth

III. Risk Assessment

Risk assessment is a qualitative and quantitative evaluation gathered from the assessment process to identify any risks to general and oral health. The data provides the clinician with the information to develop and design strategies for preventing or limiting disease and promoting health.

Examples of factors that should be evaluated to determine the level of risk (high, moderate, low):
a. Fluoride exposure
b. Tobacco exposure including smoking, smokeless/spit tobacco, and second-hand smoke
c. Nutrition history and dietary practices
d. Systemic diseases/conditions (e.g., diabetes, cardiovascular disease, autoimmune)
e. Prescriptions and OTC medications, and complementary therapies and practices (e.g., fluoride; herbal, vitamin, and other supplements; daily aspirin)
f. Salivary function and xerostomia
g. Age and gender
h. Genetics and family history
i. Habitual and lifestyle behaviors
  - Cultural issues
  - Substance abuse (recreational drugs, alcohol)
  - Eating disorders
  - Piercing and body modification
  - Oral habits (citrus, toothpicks, lip/cheek biting)
  - Sports and recreation
j. Physical disability
k. Psychological and social considerations
  - Domestic violence
  - Physical, emotional, or sexual abuse
  - Behavioral
  - Psychiatric
  - Special needs
  - Literacy
  - Economic
  - Stress
  - Neglect

Reprinted from American Dental Hygienists' Association: *Standards for clinical dental hygiene practice*, Chicago, 2008 (March 10), Author.

Standard 2: Dental Hygiene Diagnosis

The dental hygiene diagnosis is a component of the overall dental diagnosis. The dental hygiene diagnosis is the identification of an existing or potential oral health problem that a dental hygienist is educationally qualified and licensed to treat.[2,5-10,13-15] The dental hygiene diagnosis requires analysis of all available assessment data and the use of critical decision-making skills in order to reach conclusions about the patient's dental hygiene treatment needs.[5-7,15]

    I. Analyze and interpret all assessment data to evaluate clinical findings and formulate the dental hygiene diagnosis.

    II. Determine patient needs that can be improved through the delivery of dental hygiene care.

    III. Incorporate the dental hygiene diagnosis into the overall dental treatment plan.

Standard 3: Planning

Planning is the establishment of goals and outcomes based on patient needs, expectations, values, and current scientific evidence. The dental hygiene plan of care is based on assessment findings and the dental hygiene diagnosis. The dental hygiene treatment plan is integrated into the overall dental treatment plan. Dental hygienists make clinical decisions within the context of ethical and legal principles.

    I. Identify, prioritize, and sequence dental hygiene intervention (e.g., education, treatment, referral).

    II. Coordinate resources to facilitate comprehensive quality care (e.g., current technologies, pain management, adequate personnel, appropriate appointment sequencing, time management).

    III. Collaborate with the dentist and other health/dental care providers and community-based oral health programs.

    IV. Present and document dental hygiene care plan to patient.

    V. Explain treatment rationale, risks, benefits, anticipated outcomes, treatment alternatives, and prognosis.

    VI. Obtain and document informed consent and/or informed refusal.

Standard 4: Implementation

Implementation is the delivery of dental hygiene services based on the dental hygiene care plan in a manner minimizing risk and optimizing oral health.

    I. Review and implement the dental hygiene care plan with the patient/caregiver.

    II. Modify the plan as necessary and obtain consent.

    III. Communicate with patient/caregiver appropriate for age, language, culture, and learning style.

    IV. Confirm the plan for continuing care.

Standard 5: Evaluation

Evaluation is the process of reviewing and documenting the outcomes of dental hygiene care. Evaluation occurs throughout the process of care.

    I. Use measurable assessment criteria to evaluate the outcomes of dental hygiene care (e.g., probing, plaque control, bleeding points, retention of sealants).

    II. Communicate to the patient, dentist, and other health/dental care providers the outcomes of dental hygiene care.

    III. Collaborate to determine the need for additional diagnostics, treatment, referral, education, and continuing care based on treatment outcomes and self-care behaviors.

Standard 6: Documentation

Documentation is the complete and accurate recording of all collected data, treatment planned and provided, recommendations, and other information relevant to patient care and treatment.

    I. Documents all components of the dental hygiene process of care (assessment, dental hygiene diagnosis, planning, implementation, and evaluation)

    II. Objectively records all information and interactions between the patient and the practice (e.g., telephone calls, emergencies, prescriptions)

    III. Records legible, concise, and accurate information (e.g., dates and signatures, clinical information that subsequent providers can understand, ensure all components of the patient record are accurately labeled)

    IV. Recognizes ethical and legal responsibilities of record keeping including guidelines outlined in state regulations and statutes

    V. Ensures compliance with the federal Health Information Portability and Accountability Act (HIPAA)

    VI. Respects and protects the confidentiality of patient information

SUMMARY

The *Standards for Clinical Dental Hygiene Practice* is a resource for dental hygiene practitioners seeking to provide patient-centered and evidence-based care. In addition, dental hygienists are encouraged to enhance their knowledge and skill base to maintain continued competence. It is expected these *Standards* will be modified based on emerging scientific evidence, federal and state regulations, and changing disease patterns as well as other factors to assure quality care and safety.

KEY TERMS

Cultural and religious sensitivity: the ability to adjust one's perceptions, behaviors, and practice styles to effectively meet the needs of different ethnic, racial, or religious groups.[16]

Dental hygiene care plan: an organized presentation or list of interventions to promote the health or prevent disease of the patient's/client's oral condition; plan is designed by dental hygienist and consists of services that the dental hygienist is educated and licensed to provide.[5]

Evidence-based care: the integration of best research evidence with clinical expertise and patient values.[17]

Intervention: dental hygiene services rendered to clients as identified in the dental hygiene care plan. These services may be clinical, educational, or health-promotion related.

Reprinted from American Dental Hygienists' Association: *Standards for clinical dental hygiene practice,* Chicago, 2008 (March 10), Author.

Multidisciplinary teams: a group of healthcare professionals and their clients who work together to achieve shared goals. The team can consist of the dental hygienist, dentists, physician, nutritionist, smoking cessation counselor, nurse practitioner, etc.

Outcome: result derived from a specific intervention or treatment.

Patient: refers to the potential or actual recipients of dental hygiene care and includes persons, families, groups, and communities of all ages, genders, sociocultural, and economic states.

Patient-centered: approaching services from the perspective that the client is the main focus of attention, interest, and activity; the client's values, beliefs, and needs are of utmost importance in providing care.

Risk: a characteristic, behavior, or exposure that is associated with a particular disease; for example, smoking, diabetes, or poor oral hygiene.

REFERENCES

1. Standard of Applied Dental Hygiene Practice. Chicago, Ill. American Dental Hygienists' Association. 1985.
2. Accreditation Standards for Dental Hygiene Education Programs. Chicago, Ill. American Dental Association. Commission on Dental Accreditation. Revised January 2006.
3. Code of Ethics (2007-2008). Chicago, Ill. American Dental Hygienists' Association. http://www.adha.org/downloads/ADHA-Bylaws-Code-of-Ethics.pdf
4. Martin C, Daly A, McWhorter LS, Shwide-Slavine C, Kushion W. The Scope of Practice, Standards of Practice, and Standards of Professional Performance for Diabetes Educators. *Diabetes Educ.* 2005;31(4):487-512.
5. Competencies for Entry into the Profession of Dental Hygiene. *J Dent Educ.* 2004;68(7):745-9.
6. Policy Manual [Glossary, 4S-94/19-84]. Chicago, Ill. American Dental Hygienists' Association. http://www.adha.org/downloads/ADHA_Policies.pdf
7. Policy Manual [Glossary, 5S-94/19-84]. Chicago, Ill. American Dental Hygienists' Association. http://www.adha.org/downloads/ADHA_Policies.pdf
8. Darby ML, Walsh MM. *Dental Hygiene Theory and Practice.* 2nd ed. St. Louis, Mo: Saunders; 2003:2, 9, 314-217.
9. Wilkins EM. *Clinical Practice of the Dental Hygienist.* 9th ed. Philadelphia, Pa: Lippincott Williams & Wilkins; 2005:3-6, 14, 348.
10. Dental Hygiene Diagnosis [position paper]. Chicago, Ill. American Dental Hygienists' Association. http://www.adha.org/governmental_affairs/downloads/DHDx_position_paper.pdf
11. Policy Manual. Chicago, Ill. American Dental Hygienists' Association. Division of Education. http://www.adha.org/downloads/ADHA_Policies.pdf
12. Focus on Advancing the Profession. Chicago, Ill. American Dental Hygienists' Association. 2005 13. Dental Hygiene: Definition, Scope, and Practice Standards. Ottawa, ON. Canadian Dental Hygienists' Association. 2002
13. Accreditation Requirements for Dental Hygiene Programs [Standard 2.3.3]. Ottawa, ON. The Canadian Dental Association. Commission on Dental Accreditation of Canada. 2007.
14. Mueller-Joseph L, Peterson M. *Dental Hygiene Process: Diagnosis and Care Planning.* Albany, NY: Delmar Publishers; 1995:1-16, 46-63.
15. Health Careers Opportunity Program Definitions. HRSA Bureau of Health Professions. Washington, DC. US Department of Health and Human Services. http://bhpr.hrsa.gov/diversity/definitions.htm
16. Sackett DL, Haynes RB, Straus SE, Richardson WS. *Evidence-Based Medicine: How to Practice and Teach EBM.* 2nd ed. Edinburgh: Churchill Livingstone; 2000.

RESOURCES

Accreditation Standards for Dental Hygiene Education Programs. (1998). Chicago, IL: Commission on Dental Accreditation.

Policy Manual, Glossary, 18-96. Chicago, IL: American Dental Hygienists' Association.

American Dental Hygienists' Association, Education and Careers, http://www.adha.org/careerinfo/index.html, Accessed: January 15, 2008.

American Dental Hygienists' Association, *Smoking Cessation Initiative: Ask.Advise.Refer:* http://www.askadviserefer.org/.

Compendium of Curriculum Guidelines, Allied Dental Education Programs. (2005).Washington, D.C.: American Dental Education Association.

American Academy of Public Health Dentistry: http://www.aaphd.org/.

American Academy of Pediatric Dentistry: http://www.aapd.org/.

American Academy of Periodontology: http://perio.org/.

American Dental Association: http://www.ada.org/.

American Diabetes Association: http://www.diabetes.org/.

American Heart Association: http://www.americanheart.org/.

Association of State and Territorial Dental Directors: http://www.astdd.org/.

Canadian Dental Hygienists' Association: http://www.cdha.org.

Centers for Disease Control and Prevention (caries, mineralization strategies, and health protection goals): http://www.cdc.gov/

Reprinted from American Dental Hygienists' Association: *Standards for clinical dental hygiene practice*, Chicago, 2008 (March 10), Author.

http://www.cdc.gov/osi/goals/goals.html
http://www.cdc.gov/niosh/homepage.html

CDC Guidelines for Infection Control in Dental healthcare Settings. (2003). http://www.cdc.gov/OralHealth/infectioncontrol/guidelines/index.htm.

Center for Evidence-Based Dentistry: http://www.cebd.org/.

Clinical Trials: http://www.clinicaltrials.gov/.

The Cochrane Collaboration: http://www.cochrane.org/.

Forrest, J.L. & Miller, S.A. Evidence-based decision-making process. (2001). National Center for Dental Hygiene Research:
http://www.usc.edu/hsc/dental/dhnet/index.html.

Health Insurance Portability and Accountability Act (HIPAA): http://www.hipaa.org/.

National Guideline Clearing House: http://www.guidelines.gov/.

Nunn, M.E. (2003). Understanding the etiology of periodontitis: an overview of periodontal risk factors. *Periodontology 2000;*32:11-23.

Nursing Scope and Standards of Practice. (2004). Silver Spring, MD: American Nurses Association:
http://www.nursingworld.org/index.htm.

Occupational Safety and Health Administration: http://www.osha.gov/SLTC/dentistry/index.html.

The Organization for Safety and Asepsis Procedures (OSAP): http://www.osap.org/.

Special Care Dentistry: http://www.scdonline.org/.

Reprinted from American Dental Hygienists' Association: *Standards for clinical dental hygiene practice*, Chicago, 2008 (March 10), Author.

Reprinted without appendices. The entire *Standards for Clinical Dental Hygiene Practice,* including appendices, is available online at: www.adha.org/downloads/adha_standards08.pdf.

The American Dental Hygienists' Association (ADHA) acknowledges Philips Sonicare for their generous support in the printing and distribution of the *Standards for Clinical Dental Hygiene Practice.* Thanks to their generosity, every member of the ADHA will receive a copy to use in practice as a reference.

Code of Ethics for Dental Hygiene

1. PREAMBLE

As dental hygienists, we are a community of professionals devoted to the prevention of disease and the promotion and improvement of the public's health. We are preventive oral health professionals who provide educational, clinical, and therapeutic services to the public. We strive to live meaningful, productive, satisfying lives that simultaneously serve us, our profession, our society, and the world. Our actions, behaviors, and attitudes are consistent with our commitment to public service. We endorse and incorporate the Code into our daily lives.

2. PURPOSE

The purpose of a professional code of ethics is to achieve high levels of ethical consciousness, decision making, and practice by the members of the profession. Specific objectives of the Dental Hygiene Code of Ethics are:

- to increase our professional and ethical consciousness and sense of ethical responsibility.
- to lead us to recognize ethical issues and choices and to guide us in making more informed ethical decisions.
- to establish a standard for professional judgment and conduct.
- to provide a statement of the ethical behavior the public can expect from us.

The Dental Hygiene Code of Ethics is meant to influence us throughout our careers. It stimulates our continuing study of ethical issues and challenges us to explore our ethical responsibilities. The Code establishes concise standards of behavior to guide the public's expectations of our profession and supports dental hygiene practice, laws, and regulations. By holding ourselves accountable to meeting the standards stated in the Code, we enhance the public's trust on which our professional privilege and status are founded.

3. KEY CONCEPTS

Our beliefs, principles, values, and ethics are concepts reflected in the Code. They are the essential elements of our comprehensive and definitive code of ethics, and are interrelated and mutually dependent.

4. BASIC BELIEFS

We recognize the importance of the following beliefs that guide our practice and provide context for our ethics:

- The services we provide contribute to the health and well being of society.

- Our education and licensure qualify us to serve the public by preventing and treating oral disease and helping individuals achieve and maintain optimal health.
- Individuals have intrinsic worth, are responsible for their own health, and are entitled to make choices regarding their health.
- Dental hygiene care is an essential component of overall healthcare and we function interdependently with other healthcare providers.
- All people should have access to healthcare, including oral healthcare.
- We are individually responsible for our actions and the quality of care we provide.

5. FUNDAMENTAL PRINCIPLES

These fundamental principles, universal concepts, and general laws of conduct provide the foundation for our ethics.

Universality

The principle of universality expects that, if one individual judges an action to be right or wrong in a given situation, other people considering the same action in the same situation would make the same judgment.

Complementarity

The principle of complementarity recognizes the existence of an obligation to justice and basic human rights. In all relationships, it requires considering the values and perspectives of others before making decisions or taking actions affecting them.

Ethics

Ethics are the general standards of right and wrong that guide behavior within society. As generally accepted actions, they can be judged by determining the extent to which they promote good and minimize harm. Ethics compel us to engage in health promotion/disease prevention activities.

Community

This principle expresses our concern for the bond between individuals, the community, and society in general. It leads us to preserve natural resources and inspires us to show concern for the global environment.

Responsibility

Responsibility is central to our ethics. We recognize that there are guidelines for making ethical choices and accept responsibility for knowing and applying them. We accept the consequences of our actions or the failure to act and are willing to make ethical choices and publicly affirm them.

Reprinted from American Dental Hygienists' Association: *Code of ethics for dental hygiene 2007-2008*, Chicago, 2006 (August), Author.

6. CORE VALUES

We acknowledge these values as general for our choices and actions.

Individual Autonomy and Respect for Human Beings

People have the right to be treated with respect. They have the right to informed consent before treatment, and they have the right to full disclosure of all relevant information so that they can make informed choices about their care.

Confidentiality

We respect the confidentiality of client information and relationships as a demonstration of the value we place on individual autonomy. We acknowledge our obligation to justify any violation of a confidence.

Societal Trust

We value client trust and understand that public trust in our profession is based on our actions and behavior.

Non-Maleficence

We accept our fundamental obligation to provide services in a manner that protects all clients and minimizes harm to them and others involved in their treatment.

Beneficence

We have a primary role in promoting the well being of individuals and the public by engaging in health promotion/disease prevention activities.

Justice and Fairness

We value justice and support the fair and equitable distribution of healthcare resources. We believe all people should have access to high-quality, affordable oral healthcare.

Veracity

We accept our obligation to tell the truth and expect that others will do the same. We value self-knowledge and seek truth and honesty in all relationships.

7. STANDARDS OF PROFESSIONAL RESPONSIBILITY

We are obligated to practice our profession in a manner that supports our purpose, beliefs, and values in accordance with the fundamental principles that support our ethics. We acknowledge the following responsibilities:

To Ourselves as Individuals…

- Avoid self-deception, and continually strive for knowledge and personal growth.
- Establish and maintain a lifestyle that supports optimal health.
- Create a safe work environment.
- Assert our own interests in ways that are fair and equitable.

- Seek the advice and counsel of others when challenged with ethical dilemmas.
- Have realistic expectations of ourselves and recognize our limitations.

To Ourselves as Professionals…

- Enhance professional competencies through continuous learning in order to practice according to high standards of care.
- Support dental hygiene peer-review systems and quality-assurance measures.
- Develop collaborative professional relationships and exchange knowledge to enhance our own lifelong professional development.

To Family and Friends…

- Support the efforts of others to establish and maintain healthy lifestyles and respect the rights of friends and family.

To Clients…

- Provide oral healthcare utilizing high levels of professional knowledge, judgment, and skill.
- Maintain a work environment that minimizes the risk of harm.
- Serve all clients without discrimination and avoid action toward any individual or group that may be interpreted as discriminatory.
- Hold professional client relationships confidential.
- Communicate with clients in a respectful manner.
- Promote ethical behavior and high standards of care by all dental hygienists.
- Serve as an advocate for the welfare of clients.
- Provide clients with the information necessary to make informed decisions about their oral health and encourage their full participation in treatment decisions and goals.
- Refer clients to other healthcare providers when their needs are beyond our ability or scope of practice.
- Educate clients about high-quality oral heath care.

To Colleagues…

- Conduct professional activities and programs, and develop relationships in ways that are honest, responsible, and appropriately open and candid.
- Encourage a work environment that promotes individual professional growth and development.
- Collaborate with others to create a work environment that minimizes risk to the personal health and safety of our colleagues.
- Manage conflicts constructively.
- Support the efforts of other dental hygienists to communicate the dental hygiene philosophy and preventive oral care.
- Inform other healthcare professionals about the relationship between general and oral health.
- Promote human relationships that are mutually beneficial, including those with other healthcare professionals.

To Employees and Employers…

- Conduct professional activities and programs, and develop relationships in ways that are honest, responsible, open, and candid.

Reprinted from American Dental Hygienists' Association: *Code of ethics for dental hygiene 2007-2008*, Chicago, 2006 (August), Author.

- Manage conflicts constructively.
- Support the right of our employees and employers to work in an environment that promotes wellness.
- Respect the employment rights of our employers and employees.

To the Dental Hygiene Profession…

- Participate in the development and advancement of our profession.
- Avoid conflicts of interest and declare them when they occur.
- Seek opportunities to increase public awareness and understanding of oral health practices.
- Act in ways that bring credit to our profession while demonstrating appropriate respect for colleagues in other professions.
- Contribute time, talent, and financial resources to support and promote our profession.
- Promote a positive image for our profession.
- Promote a framework for professional education that develops dental hygiene competencies to meet the oral and overall health needs of the public.

To the Community and Society…

- Recognize and uphold the laws and regulations governing our profession.
- Document and report inappropriate, inadequate, or substandard care and/or illegal activities by a healthcare provider, to the responsible authorities.
- Use peer review as a mechanism for identifying inappropriate, inadequate, or substandard care provided by dental hygienists.
- Comply with local, state, and federal statutes that promote public health and safety.
- Develop support systems and quality-assurance programs in the workplace to assist dental hygienists in providing the appropriate standard of care.
- Promote access to dental hygiene services for all, supporting justice and fairness in the distribution of healthcare resources.
- Act consistently with the ethics of the global scientific community of which our profession is a part.
- Create a healthful workplace ecosystem to support a healthy environment.

- Recognize and uphold our obligation to provide pro bono service.

To Scientific Investigation…

We accept responsibility for conducting research according to the fundamental principles underlying our ethical beliefs in compliance with universal codes, governmental standards, and professional guidelines for the care and management of experimental subjects. We acknowledge our ethical obligations to the scientific community:

- Conduct research that contributes knowledge that is valid and useful to our clients and society.
- Use research methods that meet accepted scientific standards.
- Use research resources appropriately.
- Systematically review and justify research in progress to insure the most favorable benefit-to-risk ratio to research subjects.
- Submit all proposals involving human subjects to an appropriate human subject review committee.
- Secure appropriate institutional committee approval for the conduct of research involving animals.
- Obtain informed consent from human subjects participating in research that is based on specification published in Title 21 Code of Federal Regulations Part 46.
- Respect the confidentiality and privacy of data.
- Seek opportunities to advance dental hygiene knowledge through research by providing financial, human, and technical resources whenever possible.
- Report research results in a timely manner.
- Report research findings completely and honestly, drawing only those conclusions that are supported by the data presented.
- Report the names of investigators fairly and accurately.
- Interpret the research and the research of others accurately and objectively, drawing conclusions that are supported by the data presented and seeking clarity when uncertain.
- Critically evaluate research methods and results before applying new theory and technology in practice.
- Be knowledgeable concerning currently accepted preventive and therapeutic methods, products, and technology and their application to our practice.

Reprinted from American Dental Hygienists' Association: *Code of ethics for dental hygiene 2007-2008,* Chicago, 2006 (August), Author.

PART ■ I

Dental Hygiene Procedures

Copyright © 2010 by Saunders, an imprint of Elsevier Inc. All rights reserved.

Copyright © 2010 by Saunders, an imprint of Elsevier Inc. All rights reserved.

Copyright © 2010 by Saunders, an imprint of Elsevier Inc. All rights reserved.

Medical Emergencies

8

CHAPTER

Procedure **8-1**	INITIAL ASSESSMENT

EQUIPMENT

Resuscitation mask and other protective barriers

STEPS	RATIONALES
1. Tap the person on the shoulder and shout, "Are you okay? Are you okay?" (For an infant, gently tap the shoulder or flick the foot.) (Figure 8-1.)	Provides sensory stimulation to determine if the person is unconscious. Lack of response indicates the person is unconscious.

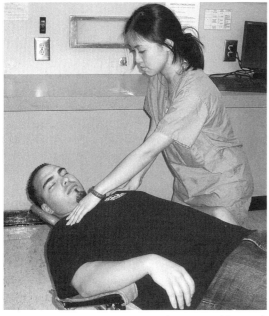

Figure 8-1. Unconsciousness is determined by performing the "shake-and-shout" maneuver, gently shaking the shoulders and calling the client's name. (From Malamed SF: *Medical emergencies in the dental office,* ed 6, St Louis, 2007, Mosby.)

(Continued)

Copyright © 2010 by Saunders, an imprint of Elsevier Inc. All rights reserved.

Procedure 8-1   INITIAL ASSESSMENT—*cont'd*

STEPS—*cont'd*	**RATIONALES**—*cont'd*

2. If no response, summon help to call emergency medical services (EMS) (e.g., 911) and to bring an automated external defibrillator (AED) in case it is needed.

Activates mechanism for higher-level emergency personnel to provide advanced life support and transport the victim to an emergency care facility.

3. Place the unconscious client in the supine position with feet slightly elevated (Figure 8-2).

A major objective in the management of unconsciousness is the delivery of oxygenated blood to the brain. The horizontal position helps the heart to deliver oxygenated blood to the brain, and elevating the feet further increases the return of blood to the heart.

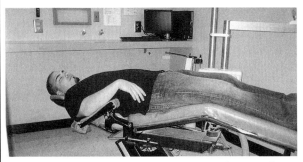

Figure 8-2. Placement of unconscious client in the supine position with feet slightly elevated. (From Malamed SF: *Medical emergencies in the dental office,* ed 6, St Louis, 2007, Mosby.)

4. Open victim's airway:
   • Tilt the head back and lift the chin. Place one hand on the victim's forehead and apply firm, backward pressure with the palm to tilt the head back. Place fingers of other hand under the bony part of the jaw near the chin, and lift to bring the chin forward and the teeth almost to occlusion (Figure 8-3).

Tilting the head back and lifting the chin maintains an open airway and allows for assessment of breathing. In an unconscious person the tongue falls backward against the wall of the pharynx, producing airway obstruction. Placing fingers under the jaw supports the jaw and helps to tilt the head back. The head tilt–chin lift technique is the most important step in maintaining an open airway.

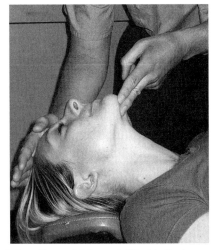

Figure 8-3. (From Malamed SF: *Medical emergencies in the dental office,* ed 6, St Louis, 2007, Mosby.)

   • If you suspect neck injury, use the jaw-thrust maneuver: Grasp angles of the victim's lower jaw and lift with both hands, thus displacing the mandible forward while tilting the head backward (Figure 8-4).

This approach opens the airway without extending the neck.

Copyright © 2010 by Saunders, an imprint of Elsevier Inc. All rights reserved.

| Procedure **8-1** | INITIAL ASSESSMENT—*cont'd* |

STEPS—*cont'd*   **RATIONALES**—*cont'd*

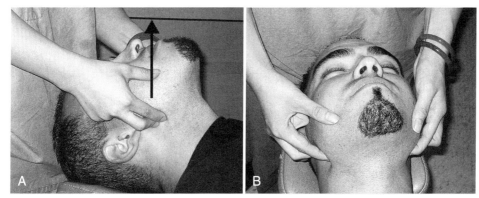

Figure 8-4. To perform the jaw-thrust technique, the clinician must grasp the angles of the mandible with both hands and displace the mandible forward. **A,** Side view. **B,** Front view. (From Malamed SF: *Medical emergencies in the dental office,* ed 6, St Louis, 2007, Mosby.)

- Look, listen, and feel for normal breathing and chest movement for no more than 10 seconds. Place your ear over victim's mouth and nose while maintaining an open airway. Look at victim's chest to check for rise and fall (Figure 8-5).

Observing chest movements and feeling or hearing air at the person's nose and mouth indicates that effective spontaneous breathing is present.

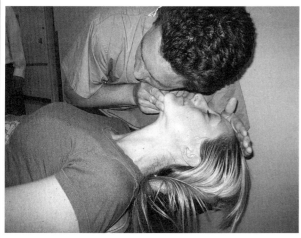

Figure 8-5. (From Malamed SF: *Medical emergencies in the dental office,* ed 6, St Louis, 2007, Mosby.)

- Irregular, gasping, or shallow breathing is not normal breathing.
5. Check the pulse:
  - For an adult or child, assess for presence of the carotid pulse for no more than 10 seconds (Figure 8-6).
  - For an infant, check the brachial pulse on the inside of the upper arm between the infant's elbow and shoulder.

Carotid artery pulse will persist when the more peripheral pulses are no longer palpable. Because of infant anatomy, the brachial pulse is easier to palpate. Performing external cardiac compressions on a victim who has a pulse may result in serious medical complications.

(Continued)

Copyright © 2010 by Saunders, an imprint of Elsevier Inc. All rights reserved.

Procedure 8-1 INITIAL ASSESSMENT—*cont'd*

STEPS—*cont'd*   **RATIONALES—*cont'd***

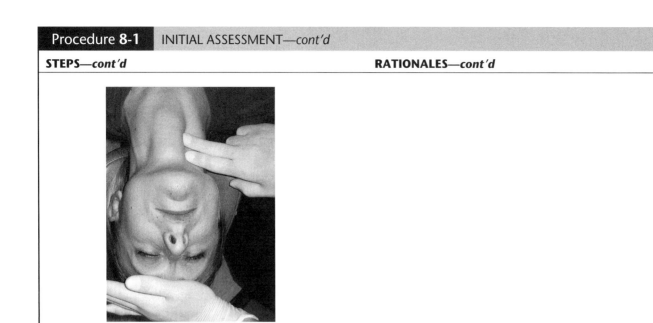

Figure 8-6. Carotid artery is located in groove between the trachea and the sternocleidomastoid muscle. Head tilt must be maintained. (From Malamed SF: *Medical emergencies in the dental office,* ed 6, St Louis, 2007, Mosby.)

6. If there is a pulse but no movement or breathing:
   • Position the resuscitation mask over the victim's nose and mouth, tilt the head back, and lift the chin to open the airway.
   • Form an airtight seal with the mask against the face, and give two rescue breaths by breathing into the mask (one breath every 5 seconds for adults) (Figure 8-7).

Resuscitation masks cover a victim's mouth and nose and allow the rescuer to breathe air into a victim without making mouth-to-mouth contact. The mask protects against disease transmission when rescue breaths are given and can be connected to emergency oxygen if it has an oxygen inlet.

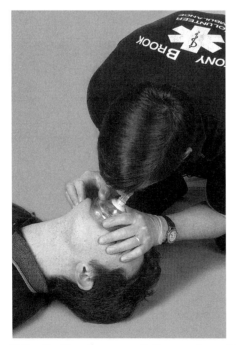

Figure 8-7. Position the resuscitation mask, and breathe into the mask while tilting the head and lifting the chin to open the airway. (From Henry M, Stapleton E: *EMT: prehospital care,* ed 3, St Louis, 2007, Mosby/JEMS.)

Copyright © 2010 by Saunders, an imprint of Elsevier Inc. All rights reserved.

Procedure 8-1   INITIAL ASSESSMENT—cont'd

STEPS—cont'd	RATIONALES—cont'd

- If there is no mask, perform two rescue breaths via mouth-to-mouth resuscitation (see Procedure 8-2).
- Each rescue breath (one breath every 5 seconds for adults) should last about 1 second and make the chest clearly rise.
- Note: For a child, the head is only slightly tilted past the neutral position. One breath is delivered every 3 seconds (Figure 8-8).

In mouth-to-mouth resuscitation the nose must be pinched closed to prevent the escape of air through the nose.

An airtight seal prevents air from escaping the mask. Breathing air into a victim provides oxygen needed to survive.

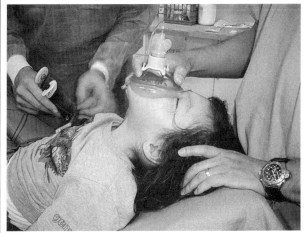

Figure 8-8. Holding pocket mask on face. (From Malamed SF: *Medical emergencies in the dental office,* ed 6, St Louis, 2007, Mosby.)

- Note: For an infant (1 to 12 months), the chin is lifted to open the airway but the head is kept in a neutral position. Also, the mask is inverted if there is no infant mask available. One slow gentle breath (a puff) is delivered every 3 seconds.
- If the chest rises and falls with delivery of two rescue breaths, remove the resuscitation mask, recheck breathing, and check for the presence of a pulse for no more than 10 seconds.

Assesses for airway, breathing, and circulation.

- If the chest does not rise and fall with delivery of two rescue breaths, remove the resuscitation mask and reposition the airway by tilting the head farther back or initiating the jaw-thrust maneuver. Then replace the mask and deliver two rescue breaths again.

Attempts to open the airway and deliver air to the victim.

7. If there is breathing and a pulse:
- Continue to monitor the ABCs until help arrives.
- Administer emergency oxygen, if available.

Keeps the client stable until EMS personnel arrive.

If there is a pulse but no movement or breathing:
- Reposition the airway by tilting the head farther back or initiating the jaw thrust maneuver.
- Replace the mask and deliver two rescue breaths again.
- If the chest rises and falls with each respiration, begin rescue breathing (see Procedure 8-2).
- If the rescue breaths still do not make the chest clearly rise, then initiate the procedure for unconscious choking (see Procedures 8-3 and 8-4).

Attempts to open the airway so the client can receive rescue breaths.
Breathes for the client and gets oxygen to the brain to prevent brain damage.
The air the clinician or rescuer exhales contains enough oxygen to keep a person alive.
Attempts to clear the airway so the client can receive rescue breaths.

(Continued)

Copyright © 2010 by Saunders, an imprint of Elsevier Inc. All rights reserved.

Procedure 8-1   INITIAL ASSESSMENT—*cont'd*

STEPS—*cont'd*	RATIONALES—*cont'd*
If there is no pulse: • CPR is initiated immediately (see Procedure 8-5).	Promotes adequate cardiac output until EMS personnel arrive.
8. After emergency care, document the situation on an incident report form (Figure 8-9) and in the client's chart. Provide a copy of incident report to EMS technician if victim is being transferred to a hospital.	Provides for continuity of care and protects rescuer from accusations of malpractice.

Client name _____   Date _____ Time _____

Address   _____   Home phone _____

_____   Work phone _____

Incident described:

Vital signs

Time	BP	Pulse	Resp	Oxygen delivery	Medications administered

Treatment administered	Healthcare provider rendering care

Client response to treatment
_____

Figure 8-9.   Medical emergency incident report form.

Copyright © 2010 by Saunders, an imprint of Elsevier Inc. All rights reserved.

Procedure 8-2   RESCUE BREATHING—ADULT, CHILD, INFANT

EQUIPMENT
Resuscitation mask (Figures 8-10 and 8-11)
Other protective barriers

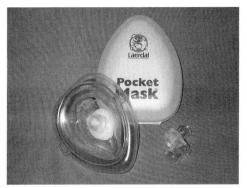

Figure 8-10. Pocket mask. (Courtesy Sedation Resource, Lone Oak, Texas, www.sedationresource.com.)

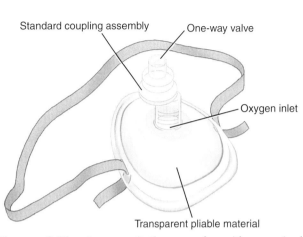

Figure 8-11. A resuscitation mask with required characteristics.

STEPS	RATIONALES
1-6. Initial assessment (see Procedure 8-1)	Initial assessment is needed to determine what basic life support is needed—positioning (P), airway maintenance (A), breathing (B), and circulation (C)—for any medical emergency victim.
7. Perform rescue breathing if there is a pulse but no movement or breathing. • Position yourself at the client's side. • Open the airway.	Positioning yourself at the client's side enables you to perform chest compressions if needed. Tilting the head back and lifting the chin maintain an open airway and allow for assessment of breathing. In an unconscious person the tongue falls backward against the wall of the pharynx, producing airway obstruction.

○ For an adult, the tip of the chin points up in the air in line with the ear lobes (Figure 8-12).

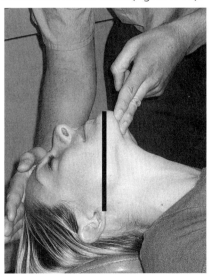

Figure 8-12. For an adult, when the unconscious person's head is extended properly, the tip of the chin points up into the air in line with the earlobes *(black line)*, lifting the mandible and tongue off the pharyngeal wall. (From Malamed SF: *Medical emergencies in the dental office,* ed 6, St Louis, 2007, Mosby.)

Copyright © 2010 by Saunders, an imprint of Elsevier Inc. All rights reserved.   *(Continued)*

Procedure 8-2   RESCUE BREATHING—ADULT, CHILD, INFANT—*cont'd*

STEPS—*cont'd*   **RATIONALES**—*cont'd*

○ For a child, the child's head is only slightly tilted past the neutral position to open the airway (Figure 8-13).

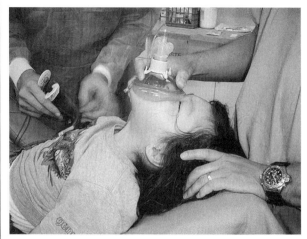

Figure 8-13. Holding pocket mask on face. (From Malamed SF: *Medical emergencies in the dental office,* ed 6, St Louis, 2007, Mosby.)

○ For an infant (1 to 12 months old), the chin is lifted to open the airway but the head is kept in a neutral position (Figure 8-14).

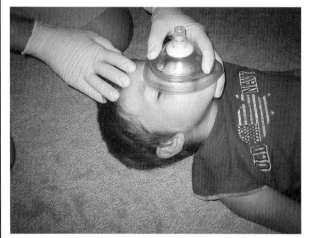

Figure 8-14. (Courtesy Sedation Resource, Lone Oak, Texas, www.sedationresource.com.)

• Mouth-to-mask resuscitation: Creates an airtight seal between the rescuer's mouth and the victim's face, preventing air from escaping from the mask.

Copyright © 2010 by Saunders, an imprint of Elsevier Inc. All rights reserved.

Procedure 8-2   RESCUE BREATHING—ADULT, CHILD, INFANT—*cont'd*

STEPS—*cont'd*

⊙ Place the resuscitation mask on the victim's face with the narrow portion over the bridge of the nose and the wider part in the cleft at the chin (Figure 8-15). (For an infant, invert the mask if no pediatric mask is available [Figure 8-16]).

RATIONALES—*cont'd*

When a pediatric resuscitation mask is not available, placing the narrow end of the mask over the mouth creates an adequate seal.

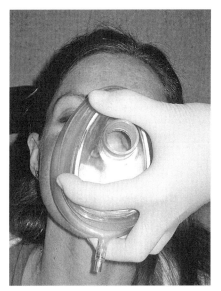

Figure 8-15. Mouth-to-mask ventilation demonstrating finger positioning. (From Malamed SF: *Medical emergencies in the dental office,* ed 6, St Louis, 2007, Mosby.)

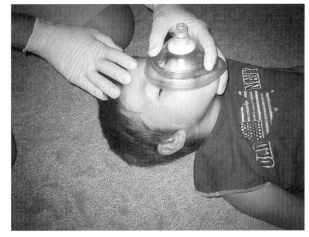

Figure 8-16. (Courtesy Sedation Resource, Lone Oak, Texas, www.sedationresource.com.)

(Continued)

Copyright © 2010 by Saunders, an imprint of Elsevier Inc. All rights reserved.

Procedure **8-2**   RESCUE BREATHING—ADULT, CHILD, INFANT—*cont'd*

STEPS—*cont'd*	**RATIONALES**—*cont'd*

○ Using the hand that is closer to the top of the victim's head, place the index finger and thumb along the border of the mask while using the other hand to place the thumb along the lower margin of the mask and grasping the mandible with the index, middle, and ring fingers (Figure 8-17).

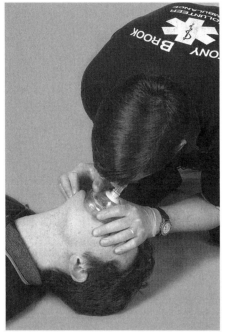

Figure 8-17.   Position the resuscitation mask, and breathe into the mask while tilting the head and lifting the chin to open the airway. (From Henry M, Stapleton E: *EMT: prehospital care,* ed 3, St Louis, 2007, Mosby/JEMS.)

○ Place your mouth on the breathing port of the mask, and breathe air into the victim's mouth and nose (Figure 8-18).

The air you exhale contains enough oxygen to keep a person alive. Slow breaths provide an adequate volume at the lowest possible pressure, thereby reducing risk of gastric distention. An excess of air volume and fast inspiratory flow rates are likely to cause pharyngeal pressures that exceed esophageal opening pressures, allowing air to enter the stomach. This air in the stomach results in gastric distention, increasing the risk of vomiting. Each breath should last about 1 second and make the chest clearly rise. Because an infant's air passages are smaller with resistance to flow quite high, the force or volume of the rescue breaths is lower than that for an adult or child.

Copyright © 2010 by Saunders, an imprint of Elsevier Inc. All rights reserved.

Procedure 8-2   RESCUE BREATHING—ADULT, CHILD, INFANT—cont'd

STEPS—cont'd

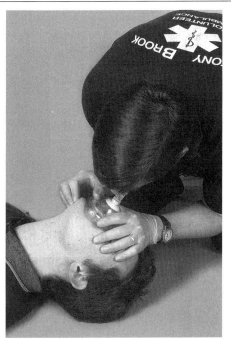

Figure 8-18. (From Henry M, Stapleton E: *EMT: prehospital care,* ed 3, St Louis, 2007, Mosby/JEMS.)

- ○ For an adult, blow one rescue breath every 5 seconds (see Figure 8-18). (Count 1001, 1002, 1003, 1004, 1005.)
- ○ For a child, blow one rescue breath every 3 seconds. (Count 1001, 1002, 1003.)
- ○ For an infant, administer a slow, shallow, gentle breath every 3 seconds (just enough to make the chest rise). (Count 1001, 1002, 1003.)
- • If there is no mask available, perform mouth-to-mouth resuscitation.
  - ○ For an adult or a child, maintain head tilt while pinching the victim's nostrils closed with the thumb and index finger, take a deep breath, form a tight seal around the victim's mouth, and blow air into the mouth. Adequate ventilation is achieved when the victim's chest visibly rises with each ventilatory effort (Figure 8-19).
  - ○ For an infant, place your mouth over the infant's nose and mouth to form an airtight seal to prevent air from escaping through the nose (Figure 8-20).
  - ○ Each rescue breath should last about 1 second and make the chest clearly rise.
- 8. Continue to give one rescue breath about every 5 seconds.
  - • Each rescue breath should last about 1 second.
  - • Watch the chest clearly rise when giving each rescue breath.

RATIONALES—cont'd

Again, an infant's air passages are smaller, with resistance to flow quite high. An appropriate volume is one that makes the chest rise and fall. Slow breaths provide an adequate volume at the lowest possible pressure, thereby reducing risk of gastric distention.

Breathing air into a victim gives him or her oxygen needed to survive. When giving rescue breaths, take a normal breath and breathe into the mask.

Observing chest wall movement ensures that artificial respirations enter the lungs.

(Continued)

Copyright © 2010 by Saunders, an imprint of Elsevier Inc. All rights reserved.

Procedure 8-2	RESCUE BREATHING—ADULT, CHILD, INFANT—*cont'd*

STEPS—*cont'd* | **RATIONALES—*cont'd***

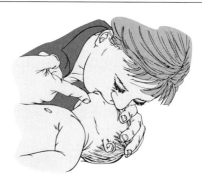

Figure 8-20. (From Potter PA, Perry AG: *Fundamentals of nursing,* ed 7, St Louis, 2009, Mosby.)

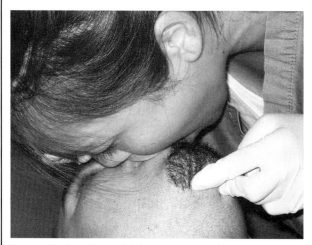

Figure 8-19. (From Malamed SF: *Medical emergencies in the dental office,* ed 6, St Louis, 2007, Mosby.)

- Do this for about 2 minutes, then recheck the pulse.
9. • Remove the resuscitation mask, look for movement, and recheck for breathing (Figure 8-21).

The presence of a pulse indicates the heart is beating.

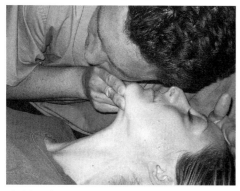

Figure 8-21. (From Henry M, Stapleton E: *EMT: prehospital care,* ed 3, St Louis, 2004, Saunders.)

- Check for a pulse for at least 5 seconds but no more than 10 seconds (Figure 8-22).

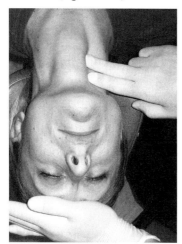

Figure 8-22. (From Malamed SF: *Medical emergencies in the dental office,* ed 6, St Louis, 2007, Mosby.)

Copyright © 2010 by Saunders, an imprint of Elsevier Inc. All rights reserved.

Procedure 8-2   RESCUE BREATHING—ADULT, CHILD, INFANT—cont'd

STEPS—cont'd	RATIONALES—cont'd

10. If there is a pulse but still no movement or breathing:
  • Replace the mask and continue rescue breathing.
  • Look for movement and recheck for breathing and a pulse about every 2 minutes.
	Keeps the client stable until EMS personnel arrive.

If movement, breathing, and a pulse are present: • Continue to monitor the ABCs.	Promotes adequate cardiac output until EMS personnel arrive.
• Administer emergency oxygen, if available. If there is no movement, breathing, or pulse: • Perform cardiopulmonary resuscitation (CPR) (see Procedure 8-3).	
11. After emergency care, document the situation on an incident report form (Figure 8-23) and in the client's chart. Provide a copy of incident report to EMS technician if victim is being transferred to a hospital.	Provides for continuity of care and protects rescuer from accusations of malpractice.

Client name _____   Date _____ Time _____

Address   _____   Home phone _____

         _____   Work phone _____

Incident described:

Vital signs

Time	BP	Pulse	Resp	Oxygen delivery	Medications administered

Treatment administered	Healthcare provider rendering care

Client response to treatment
_____

Figure 8-23. Medical emergency incident report form.

Copyright © 2010 by Saunders, an imprint of Elsevier Inc. All rights reserved.

| Procedure 8-3 | ONE-RESCUER CARDIOPULMONARY RESUSCITATION (CPR) FOR ADULT, CHILD, AND INFANT |

EQUIPMENT
Resuscitation mask
Other protective barriers
Automated external defibrillator (AED)

STEPS	RATIONALES
1-6. Complete Steps 1-6, Initial Assessment (see Procedure 8-1).	Initial assessment is needed to determine what to do regarding applying, as needed, the procedures of positioning (P), airway maintenance (A), breathing (B), and circulation (C) to any medical emergency victim.
If the victim has no pulse, begin CPR.	Effective chest compressions circulate blood to the victim's brain and other vital organs. Chest compression causes the heart muscle to contract, forcing blood out of the heart. When the chest recoils, the heart muscle relaxes and blood refills the heart chambers. CPR helps supply oxygen to the brain and other vital organs to keep the victim alive until an AED is used or advanced medical care is given.
7. Find the correct hand position to give compressions.	
• Remove clothing covering the victim's chest.	Facilitates proper hand positioning.
• Place the heel of one hand on the center of the chest between the nipples.	Proper hand positioning results in maximal compression of the heart between the sternum and the vertebrae.
• Place the other hand on top and intertwine the fingers. Keep fingers off the chest when giving compressions.	Reduces risk of rib fracture during compressions.
• Position your shoulders over your hands with your elbows locked (Figure 8-24).	With this technique each compression is performed straight down on the sternum. Bending of the elbows greatly decreases effectiveness and leads to rapid rescuer fatigue.

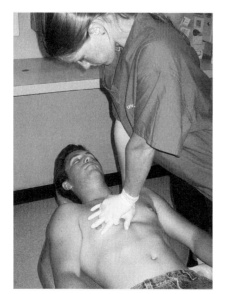

Figure 8-24. (From Malamed SF: *Medical emergencies in the dental office,* ed 6, St Louis, 2007, Mosby.)

• Use your body weight, not your arms, to compress the chest.	Decreases rescuer fatigue.

Copyright © 2010 by Saunders, an imprint of Elsevier Inc. All rights reserved.

Procedure 8-3	ONE-RESCUER CARDIOPULMONARY RESUSCITATION (CPR) FOR ADULT, CHILD, AND INFANT—*cont'd*

STEPS—*cont'd*	RATIONALES—*cont'd*

8. Give 30 chest compressions.
  • For an adult, compress the chest about 1½ to 2 inches.
  • For a child, compress the chest about 1 to 1½ inches.
  • Let the chest fully recoil to its normal position after each compression.
  • Compress at a rate of about 100 compressions per minute.
  • Count out loud to keep an even pace ("1 and 2 and 3 and…").
9. Replace the resuscitation mask and give two rescue breaths.
  • Each rescue breath should last about 1 second.
  • Give rescue breaths that make the chest clearly rise (Figure 8-25).
	Supplies oxygen to the brain and other vital organs.
	Faster rate increases blood flow with an increased flow to the brain and heart.
	
	Breathing air into a victim provides oxygen needed to survive.

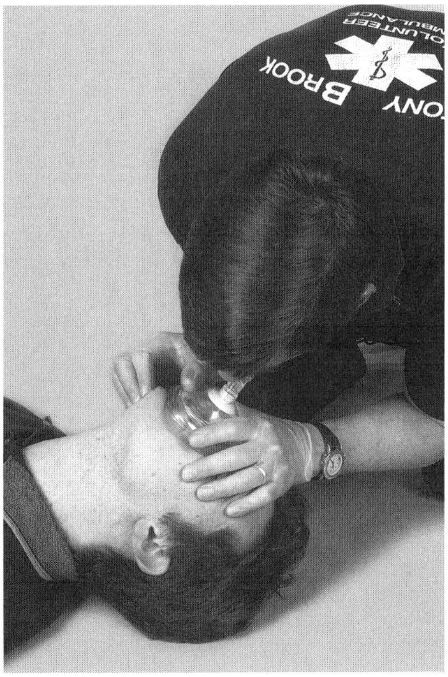

Figure 8-25.   (From Henry M, Stapleton E: *EMT: prehospital care,* ed 3, St Louis, 2007, Mosby/JEMS.)

STEPS—*cont'd*	RATIONALES—*cont'd*
10. Do cycles of 30 compressions and two rescue breaths. Reassess victim after four cycles (i.e., two ventilations, 30 compressions each cycle).	A compression-ventilation ratio of 30 compressions to two breaths is currently recommended for one-rescuer resuscitation.

(Continued)

Copyright © 2010 by Saunders, an imprint of Elsevier Inc. All rights reserved.

Procedure 8-3	ONE-RESCUER CARDIOPULMONARY RESUSCITATION (CPR) FOR ADULT, CHILD, AND INFANT—*cont'd*

STEPS—*cont'd*

RATIONALES—*cont'd*

11. • If there is a pulse, continue rescue breathing at one breath every 5 seconds.
    • If there is no pulse, continue CPR until:
      ○ Another trained rescuer arrives and takes over
      ○ An AED is available and ready to use
      ○ You are too exhausted to continue
      ○ You notice an obvious sign of life

Breathing air into a victim gives him or her oxygen needed to survive.

A 30:2 compression-ventilation ratio is tiring. Therefore when an additional rescuer is available, two-rescuer CPR is administered (see Procedure 8-4). In two-rescuer CPR, one rescuer gives rescue breaths and the other rescuer gives chest compressions. It is recommended to switch the compressor every 2 minutes (or after five cycles of compressions.

In many cases, CPR by itself cannot correct the underlying heart problem, but ventricular fibrillation ("V-fib") and ventricular tachycardia ("V-tach") can be corrected by early defibrillation.

12. After emergency care, document the situation on an incident report form (Figure 8-26) and in the client's chart. Provide a copy of incident report to EMS technician if victim is being transferred to a hospital.

Provides for continuity of care and protects rescuer from accusations of malpractice.

Client name _____   Date _____ Time _____

Address   _____   Home phone _____

           _____   Work phone _____

Incident described:

Vital signs

Time	BP	Pulse	Resp	Oxygen delivery	Medications administered

Treatment administered	Healthcare provider rendering care

Client response to treatment

Figure 8-26.   Medical emergency incident report form.

Copyright © 2010 by Saunders, an imprint of Elsevier Inc. All rights reserved.

Procedure 8-4   TWO-RESCUER CARDIOPULMONARY RESUSCITATION (CPR)—ADULT AND CHILD

EQUIPMENT
Resuscitation mask
Other protective barriers
Automated external defibrillator (AED)

STEPS	RATIONALES
1-10. Completed by Rescuer 1 (see Procedure 8-3).	A person who is unconscious, is not moving or breathing, and has no pulse is in cardiac arrest and needs CPR. A 30:2 compression-ventilation ratio is tiring. Therefore when an additional rescuer is available, two-rescuer CPR is provided Having another trained rescuer assist with CPR prevents the initial rescuer from becoming too exhausted to continue.
11. Rescuer 2 finds the correct hand position to give compressions. • Places the heel of one hand on the center of the chest • Places the other hand on top	Rescuer 2 is preparing to take over chest compressions.
12. Rescuer 2 gives chest compressions when Rescuer 1 says, "Victim has no pulse. Begin CPR." • Adult: 30 compressions; compress the chest about 1½ to 2 inches • Child: 15 compressions; compress the chest about 1 to 1½ inches • Lets the chest fully recoil to its normal position after each compression • Compresses at a rate of about 100 compressions per minute	Effective chest compressions circulate blood to the victim's brain and other vital organs. Chest compression causes the heart muscle to contract, forcing blood out of the heart. When the chest recoils, the heart muscle relaxes and blood refills the heart chambers.
13. Rescuer 1 replaces the mask on the victim's face and gives two rescue breaths. • Each rescue breath should last about 1 second. • Gives rescue breaths that make the chest clearly rise.	Breathing air into a victim provides oxygen needed to survive. Indicates the airway is open.
14. Do about 2 minutes of compressions and breaths.	
15. Change positions: • Rescuer 2 calls for a position change by using the word "change" at the end of the last compression cycle. • Rescuer 1 gives two rescue breaths. • Rescuer 2 moves to the victim's head with his or her own mask. • Rescuer 1 moves into position at the victim's chest and locates correct hand position on the victim's chest. • Changing positions should take less than 5 seconds.	Changing positions prevents the rescuer providing compressions from becoming too exhausted to continue.

(Continued)

Copyright © 2010 by Saunders, an imprint of Elsevier Inc. All rights reserved.

Procedure 8-4   TWO-RESCUER CARDIOPULMONARY RESUSCITATION (CPR)—ADULT AND CHILD—*cont'd*

STEPS—*cont'd*	RATIONALES—*cont'd*

16. Continue CPR until:
  • Help arrives
  • An AED is available and ready to use
  • You are too exhausted to continue
  • You notice signs of life	

17. After emergency care, document the situation on an incident report form (Figure 8-27) and in the client's chart. Provide a copy of incident report to EMS technician if victim is being transferred to a hospital.	Provides for continuity of care and protects rescuer from accusations of malpractice.

Client name _____   Date _____ Time _____

Address   _____   Home phone _____

          _____   Work phone _____

Incident described:

Vital signs

Time	BP	Pulse	Resp	Oxygen delivery	Medications administered

Treatment administered	Healthcare provider rendering care

Client response to treatment
_____

Figure 8-27.   Medical emergency incident report form.

Copyright © 2010 by Saunders, an imprint of Elsevier Inc. All rights reserved.

Procedure 8-5	SINGLE RESCUER USING AN AUTOMATED EXTERNAL DEFIBRILLATOR (AED)—ADULT AND CHILD*

EQUIPMENT

Automated external defibrillator (AED) (Figure 8-28)

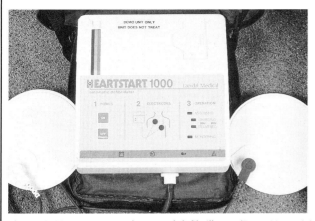

Figure 8-28. Automated external defibrillator. (From Henry M, Stapleton E: *EMT: prehospital care,* ed 3, St Louis, 2007, Mosby/JEMS.)

STEPS	RATIONALES
1-6. Complete Initial Assessment (see Procedure 8-1); verify the absence of breathing and pulse (Figure 8-29).	Initial assessment is needed to determine what to do regarding applying, as needed, the procedures of positioning (P), airway maintenance (A), breathing (B), and circulation (C) to any medical emergency victim.

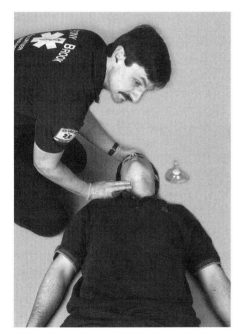

Figure 8-29. (From Henry M, Stapleton E: *EMT: prehospital care,* ed 3, St Louis, 2007, Mosby-JEMS.)

(Continued)

Copyright © 2010 by Saunders, an imprint of Elsevier Inc. All rights reserved.

Procedure 8-5	SINGLE RESCUER USING AN AUTOMATED EXTERNAL DEFIBRILLATOR (AED)— ADULT AND CHILD*—*cont'd*

STEPS—*cont'd*	**RATIONALES—*cont'd***

7. • Begin CPR (see Procedure 8-3).
   • After five cycles, stop CPR.
   • Position the defibrillator machine on the left side of the victim's head.
   • Turn on the AED.
	The heart's electrical system controls the pumping action of the heart. Damage to the heart from disease or injury can disrupt the heart's electrical system, resulting in an abnormal heart rhythm that can stop circulation. The two most common treatable abnormal rhythms initially present in sudden cardiac arrest victims are ventricular fibrillation ("V-fib") and ventricular tachycardia ("V-tach"). An AED is a device that provides an electrical shock to the heart, called *defibrillation*. Defibrillation disrupts the electrical activity of V-fib and V-tack long enough to allow the heart to spontaneously develop an effective rhythm on its own. The sooner the shock is administered, the greater the likelihood of the victim's survival.
	If V-fib or V-tach is not interrupted, all electrical activity will eventually cease (asystole), a condition that cannot be corrected by defibrillation.

8. Wipe the chest dry.	A dry environment must be provided before electrical current of an AED is delivered. Therefore the victim's chest must be wiped dry before the AED is attached. If the victim was removed from water, be sure there are no puddles of water around you, the victim, or the AED.
9. Attach the electrode lines to the pads (Figure 8-30).	

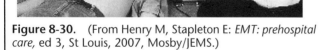

Figure 8-30.   (From Henry M, Stapleton E: *EMT: prehospital care,* ed 3, St Louis, 2007, Mosby/JEMS.)

| 10. Attach the pads to the victim.
   • Remove the cover from the adhesive side of the pads.
   • Place one pad on the upper right side of the victim's chest above the nipple area. | Enables the application of a shock. |

Copyright © 2010 by Saunders, an imprint of Elsevier Inc. All rights reserved.

Procedure **8-5**	SINGLE RESCUER USING AN AUTOMATED EXTERNAL DEFIBRILLATOR (AED)— ADULT AND CHILD*—*cont'd*

STEPS—*cont'd*

RATIONALES—*cont'd*

- Place the other pad on the victim's lower left side at the left sterna border (Figure 8-31). Make sure the pads are not touching.

The electrical current of an AED is very directional between the pads. If the pads touch, it will interfere with the analysis of the heart rhythm and may interfere with the delivery of the shock.

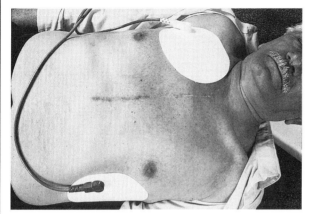

Figure 8-31. (From Henry M, Stapleton E: *EMT: prehospital care,* ed 3, St Louis, 2007, Mosby-JEMS.)

- For a child, use pediatric AED pads if available. Make sure the pads are not touching.

Note: If the pads risk touching each other on a child, place one pad on the child's chest and the other pad on the child's back (between the shoulder blades).

11. Plug the connector into the AED, if necessary.
12. Clear the victim.
    - Make sure that nobody, including you, is touching the victim.
    - Tell everyone to "stand clear."
13. Push the "analyze" button. Let the AED analyze the heart rhythm (Figure 8-32).

It is important that no one be touching the victim because the heart rhythms of individuals touching the victim also may be analyzed, which may affect the AED's analysis.

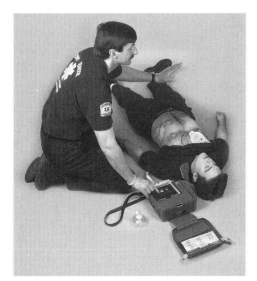

Figure 8-32. (From Henry M, Stapleton E: *EMT: prehospital care,* ed 3, St Louis, 2007, Mosby/JEMS.)

(Continued)

Copyright © 2010 by Saunders, an imprint of Elsevier Inc. All rights reserved.

Procedure 8-5	SINGLE RESCUER USING AN AUTOMATED EXTERNAL DEFIBRILLATOR (AED)—ADULT AND CHILD*—cont'd

STEPS—*cont'd*	**RATIONALES**—*cont'd*
14. If a shock is advised, push the "shock" button. • Look to see that nobody is touching the victim. • Tell everyone to "stand clear." 15. After the shock or if no shock is indicated: • Give five cycles (about 2 minutes) of CPR before analyzing the heart rhythm again. • If no shock advised, give 5 cycles or about 2 minutes of CPR. • If at any time you notice an obvious sign of life, stop CPR and monitor the ABCs. Administer emergency oxygen, if it is available and you are trained to do so. 16. After emergency care, document the situation on an incident report form (Figure 8-33) and in the client's chart. Provide a copy of incident report to EMS technician if victim is being transferred to a hospital.	Anyone touching the victim during the shock also will receive a shock. Provides for continuity of care and protects rescuer from accusations of malpractice.

Client name _____   Date _____ Time _____

Address   _____   Home phone _____

_____   Work phone _____

Incident described:

Vital signs

Time	BP	Pulse	Resp	Oxygen delivery	Medications administered

Treatment administered	Healthcare provider rendering care

Client response to treatment
_____

Figure 8-33. Medical emergency incident report form.

Adapted from American Red Cross: *Skill sheet using an AED—adult and child*, Washington, DC, American Red Cross.
*Note: If two trained responders are present, one should perform CPR while the second responder operates the AED.

Copyright © 2010 by Saunders, an imprint of Elsevier Inc. All rights reserved.

Procedure 8-6	CONSCIOUS CHOKING—ADULT AND CHILD

EQUIPMENT
Resuscitation mask
Other protective barriers

STEPS	RATIONALES
1. Ask the person, "Are you choking?" • If the person is coughing forcefully, encourage continued coughing. • A conscious victim who is clutching his or her throat with one or both hands is usually choking. (Figure 8-34).	If the victim has a partial airway obstruction with good air exchange and can cough forcefully, the hygienist should not interfere with attempts to dislodge the object but should remain with the victim until it is dislodged or help arrives. This is the universal sign of choking.

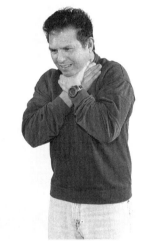

Figure 8-34. (From Chapleau W: *Emergency first responder: making the difference,* St Louis, 2004, Mosby.)

STEPS	RATIONALES
2. If the person cannot cough, speak, or breathe, have someone else summon advanced medical personnel.	Activates mechanism for higher-level emergency personnel to provide advanced life support and transport the victim to an emergency care facility.
3. Get consent before helping a conscious choking victim (e.g., "Is it OK if I try to help you?").	Protects rescuer from accusations of malpractice.
4. Lean the victim forward and give five back blows with the heel of your hand. • Position yourself slightly behind the victim. • Provide support by placing one arm diagonally across the chest, and lean the victim forward. • Firmly strike the victim between the shoulder blades with the heel of your hand.	Having the victim lean forward allows gravity to help with the displacement of the obstruction. Each blow is a distinct attempt to dislodge the object. Use less force when giving back blows to a child because children have smaller bodies.
5. Give five abdominal thrusts. • Adult: Stand behind the victim. • Child: Stand or kneel behind the child depending on the child's height. Use less force on a child than you would on an adult. • Use one hand to find the navel.	Maximizes hand positioning.

(Continued)

Copyright © 2010 by Saunders, an imprint of Elsevier Inc. All rights reserved.

Procedure 8-6   CONSCIOUS CHOKING—ADULT AND CHILD—*cont'd*

STEPS—*cont'd*	**RATIONALES**—*cont'd*
• Make a fist with your other hand and place the thumb side of your fist against the middle of the victim's abdomen, just above the navel and well below the tip of the xiphoid process (Figure 8-35).	Avoids fracture of the xiphoid process.

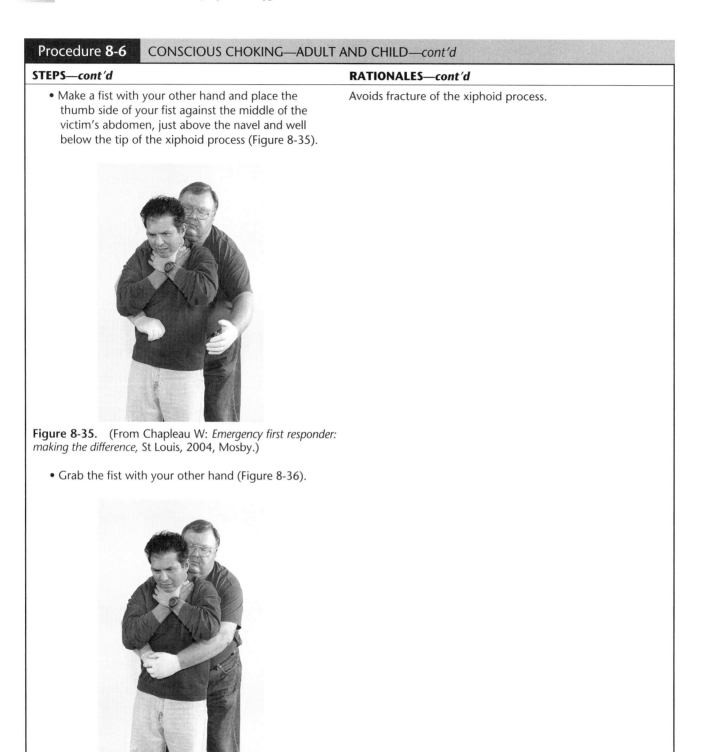

Figure 8-35.   (From Chapleau W: *Emergency first responder: making the difference,* St Louis, 2004, Mosby.)

• Grab the fist with your other hand (Figure 8-36).

Figure 8-36.   (From Chapleau W: *Emergency first responder: making the difference,* St Louis, 2004, Mosby.)

Copyright © 2010 by Saunders, an imprint of Elsevier Inc. All rights reserved.

Procedure 8-6   CONSCIOUS CHOKING—ADULT AND CHILD—*cont'd*

STEPS—*cont'd*

- Press the fist into the victim's abdomen with a brisk inward and upward motion. Give quick upward thrusts. Each thrust should be a distinct attempt to dislodge the object (Figure 8-37).

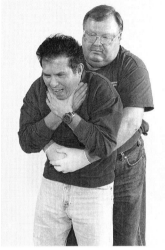

Figure 8-37. (From Chapleau W: *Emergency first responder: making the difference,* St Louis, 2004, Mosby.)

- Note: Use chest thrusts if:
    - You cannot reach far enough around the victim to give abdominal thrusts
    - The victim is pregnant (Figure 8-38)

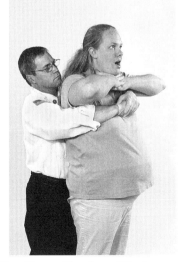

Figure 8-38. (From Chapleau W: *Emergency first responder: making the difference,* St Louis, 2004, Mosby.)

RATIONALES—*cont'd*

Each of these subdiaphragmatic abdominal thrusts (the Heimlich maneuver) should be distinct to facilitate removal of the foreign body.

Increased intra-abdominal pressure from the Heimlich maneuver pushes up the diaphragm, which results in increased outflow of air from the lungs. The repeated abdominal thrust forces short bursts of air from the lungs. This dislodges the foreign body.

Placement on midsternum avoids fracture of xiphoid process and ribs and protects an unborn baby.

(Continued)

Copyright © 2010 by Saunders, an imprint of Elsevier Inc. All rights reserved.

Procedure 8-6   CONSCIOUS CHOKING—ADULT AND CHILD—*cont'd*

STEPS—*cont'd*	RATIONALES—*cont'd*
6. Continue giving five back thrusts and five abdominal thrusts until: • The foreign body is forced out. • The victim begins to breathe or cough forcefully. • The victim becomes unconscious.	A victim whose airway is blocked can quickly stop breathing, lose consciousness, and die.
7. After emergency care, document the situation on an incident report form (Figure 8-39) and in the client's chart. Provide a copy of incident report to EMS technician if victim is being transferred to a hospital.	Provides for continuity and protects rescuer from accusations of malpractice.

Client name _____   Date _____Time _____

Address   _____   Home phone _____

    _____   Work phone _____

Incident described:

Vital signs

Time	BP	Pulse	Resp	Oxygen delivery	Medications administered

Treatment administered	Healthcare provider rendering care

Client response to treatment

Figure 8-39.   Medical emergency incident report form.

Copyright © 2010 by Saunders, an imprint of Elsevier Inc. All rights reserved.

Procedure 8-7   UNCONSCIOUS CHOKING—ADULT AND CHILD

SITUATION
The victim is unconscious, and rescue breaths do not make the chest clearly rise.

STEPS	RATIONALES
1. Place the victim in the supine position with his or her head in neutral position. • For adult: Reposition the airway by tilting the head farther back, and try two rescue breaths again. • For child: Reposition the airway by retilting the child's head slightly past the neutral position, and try two rescue breaths again.	Lack of response to sensory stimulation indicates the person is unconscious. It is always necessary to reposition if unable to ventilate, because the tongue and/or soft tissue may be the cause of the airway obstruction.
2. If rescue breaths still do not make the chest clearly rise, give five chest thrusts. • If victim is not in the dental chair, straddle the victim's legs or thighs (Figure 8-40).	Provides stable access to victim's chest.

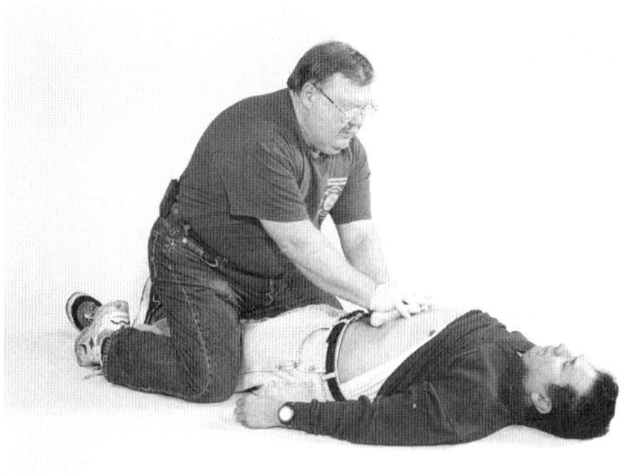

Figure 8-40. (From Chapleau W: *Emergency first responder: making the difference,* St Louis, 2004, Mosby.)

(Continued)

Copyright © 2010 by Saunders, an imprint of Elsevier Inc. All rights reserved.

Procedure 8-7 · UNCONSCIOUS CHOKING—ADULT AND CHILD—*cont'd*

STEPS—*cont'd*	**RATIONALES**—*cont'd*
• If victim is in the dental chair, place your knees close to the victim's hip either on the left or the right side of the chair (Figure 8-41).	Provides stabilization.

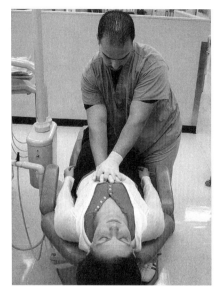

Figure 8-41. (From Malamed SF: *Medical emergencies in the dental office,* ed 6, St Louis, 2007, Mosby.)

• Place the heel of one hand against the victim's abdomen, on the center of the chest above the navel and well below the tip of the xiphoid process.	Provides stabilization and access. Avoids fracture of the xiphoid process.
• Place the other hand directly on top of the first hand.	
• Press into the victim's abdomen with a quick inward and upward motion. (Do not direct the force laterally.)	Each of these subdiaphragmatic abdominal thrusts (the Heimlich maneuver) should be distinct to facilitate removal of the foreign body.
○ Keep your fingers off the chest when giving chest thrusts.	Increased intra-abdominal pressure from the Heimlich maneuver pushes up the diaphragm, which results in increased outflow of air from the lungs. The repeated abdominal thrust forces short bursts of air from the lungs. This dislodges the foreign body.
○ Use your body weight, not your arms, to compress the abdomen.	

Copyright © 2010 by Saunders, an imprint of Elsevier Inc. All rights reserved.

Procedure 8-7   UNCONSCIOUS CHOKING—ADULT AND CHILD—*cont'd*

STEPS—*cont'd*	**RATIONALES**—*cont'd*
○ Position your shoulders over your hands with your elbows locked (Figure 8-42).	Locked elbows provide stabilization and strength to prevent fatigue.

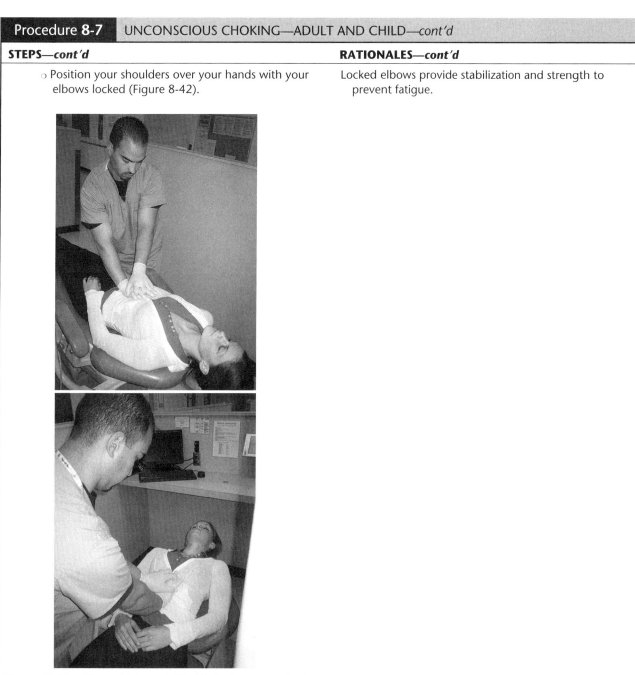

Figure 8-42.   (From Malamed SF: *Medical emergencies in the dental office,* ed 6, St Louis, 2007, Mosby.)

○ For a child, use one hand to compress the abdomen and place the other hand on the child's forehead.	
• Perform up to five abdominal thrusts.	Each thrust is a distinct attempt to dislodge the object.

(Continued)

Copyright © 2010 by Saunders, an imprint of Elsevier Inc. All rights reserved.

Procedure 8-7	UNCONSCIOUS CHOKING—ADULT AND CHILD—*cont'd*

STEPS—*cont'd*	**RATIONALES—*cont'd***
3. Look inside the victim's mouth. Grasp the tongue and lower jaw between your thumb and fingers and the jaw. Look to see if the object has been dislodged and is visible. If the object is visible it should be removed. (New guidelines do not recommend a blind finger sweep.) (Figure 8-43.)	Rescuer attempts to see a foreign body.

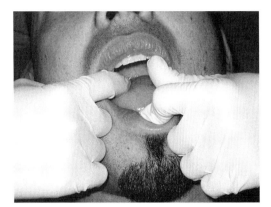

Figure 8-43.   (From Malamed SF: *Medical emergencies in the dental office*, ed 6, St Louis, 2007, Mosby.)

• For an adult, remove the object with your index finger by sliding the finger along the inside of the cheek, using a hooking motion to sweep the object out. • For a child, remove the object with your little finger by sliding it along the inside of the cheek, using a hooking motion to sweep the object out.	Attempts removal of a visualized foreign body.
4. Replace the resuscitation mask and give two rescue breaths.	Determines if airway obstruction still exists. Breathing air into a victim provides oxygen needed to survive.
5. • If the rescue breaths still do not make the chest clearly rise, repeat steps 1 to 4.	Attempts to open the airway so the client can receive rescue breaths.
• If the rescue breaths make the chest clearly rise, remove the mask, look for movement, and check for breathing and a pulse for no more than 10 seconds.	Assesses for respiration and circulation.

• If there is movement, breathing, and a pulse:
  ○ Continue to monitor ABCs.
  ○ Administer emergency oxygen if available.
	Keeps the client stable until emergency medical services (EMS) personnel arrive.

• If there is a pulse but no movement or breathing, give rescue breathing (see Procedure 8-2).	Delivers oxygenated blood to the brain to promote victim survival.
• If there is no movement, breathing, or pulse, perform CPR (see Procedure 8-3 for one-rescuer CPR; see Procedure 8-4 for two-rescuer CPR).	Promotes adequate cardiac output until EMS personnel arrive.

Copyright © 2010 by Saunders, an imprint of Elsevier Inc. All rights reserved.

| Procedure 8-7 | UNCONSCIOUS CHOKING—ADULT AND CHILD—*cont'd* |

STEPS—*cont'd*

6. After emergency care, document the situation on an incident report form (Figure 8-44) and in the client's chart. Provide a copy of incident report to EMS technician if victim is being transferred to a hospital.

RATIONALES—*cont'd*

Provides for continuity of care and protects rescuer from accusations of malpractice.

Client name _____   Date _____ Time _____

Address _____   Home phone _____

_____   Work phone _____

Incident described:

Vital signs

Time	BP	Pulse	Resp	Oxygen delivery	Medications administered

Treatment administered	Healthcare provider rendering care

Client response to treatment
_____

Figure 8-44. Medical emergency incident report form.

Copyright © 2010 by Saunders, an imprint of Elsevier Inc. All rights reserved.

Procedure **8-8**	CONSCIOUS CHOKING—INFANT

SITUATION

The infant cannot cough, cry, or breathe.

STEPS	RATIONALES
1. • Carefully position the infant face down along your forearm.	Position allows gravity to facilitate displacement of the obstruction.
• Support the infant's head and neck with your hand.	Helps to stabilize the infant physically and prevent neck injuries.
• Lower the infant onto your thigh, keeping the infant's head lower than his or her chest.	Your thigh provides additional support for the infant physically, and the position allows gravity to help with the displacement of the obstruction.
2. Give five back blows.	Each back blow should be a distinct attempt to dislodge the object.
• Use the heel of your hand.	
• Give five back blows between the infant's shoulder blades (Figure 8-45).	

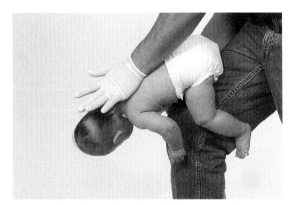

Figure 8-45. (From Chapleau W: *Emergency first responder: making the difference,* St Louis, 2004, Mosby.)

STEPS	RATIONALES
• Note: Use less force when giving back blows to an infant than would be given to a child.	Infants have smaller bodies than children.
3. Position the infant face-up along your forearm.	
• Before turning the infant, position the infant between both of your forearms, supporting the infant's head and neck.	Provides maximum stabilization and support for the infant's head and neck.
• Turn the infant face-up.	Positions the infant to receive chest compressions.
• Lower the infant onto your thigh with the infant's head lower than his or her chest.	Allows gravity to help with the displacement of the obstruction.
4. Give five chest thrusts.	Each of these chest compressions creates increased intra-abdominal pressure and pushes up the diaphragm, which results in increased outflow of air from the lungs. The repeated compression forces short bursts of air from the lungs, which may dislodge the foreign body.
• Put two or three fingers on the center of the chest just below the nipple line (Figure 8-46).	Avoids fracture of xiphoid process.
• Compress the chest five times about ½ to 1 inch.	
• Each chest thrust should be a distinct attempt to dislodge the object.	Attempts to dislodge the object.
5. Look for object in the mouth. Grasp the tongue and lower jaw between your thumb and fingers and lift the jaw.	Lifting the jaw enhances vision of the area once the mouth is opened.

Copyright © 2010 by Saunders, an imprint of Elsevier Inc. All rights reserved.

Procedure 8-8   CONSCIOUS CHOKING—INFANT—*cont'd*

STEPS—*cont'd*   **RATIONALES**—*cont'd*

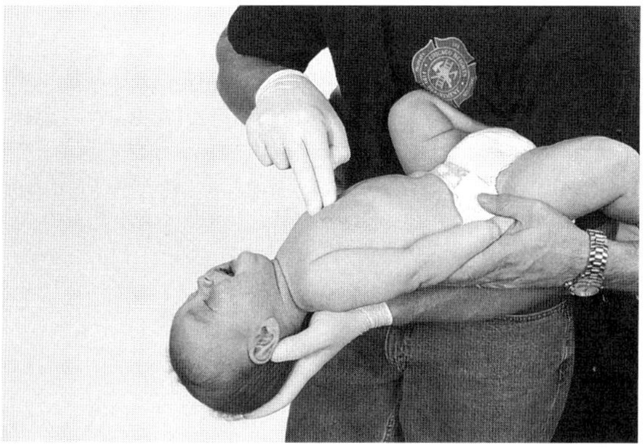

Figure 8-46.   (From Chapleau W: *Emergency first responder: making the difference,* St Louis, 2004, Mosby.)

6. If you see an object, remove it with your little finger by sliding it along the inside of the cheek, using a hooking motion to sweep the object out.

7. Continue giving five back blows and five chest thrusts until:
   • The object is forced out.
   • The infant begins to cough or breathe on his or her own.
   • The infant becomes unconscious (see Procedure 8-9).

8. After emergency care, document the situation on an incident report form (Figure 8-47) and in the client's chart. Provide a copy of incident report to EMS technician if victim is being transferred to a hospital.

Do not perform blind finger sweep in an infant, as it may force the foreign body down farther.

Indicates removal of foreign body.
Indicates infant can breathe.

Provides for continuity of care and protects rescuer from accusations of malpractice.

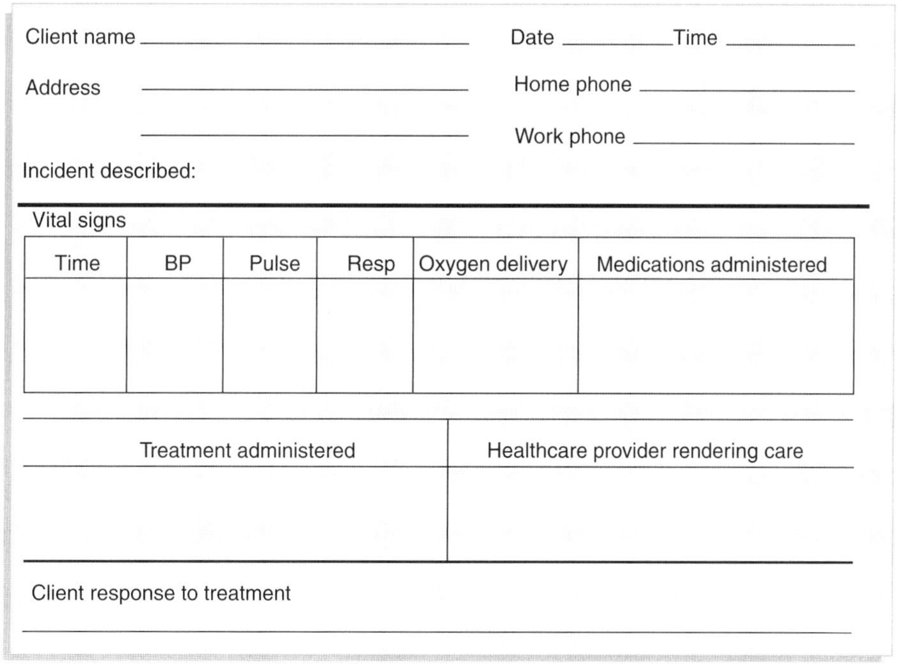

Client name _____	Date _____ Time _____
Address _____	Home phone _____
_____	Work phone _____

Incident described:

Vital signs

Time	BP	Pulse	Resp	Oxygen delivery	Medications administered

Treatment administered	Healthcare provider rendering care

Client response to treatment

Figure 8-47.   Medical emergency incident report form.

Copyright © 2010 by Saunders, an imprint of Elsevier Inc. All rights reserved.

Procedure 8-9   UNCONSCIOUS CHOKING—INFANT

SITUATION

The infant does not move or breathe and does not respond to sensory stimulation.

STEPS	RATIONALES
1. If rescue breaths do not make the chest clearly rise, reposition the airway by retilting the infant's head and try two rescue breaths again.	It is always necessary to reposition if unable to ventilate, because the tongue and/or soft tissue may be the cause of the airway obstruction.
• Keep one hand on the infant's forehead to maintain an open airway, and seal the nose and mouth with your mouth or a resuscitation mask (Figure 8-48).	Maintains an open airway to breathe air into the victim to provide oxygen needed to survive.

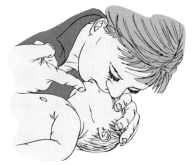

Figure 8-48. (From Potter PA, Perry AG: *Fundamentals of nursing,* ed 7, St Louis, 2009, Mosby.)

STEPS	RATIONALES
2. If rescue breaths still do not make the chest clearly rise, remove the resuscitation mask (if available) and give five chest thrusts.	Attempts to dislodge obstruction.
• Put two or three fingers on the center of the chest just below the nipple line (Figure 8-49).	Avoids fracture of the xiphoid process.

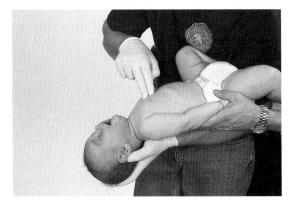

Figure 8-49. (From Chapleau W: *Emergency first responder: making the difference,* St Louis, 2004, Mosby.)

STEPS	RATIONALES
• Compress the chest approximately ½ to 1 inch.	Each of these chest compressions creates increased intra-abdominal pressure and pushes up the diaphragm, which results in increased outflow of air from the lungs. The repeated compressions force short bursts of air from the lungs, which may dislodge the foreign body.
• Each chest compression should be a distinct attempt to dislodge the object.	
• Compress at a rate of approximately 100 compressions per minute.	

Copyright © 2010 by Saunders, an imprint of Elsevier Inc. All rights reserved.

Procedure **8-9**	UNCONSCIOUS CHOKING—INFANT—*cont'd*

STEPS—*cont'd*	**RATIONALES**—*cont'd*
3. Look for object in the mouth. Grasp the tongue and lower jaw between your thumb and fingers and lift the jaw.	Attempts to remove a visualized foreign body. Lifting the jaw enhances visualization.
4. If you see an object, remove it with your little finger by sliding it along the inside of the cheek, using a hooking motion to sweep the object out.	Do not perform a blind finger sweep, as it may force the foreign body down farther.
5. Replace the resuscitation mask (if available) and give two rescue breaths.	Determines whether airway obstruction still exists. Breathing air into a victim provides oxygen needed to survive.
6. • If the rescue breaths still do not make the chest clearly rise and there is still a pulse, repeat steps 1 to 5.	Attempts to open the airway so the client can receive rescue breaths.
• If the rescue breaths make the chest clearly rise, remove the mask, look for movement, and check for breathing and a pulse for no more than 10 seconds.	Assesses for respiration and circulation.
• If there is movement, breathing, and a pulse: ○ Continue to monitor ABCs. ○ Administer emergency oxygen if available.	Keeps the client stable until emergency medical services (EMS) personnel arrive.
• If there is a pulse but no movement or breathing, give rescue breathing (see Procedure 8-2).	Delivers oxygenated blood to the brain to promote victim survival.
• If there is no movement, breathing, or pulse, perform CPR (see Procedures 8-3 and 8-4).	Promotes adequate cardiac output until EMS personnel arrive.
7. After emergency care, document the situation on an incident report form (Figure 8-50) and in the client's chart. Provide a copy of incident report to EMS technician if victim is being transferred to a hospital.	Provides for continuity of care and protects rescuer from accusations of malpractice.

Client name _____   Date _____ Time _____

Address   _____   Home phone _____

              _____   Work phone _____

Incident described:

Vital signs

Time	BP	Pulse	Resp	Oxygen delivery	Medications administered

Treatment administered	Healthcare provider rendering care

Client response to treatment
_____

Figure 8-50. Medical emergency incident report form.

Please refer to the Evolve website (http://evolve.elsevier.com/Darby/hygiene) for competency forms to help evaluate your mastery of each procedure in this chapter.

Copyright © 2010 by Saunders, an imprint of Elsevier Inc. All rights reserved.

Vital Signs

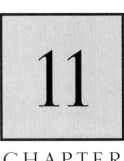

11

CHAPTER

Procedure 11-1	TAKING AN ORAL TEMPERATURE MEASUREMENT WITH A MERCURY-IN-GLASS THERMOMETER

EQUIPMENT
Personal protective equipment for the clinician
Mercury-in-glass thermometer, disposable sheath
Accurate timepiece

STEPS	RATIONALES
1. Wash hands with antimicrobial soap.	Reduces chances of transmitting infectious microorganisms.
2. Explain procedure to client.	Inform client of the hygienist's intent.
3. Ask client if hot or cold substances were ingested or if tobacco was smoked within the previous 30 minutes.	Hot and cold fluids or food or recent smoking may alter the client's true temperature; therefore wait 20 to 30 minutes before taking temperature.
4. Hold end of the thermometer opposite the mercury end with your fingertips.	This prevents contamination of the bulb to be inserted into the client's mouth.
5. Before inserting the thermometer into client's oral cavity, read the mercury level.	Mercury is to be below 35.5° C (96° F); thermometer reading must be below the client's actual temperature before use.
6. If mercury is above the desired level, shake the thermometer so that the mercury moves toward the bulb. Grasp tip of the thermometer securely and stand away from any solid objects. Sharply flick the wrist downward as though you were cracking a whip. Continue until the reading is below 35.5° C (96° F).	Brisk shaking lowers the mercury level in the glass tube; stand in an open area to prevent thermometer from breaking.
7. Place disposable cover or sheath on thermometer.	Prevents cross-contamination.
8. Ask client to open mouth, and gently place the thermometer under the tongue lateral to the lower jaw. Avoid area directly under tongue.	The area directly under the tongue has a significantly higher temperature owing to vascular supply; the client's true temperature is taken from the posterior sublingual arteries under the tongue.
9. Ask client to hold the thermometer with the lips closed. Warn client to avoid biting down on the thermometer.	The lips hold the thermometer in place and prevent the thermometer from breaking.
10. Leave the thermometer in place for 3 full minutes or as directed by the manufacturer.	The thermometer should remain in place for a minimum of 3 minutes, but no longer than 6 minutes.

Copyright © 2010 by Saunders, an imprint of Elsevier Inc. All rights reserved.

Procedure **11-1**	TAKING AN ORAL TEMPERATURE MEASUREMENT WITH A MERCURY-IN-GLASS THERMOMETER—*cont'd*

STEPS—*cont'd*	RATIONALES—*cont'd*
11. Carefully remove the thermometer.	Prevents breakage.
12. Remove and discard the disposable cover.	The cover should be removed to allow maximum visibility and should be discarded in the appropriate manner to prevent cross-contamination.
13. Read thermometer as it is held in a horizontal position at eye level.	Yields an accurate reading.
14. Wash thermometer in soap and water, and disinfect.	Prevents cross-contamination in the event that the disposable cover breaks or tears.
15. Store thermometer in its proper container.	Proper storage prevents breakage and contamination.
16. Inform dentist of readings above 37.5° C (99.6° F).	A client experiencing fluctuations in temperature should be referred to his or her physician for immediate consultation.
17. Document in ink the completion of this service in the client's record under "Services Rendered," with the time of day, and date the entry. For example: "12/1/09 client stated that she was not feeling well and felt that she was running a fever. Client's temperature taken at 2:00 PM was 101.5° F. Dentist consulted and client appointment rescheduled."	Ensures the integrity of the client's record for both the client's health and practitioner's protection from legal risks.

Adapted from Potter PA, Perry AG: *Fundamentals of nursing,* ed 7, St Louis, 2009, Mosby.

Copyright © 2010 by Saunders, an imprint of Elsevier Inc. All rights reserved.

Procedure 11-2   TAKING AN ORAL TEMPERATURE MEASUREMENT WITH AN ELECTRONIC THERMOMETER

EQUIPMENT
Personal protective equipment for the clinician
Electronic thermometer, disposable sheath

STEPS	RATIONALES
1. Wash hands with antimicrobial soap.	Reduces chances of transmitting infectious microorganisms.
2. Explain procedure to client.	Inform client of the hygienist's intent.
3. Ask client if hot or cold substances were ingested or if tobacco was smoked within the previous 30 minitus.	Hot or cold fluids or food or recent smoking may alter the client's true temperature; therefore wait 20 to 30 minutes before taking temperature.
4. Remove thermometer pack from charging unit, check to make sure the oral probe is attached to the unit.	To prepare the unit.
5. Insert the oral probe into the plastic, disposable cover until it locks into place.	Prevents cross-contamination.
6. Ask the client to open his or her mouth, and gently place the probe under the tongue, posterior and lateral to the lower jaw. Avoid placing probe directly under tongue.	Body heat from the posterior sublingual arteries under the tongue produces the most accurate readings.
7. Ask client to hold the probe with the lips closed.	The lips hold the probe in the proper position.
8. An audible tone will signal that the temperature has been taken; note display.	
9. Remove the probe and discard the disposable cover by pushing the ejection button.	Prevents cross-contamination.
10. Place probe back into original storage well in the unit.	Prevents damage to probe and clears digital readout.
11. Return the thermometer to the charger.	Keeps unit charged and ready for use.
12. Record the client's temperature, the date, and the time of day on the chart.	Vital signs should be recorded immediately to ensure accuracy.
13. Inform dentist of readings above 37.5° C (99.6° F).	A client experiencing fluctuations in temperature should be referred to the physician of record for immediate consultation.
14. Document in ink the completion of this service in the client's record under "Services Rendered," with the time of day, and date the entry. For example: "12/1/09 client stated that she was not feeling well and felt that she was running a fever. Client's temperature taken at 2:00 PM was 101.5° F. Dentist consulted and client appointment rescheduled."	Ensures integrity of the client's record for both the client's health and practitioner protection from legal risks.

Adapted from Potter PA, Perry AG: *Fundamentals of nursing,* ed 7, St Louis, 2009, Mosby.

Copyright © 2010 by Saunders, an imprint of Elsevier Inc. All rights reserved.

Procedure **11-3**   MEASURING THE RADIAL PULSE

EQUIPMENT
Wristwatch with a second hand

STEPS	RATIONALES
1. Use a wristwatch with a second hand.	Allows for an accurate assessment.
2. Wash hands with antimicrobial soap.	Reduces chances of transmitting infectious microorganisms.
3. Explain purpose and method of procedure to the client. Advise client to relax and not to speak.	Activity and anxiety can elevate heart rate. Client's voice may interfere with the dental hygienist's ability to concentrate.
4. Have client assume a sitting position, bend the client's elbow 90 degrees, and support the client's lower arm on the armrest of the chair. Extend the wrist with the palm down.	Proper positioning exposes the radial artery for palpation without restriction.
5. Place first two fingers of hand along the client's radial artery (thumb side of wrist) and lightly compress (Figure 11-1).	Fingertips are the most sensitive part of the hand.

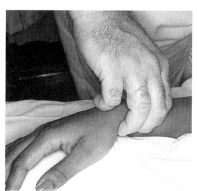

Figure 11-1. Position of the fingers in measuring the radial pulse. (From Potter PA, Perry AG: *Fundamentals of nursing,* ed 6, St Louis, 2005, Mosby.)

STEPS	RATIONALES
6. Obliterate the pulse initially, then relax pressure so that the pulse is easily palpable.	Pulse is more accurately assessed with moderate finger pressure; too much pressure occludes the pulse, and too little prevents the examiner from feeling the pulse with regularity.
7. Determine rhythm and quality of the pulse (regular, regularly irregular, full and strong, weak and thready).	Pulse quality reflects volume of blood ejected against arterial wall with each heart contraction. Alternating strong and weak beats may indicate ventricular failure, high blood pressure, or coronary heart disease. A full, bounding pulse may indicate high blood pressure. Hypotension and shock produce a weak, thready pulse.
8. When pulse can be felt regularly, use the watch's second hand and begin to count the rate, starting with 0 and then 1, and so on.	Rate is determined accurately only after the examiner is certain that the pulse can be palpated. Timing should begin with 0. The count of 1 is the first beat felt after timing begins.
9. If the pulse is regular, count for 30 seconds and multiply the total by 2.	Thirty-second count is accurate for rapid, slow, or regular pulse rates.
10. If the pulse is irregular, count for a full minute.	The longer time ensures an accurate count.
11. Record heart rate (beats per minute [BPM]), rhythm of the heart (regular or irregular), the quality of the pulse (thready, strong, weak, bounding), and the date in the chart. Pulse rates outside the normal range should be evaluated by the client's physician.	Vital signs should be recorded immediately on the client's record.

(Continued)

Copyright © 2010 by Saunders, an imprint of Elsevier Inc. All rights reserved.

Procedure **11-3**   MEASURING THE RADIAL PULSE—*cont'd*

STEPS—*cont'd*	RATIONALES—*cont'd*
12. Document in ink the completion of this service in the client's record under "Services Rendered." Record heart rate (BPM), rhythm of the heart (regular, regularly irregular, or irregularly irregular), the quality of the pulse (thready and weak [not easily felt], strong and full [easily felt]), and the date in the chart. For example: "12/1/09 Client's pulse has a regular rhythm and strong quality with rate of 65 BPM."	Ensures the integrity of the client's record for both the client's health and the practitioner's protection from legal risks.

Adapted from Potter PA, Perry AG: *Fundamentals of nursing,* ed 7, St Louis, 2009, Mosby.

Procedure **11-4**   MEASURING RESPIRATIONS

EQUIPMENT
Wristwatch with a second hand

STEPS	RATIONALES
1. Use a wristwatch with a second hand.	Allows the clinician to make an accurate assessment.
2. Place hand along the client's radial artery and inconspicuously observe the client's chest.	Allows the dental hygienist to make the assessment without the client's awareness of the process.
3. Observe the rise and fall of client's chest. Count complete respiratory cycles (one inspiration and one expiration).	
4. For an adult, count the number of respirations in 30 seconds and multiply that number by 2. For a young child, count respirations for a full minute.	Respiratory rate is equivalent to the number of respirations per minute; young infants and children breathe in an irregular rhythm.
5. If an adult has respirations with an irregular rhythm, or if respirations are abnormally slow or fast (<12 or >20 breaths/minute), count for a full minute.	Accurate interpretation requires assessment for at least a minute.
6. While counting, note whether depth is shallow, normal, or deep and whether rhythm is normal or one of the altered patterns.	The character of ventilatory movements may reveal specific alterations or disease states.
7. Document in ink the completion of this service in the client's record under "Services Rendered." Record the date and the client's respirations per minute (RPM) in the chart; a respiration rate with an irregular pattern or that is outside of the normal range should be evaluated by the physician. For example: "12/1/09 Client's respiration has a regular rhythm with rate of 18 RPM."	Ensures the integrity of the client's record for both the client's health and the legal protection of the practitioner.

Adapted from Potter PA, Perry AG: *Fundamentals of nursing,* ed 7, St Louis, 2009, Mosby.

Copyright © 2010 by Saunders, an imprint of Elsevier Inc. All rights reserved.

Procedure 11-5 | ASSESSING BLOOD PRESSURE BY AUSCULTATION

EQUIPMENT
Blood pressure cuff or sphygmomanometer
Stethoscope

STEPS	RATIONALES
1. Ask client about recent activities that could alter the client's normal blood pressure.	Recent activities, e.g., tobacco use, exercise, and caffeine consumption, can elevate blood pressure.
2. Determine proper cuff size. Inspect the parts of the release valve and the pressure bulb. The valve should be clean and freely movable in either direction.	Proper cuff size is necessary so that the correct amount of pressure is applied over the artery. Cuffs that are too small for a client's arm produce artificially high blood pressure readings; cuffs that are too large produce artificially low readings. If the valve sticks or becomes too tightly closed, the deflation of the pressure cuff will be hard to regulate.
3. Wash hands with antimicrobial soap.	Washing reduces chance of transmitting infectious microorganisms.
4. Explain purpose of the procedure, but avoid talking to client for at least a minute before taking the client's blood pressure.	Explanations reassure the client and increase the likelihood of compliance in the event of an abnormal reading. Talking to a client while taking blood pressure can increase the client's blood pressure by 10% to 40%.
5. Assist client to a comfortable sitting position, with arm slightly flexed, forearm supported, and palm turned up.	Facilitates cuff application. Having arm above heart level would produce a falsely low reading.
6. Expose the upper arm fully.	Ensures proper cuff application.
7. Palpate brachial artery. Position the cuff approximately 1 inch above the brachial artery.	Proper positioning of cuff facilitates an accurate reading.
8. Center arrows marked on the cuff over the brachial artery.	Inflating bladder directly over brachial artery ensures that proper pressure is applied during inflation.
9. Be sure cuff is fully deflated. Wrap cuff evenly and snugly around the upper arm. Center arrow on cuff over artery. If there is no arrow, estimate center of bladder and place over artery.	Ensures that proper pressure will be applied over the artery.
10. Be sure manometer is positioned for easy reading.	Eye-level placement ensures accurate reading of the mercury level.
11. If client's normal systolic pressure is unknown, palpate the radial artery and rapidly inflate cuff to a pressure 30 mm Hg above the point at which radial pulsation disappears. Deflate the cuff and wait 30 seconds.	This determines the maximal inflation point and prevents auscultatory gap; 30-second delay prevents venous congestion and falsely high readings.
12. Place stethoscope earpieces in ears and be sure sounds are clear, not muffled.	Each earpiece should follow angle of examiner's ear canal to facilitate hearing.
13. Place diaphragm (or the bell) of the stethoscope over the brachial artery in the antecubital fossa. The antecubital fossa is the depression in the underside of the arm at the bend of the elbow. Avoid contact with blood pressure cuff or clothing.	Proper stethoscope placement ensures optimal sound reception. A stethoscope that is not positioned properly produces muffled sounds resulting in falsely low systolic and falsely high diastolic readings.
14. Close valve of pressure bulb clockwise until tight.	Tightening valve prevents air leaks during inflation.
15. Inflate cuff to 30 mm Hg above client's normal systolic level.	Proper cuff inflation ensures accurate pressure measurement.
16. Slowly release valve, allowing mercury (or needle of the aneroid gauge) to fall at a rate of 2 to 3 mm Hg per second.	Too rapid or slow a decline in pressure may lead to an inaccurate reading.
17. Note point on manometer at which the first clear sound is heard.	First Korotkoff sound indicates the systolic pressure. Blood pressure levels should be recorded in even numbers.
18. Continue cuff deflation, noting point on the manometer at which the sound muffles (phase IV) and disappears (phase V).	Fifth Korotkoff sound is the diastolic pressure in adults. Children may have a 0–mm Hg reading using the fifth Korotkoff sound; therefore record the fourth Korotkoff sound as well (e.g., 100/50/0 mm Hg).

(Continued)

Copyright © 2010 by Saunders, an imprint of Elsevier Inc. All rights reserved.

Procedure **11-5**	ASSESSING BLOOD PRESSURE BY AUSCULTATION—*cont'd*
STEPS—*cont'd*	**RATIONALES—***cont'd*
19. Deflate cuff rapidly. To determine an average blood pressure and ensure a correct reading, wait 2 minutes, then repeat procedure for the same arm.	Continuous cuff inflation causes arterial occlusion, resulting in arm numbness and tingling. Blood pressure reading is repeated on same arm because there may be as much as 10 mm Hg difference in readings between arms.
20. Remove cuff from client's arm. Assist client to a comfortable position and cover upper arm.	Maintains client's comfort.
21. Disinfect earpieces of stethoscope and fold cuff, and store properly in a cool, dry place.	Proper maintenance of supplies contributes to instrument accuracy. Sunlight and heat may compromise rubber tubing.
22. Discuss findings with client.	Gives immediate client feedback and assists client in understanding his or her current health status.
23. Document in ink the completion of this service in client's record under "Services Rendered." Record in client's chart the systolic over the diastolic blood pressure reading in mm Hg, the date, cuff size if it was an atypical size, and arm used for measurement (use guidelines in Tables 11-6 to 11-9 on pp. 187-189 to determine need for a physician referral). For example: "12/1/09 Client's blood pressure measured with adult size cuff is 110/75 mm Hg right arm sitting."	Ensures integrity of the client's record for both the client's health and the practitioner's protection from legal risks.

Adapted from Potter PA, Perry AG: *Fundamental of nursing,* ed 7, St Louis, 2009, Mosby.

Please refer to the Evolve website (http://evolve.elsevier.com/Darby/hygiene) for competency forms to help evaluate your mastery of each procedure in this chapter.

Copyright © 2010 by Saunders, an imprint of Elsevier Inc. All rights reserved.

Extraoral and Intraoral Clinical Assessment

Procedure **13-1**	CONDUCTING EXTRAORAL ASSESSMENTS	
EXTRAORAL REGIONS	**STEPS**	**RATIONALES**
Overall evaluation of the face, head, and neck including skin (Figure 13-1) **Figure 13-1.**	Visually observe symmetry and coloration of face and neck.	Allows the clinician to check for signs of nutritional deficiency and signs of systemic disease, possible asymmetry from neoplasm, or abnormal growth and development. Be aware that signs of physical abuse often occur in the head, face, and neck region.
Parietal and occipital regions, including scalp (Figure 13-2, *A*), hair, and occipital nodes (Figure 13-2, *B*) A B **Figure 13-2.** **A,** Parietal and occipital regions including scalp, hair, and occipital nodes. **B,** Palpating the occipital lymph nodes by bending the client's head forward.	Visually inspect the entire scalp by moving the hair, especially around the hairline, starting from around one ear and proceeding to the other ear. Standing behind, have the client bend the head forward, and bilaterally palpate the occipital nodes.	Allows the clinician to inspect the scalp, where many lesions may be hidden by hair, and inspect the occipital nodes to check for tender, enlarged nodes or masses indicating local or systemic involvement. These nodes drain the area and may indicate a disease state in that area.
Temporal region, including auricular nodes (Figure 13-3, *A* and *B*) and ears (Figure 13-3, *C*)	Standing near the client on one side then the other, visually inspect and bilaterally palpate the auricular nodes and the scalp and face around each ear. Visually inspect and palpate each ear.	Allows the clinician to check for tender, enlarged nodes or massing indicating local or systemic involvement. These nodes drain the areas around the ear and may indicate a disease state in that area. Also allows for inspection of the ear itself to check for infection or skin cancer.

(Continued)

Copyright © 2010 by Saunders, an imprint of Elsevier Inc. All rights reserved.

Procedure 13-1 | CONDUCTING EXTRAORAL ASSESSMENTS—*cont'd*

EXTRAORAL REGIONS—*cont'd*	STEPS—*cont'd*	RATIONALES—*cont'd*

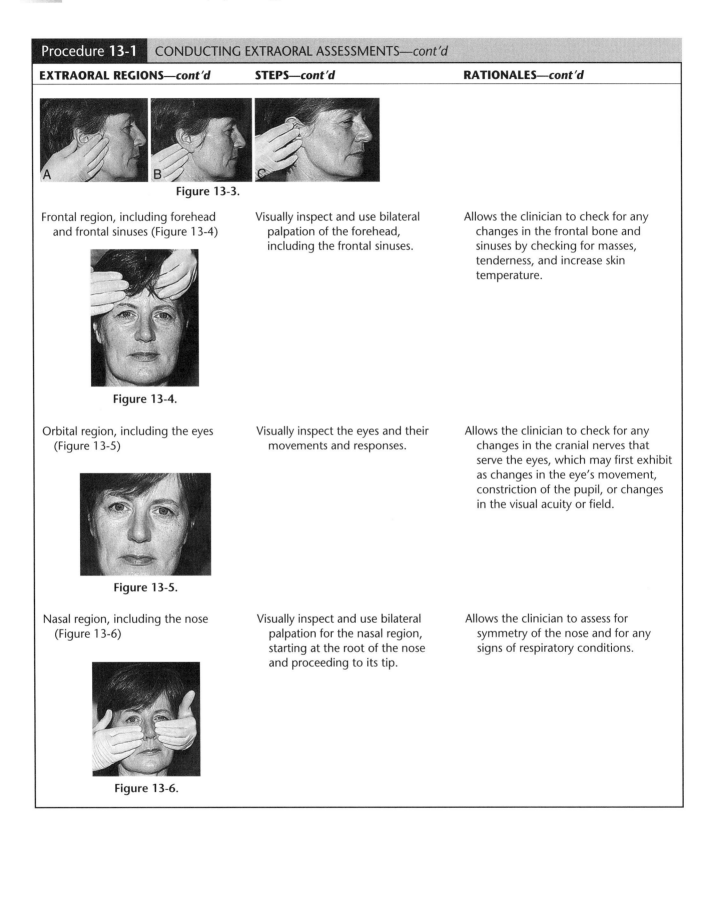

Figure 13-3.

EXTRAORAL REGIONS	STEPS	RATIONALES
Frontal region, including forehead and frontal sinuses (Figure 13-4)	Visually inspect and use bilateral palpation of the forehead, including the frontal sinuses.	Allows the clinician to check for any changes in the frontal bone and sinuses by checking for masses, tenderness, and increase skin temperature.

Figure 13-4.

Orbital region, including the eyes (Figure 13-5)	Visually inspect the eyes and their movements and responses.	Allows the clinician to check for any changes in the cranial nerves that serve the eyes, which may first exhibit as changes in the eye's movement, constriction of the pupil, or changes in the visual acuity or field.

Figure 13-5.

Nasal region, including the nose (Figure 13-6)	Visually inspect and use bilateral palpation for the nasal region, starting at the root of the nose and proceeding to its tip.	Allows the clinician to assess for symmetry of the nose and for any signs of respiratory conditions.

Figure 13-6.

Copyright © 2010 by Saunders, an imprint of Elsevier Inc. All rights reserved.

Procedure 13-1 CONDUCTING EXTRAORAL ASSESSMENTS—*cont'd*

EXTRAORAL REGIONS—*cont'd*	STEPS—*cont'd*	RATIONALES—*cont'd*
Infraorbital and zygomatic regions, including the muscles of facial expression (Figure 13-7, *A*), facial nodes (Figure 13-7, *B*), maxillary sinuses (Figure 13-7, *C*), and temporomandibular joints (TMJs) (Figure 13-7, *D* and *E*)	Visually inspect the under eye and cheek areas, noting the use of the muscles of facial expression. Visually inspect and use bilateral palpitation of the facial nodes by moving from infraorbital region to the labial commissure and then to the surface of the mandible. Visually inspect and use bilateral palpitation of the maxillary sinuses. Gently place a finger into the outer portion of the external acoustic meatus. To access the TMJ and its associated muscles, use bilateral palpitation and ask the client to open and close the mouth several times. Then ask client to move the opened jaw left, then right, and then forward. Ask the client if they experienced any pain or tenderness. Note any sounds made by the joint.	Checks for a lack of expression, which may indicate a change in the cranial nerve that serves the facial muscles. Also checks the maxillary sinus for tenderness and increased skin temperature. Allows the clinician to assess for temporomandibular disorders (TMDs).

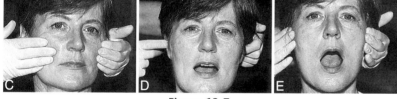

Figure 13-7.

| Buccal region, including the masseter muscle (Figure 13-8, *A*) and parotid salivary glands (Figure 13-8, *B*) | Standing near the client on each side, visually inspect and use bilateral palpation of the masseter muscle and parotid gland by starting in front of each ear and moving to the cheek area and down to the angle of the mandible. Place the fingers of each hand over the masseter muscle and ask client to clench the teeth together several times. | Allows the clinician to check for tender, enlarged nodes or masses indicating local or systemic infection. These nodes drain the area of the cheek and may indicate a disease state in that area. Also allows the clinician to check the masseter muscle for development and that the parotid glands are free of tenderness and enlargement. |

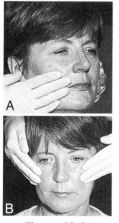

Figure 13-8.

(Continued)

Copyright © 2010 by Saunders, an imprint of Elsevier Inc. All rights reserved.

EXTRAORAL REGIONS—*cont'd*	STEPS—*cont'd*	RATIONALES—*cont'd*
Mental region, including the chin (Figure 13-9) 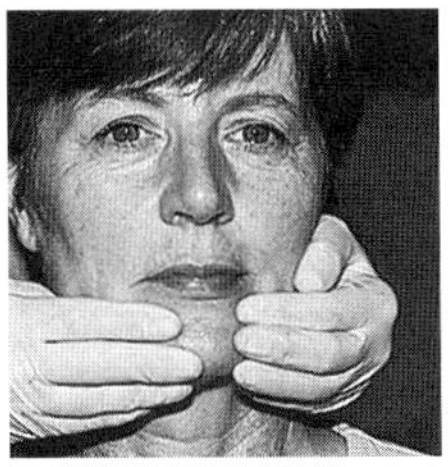 **Figure 13-9.**	Standing near the client on each side, visually inspect and use bilateral palpitation of the chin.	Allows the clinician to detect enlargement or masses, as well as any abnormal growth of soft tissue or bone, surface lesions, and tenderness.
Anterior and posterior cervical regions, including sternocleidomastoid muscle (SCM) and associated nodes (Figure 13-10) 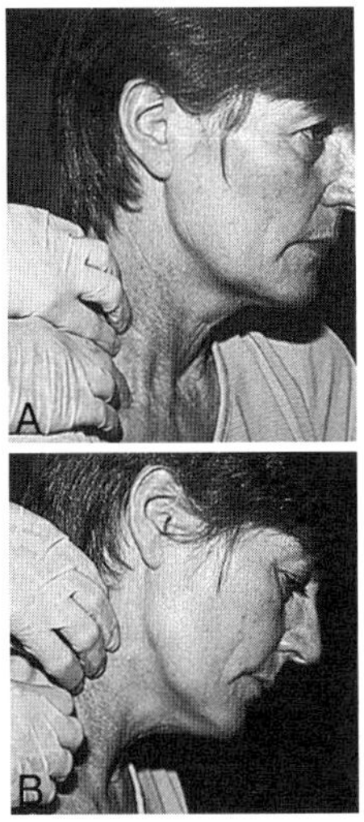 **Figure 13-10.**	With the client looking straight ahead, use manual palpation with two hands on each side of the neck to assess the superficial cervical nodes. Start below the ear and continue the whole length of the SCM surface to the clavicles (see Figure 13-18, *A*). Then have the client tilt the head to the side and palpate the deep cervical nodes on the underside of the anterior and posterior aspects of the SCM.	Allows the clinician to check for enlarged nodes or masses indicating local or systemic disease.
Submandibular and submental triangle regions, including submandibular and sublingual salivary glands and associated nodes (Figure 13-11) 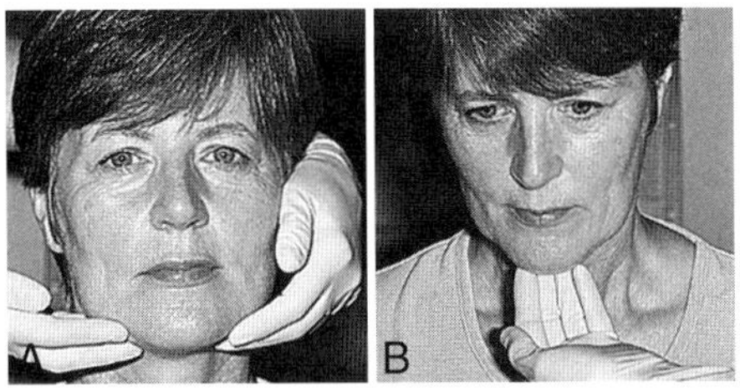 **Figure 13-11.**	Standing slightly behind the client on each side, have the client lower chin for palpation underneath the chin and sides of the mandible. Roll the tissue on each side over the angle of the mandible.	Allows the clinician to assess the submental, sublingual, and submandibular glands; associated lymph nodes; and mandible.

Copyright © 2010 by Saunders, an imprint of Elsevier Inc. All rights reserved.

Procedure 13-1 | CONDUCTING EXTRAORAL ASSESSMENTS—*cont'd*

EXTRAORAL REGIONS—*cont'd*	STEPS—*cont'd*	RATIONALES—*cont'd*
Anterior midline cervical region, including hyoid bone, thyroid cartilage and gland (Figure 13-12) **Figure 13-12.**	Standing near the client, place one hand on each side of the trachea. Then gently displace the thyroid tissue to the other side of the neck while the other hand manually palpates the displaced glandular tissue. Then compare the two lobes of the thyroid using visual inspection and bimanual or manual palpation. Ask the client to swallow to check for mobility of the gland by visually inspecting it while it moves superiorly. Client may need to use a glass of water to swallow.	This neck position relaxes the muscles and allows the clinician to check the thyroid for masses. Enlargement or immobility may be a manifestation of thyroid disease.

Steps from Fehrenbach MJ, Herring SW: *Illustrated anatomy of the head and neck*, ed 3, St Louis, 2007, Saunders. Figures courtesy Dr. Margaret Walsh, University of California–San Francisco.

Copyright © 2010 by Saunders, an imprint of Elsevier Inc. All rights reserved.

Procedure **13-2**   CONDUCTING INTRAORAL ASSESSMENTS

EQUIPMENT
Mouth mirror
Explorer
Periodontal probe
Hand mirror
2 × 2 gauze
Air and water syringe
Personal protective equipment

INTRAORAL REGIONS	STEPS	RATIONALES
Lips (Figure 13-13) 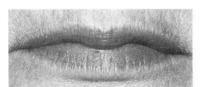 **Figure 13-13.**	Visually inspect the lips, including the commissures. Ask the patient to close and then to smile. Use bidigital palpation on the lower lip in a systematic manner from one corner of the mouth to the other. Use same technique for the upper lip.	Allows the clinician to observe the lips and vermilion border and surrounding skin and the relationship between lips and teeth.
Oral cavity (Figure 13-14) 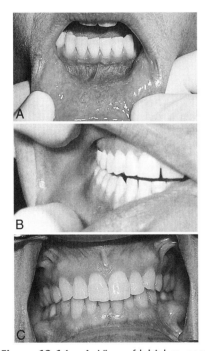	Have the client open the mouth slightly, and gently pull the lower lip away from the teeth to observe the labial mucosa. Then gently pull the buccal mucosa slightly away from the teeth to palpate bidigitally, using circular compression. Dry the area and observe the flow of saliva from each duct. Retract mucosa enough to visually inspect the vestibular area. Palpate and visually examine the alveolar ridges and attached gingiva. Palpate the maxillary tuberosity and retromolar area using digital compression.	Allows the clinician to further assess lips, as well as the oral mucosa, for changes in color, form, and texture and signs of nutritional deficiency or fungal infection and to check the labial frena for tightness, tissue tags, or scarring. Allows assessment for enlargements or masses within the gland or duct. Also allows the clinician to observe swelling, lesions, and color changes of the attached gingival tissue and gross signs of periodontal disease. Be aware that signs of physical abuse often occur in the oral cavity.

Figure 13-14. A, View of labial mucosa, labial frenum, mucogingival junction, and attached gingiva. **B,** View of the buccal mucosa, parotid papilla, maxillary vestibule, mandibular vestibule, and alveolar mucosa. **C,** Frontal view of periodontium.

Copyright © 2010 by Saunders, an imprint of Elsevier Inc. All rights reserved.

Procedure **13-2** CONDUCTING INTRAORAL ASSESSMENTS—*cont'd*

INTRAORAL REGIONS—*cont'd*	STEPS—*cont'd*	RATIONALES—*cont'd*
Palate and pharynx, including the hard and soft palates, faucial arches, palatine tonsils, uvula, oropharynx, and nasopharynx (Figure 13-15) 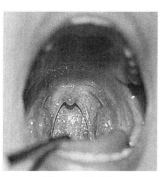 **Figure 13-15.**	Have client tilt the head back slightly. Use mouth mirror to intensify light source and view the palatal and pharyngeal regions. Have client extend the tongue; observe the soft palate. Gently place the mouth mirror (mirror side down) on the middle of the tongue and ask the client to say "ah." As this is done, visually observe the uvula and the visible portions of the pharynx. Compress hard and soft palates with first or second finger of one hand. Avoid circular compression on the soft palate to prevent initiating the gag reflex.	Allows the clinician to check palatal and pharyngeal tissues for changes in color, form, and texture.
Tongue (Figure 13-16) 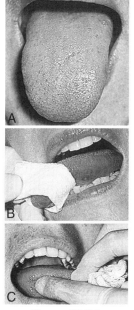 **Figure 13-16.**	To assess the dorsal and lateral surfaces of the tongue, wrap a gauze square around the anterior third of the tongue to obtain a firm grasp. Digitally palpate dorsal surface. (If the client is forced to extend the tongue too far, the gag reflex is triggered). Turn the tongue slightly on its side to inspect its base and lateral borders. Bidigitally palpate the lateral surfaces of the tongue. To assess the ventral surface, have the client lift the tongue to permit inspection and digital palpation of the surface. Release the tongue.	Allows the clinician to assess the tongue, especially its base and lateral borders, for abnormal color, swellings, masses, or lesion. Allows for the labial frena to be checked for tightness, tissue tags, or scarring. Allows the clinician to check lingual papilla, foramen cecum, and lingual tonsils. Allows evaluation of swallowing pattern.

(Continued)

Copyright © 2010 by Saunders, an imprint of Elsevier Inc. All rights reserved.

Procedure **13-2**	CONDUCTING INTRAORAL ASSESSMENTS—*cont'd*	
INTRAORAL REGIONS—*cont'd*	**STEPS—*cont'd***	**RATIONALES—*cont'd***
Floor of the mouth, including the submandibular and sublingual salivary glands and ducts (Figure 13-17) 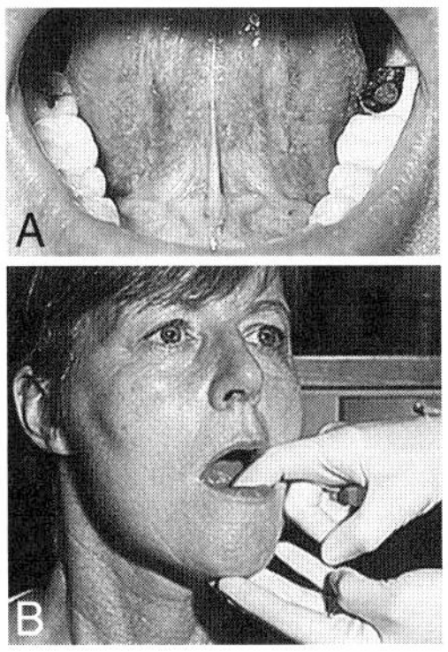 **Figure 13-17.**	Use the mouth mirror to facilitate lighting and direct observation. While the client lifts the tongue to the roof of the mouth, observe the mucosa of the floor of the mouth for lesions, swelling, or color change. Check the lingual frenum. Wipe the sublingual caruncle with gauze and observe the saliva flow from the duct. Bimanually palpate the sublingual area by placing the right index finger intraorally and the fingertips of the left hand extraorally under the chin to feel the tissue between the two hands. Use bidigital palpation for the sublingual gland on the floor of the mouth, behind each mandibular canine, by placing the index finger of one hand intraorally and the index finger of the other hand extraorally, with the gland compressed between.	Allows the clinician to detect enlargement or masses and to note any abnormal growth of soft tissue, gland, or bone; surface lesions; and tenderness.

Steps from Fehrenbach MJ, Herring SW: *Illustrated anatomy of the head and neck*, ed 3, St Louis, 2007, Saunders. Figures courtesy Dr. Margaret Walsh, University of California–San Francisco.

Copyright © 2010 by Saunders, an imprint of Elsevier Inc. All rights reserved.

Procedure 13-3 | CONDUCTING AN ORALCDx BRUSH BIOPSY

EQUIPMENT
OralCDx test kit with instructions, return mailing box, barcoded specimen slide and holder, sterile brush instrument, fixative packet (Figure 13-18)
Personal protective equipment

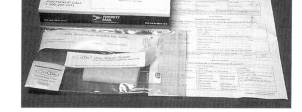

Figure 13-18. OralCDx test kit. (Courtesy CDx Laboratories, Suffern, New York.)

STEPS	RATIONALES
1. Put on personal protective equipment before handling brush instrument and slide.	Prevents contamination of the slide and maintains infection control protocol.
2. Remove brush from kit (Figure 13-19). Slightly moisten the brush with the client's saliva if the lesion is dry. Neither local nor topical anesthetic is required and should not be used because it may distort the sample.	Prevents the cells from drying and becoming distorted.

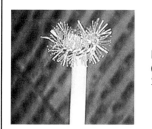

Figure 13-19. OralCDx brush. (Courtesy CDx Laboratories, Suffern, New York.)

3. Press the brush firmly against the lesion, and rotate 5 to 10 times (depending on the thickness of the lesion) until pink tissue or pinpoint microbleeding is observed (Figure 13-20).

Allows a full transepithelial collection of sample cells from the lesion.

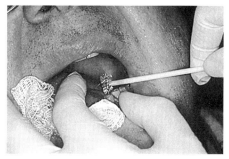

Figure 13-20. Pressing the brush firmly against the lesion. (Courtesy CDx Laboratories, Suffern, New York.)

(Continued)

Copyright © 2010 by Saunders, an imprint of Elsevier Inc. All rights reserved.

Procedure 13-3   CONDUCTING AN ORALCDx BRUSH BIOPSY—*cont'd*

STEPS—*Cont'd*	**RATIONALES**—*Cont'd*
4. Spread the cellular sample from the brush onto the slide by rotating and dragging the brush lengthwise (Figure 13-21).	Ensures that the greatest possible amount of material is transferred from the brush to the slide.

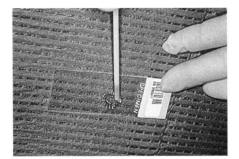

Figure 13-21. Spreading cellular sample on OralCDx slide. (Courtesy CDx Laboratories, Suffern, New York.)

5. Immediately fix the cells by squeezing the entire contents of one fixative package onto the slide, flooding the slide. Set the slide aside to dry for 15 minutes, and then place in slide holder.	Ensures that the cells do not dry out and become distorted.
6. Complete the test requisition form, and send the specimen to the laboratory in the box provided.	Allows for completion of information such as the dentist's name and address, client's name and address, and a complete clinical description of the lesion necessary for documentation.
7. Document procedure in the client record, and note on calendar when the pathology report is due back.	Done for legal purposes and to facilitate continuity of care and ensure that the report is not overlooked or ignored.
8. Read the pathology report from the laboratory, and make sure that findings are shared with the client.	Ensures that the client is information and that appropriate follow-up care is obtained.
9. Guide the client to receive the appropriate follow-up care as recommended by the supervising dentist.	Increases the likelihood that the client will adhere to the recommendations.

Please refer to the Evolve website (http://evolve.elsevier.com/Darby/hygiene) for competency forms to help evaluate your mastery of each procedure in this chapter.

Copyright © 2010 by Saunders, an imprint of Elsevier Inc. All rights reserved.

Assessment of the Dentition

14

| Procedure 14-1 | USE OF AN ELECTRIC PULP TESTER TO DETERMINE PULP VITALITY |

EQUIPMENT
Personal protective equipment
2 × 2 gauze
Saliva ejector
Cotton rolls
Toothpaste
Electric pulp tester

STEPS	RATIONALES
1. Assemble equipment.	Manufacturers' instructions must be followed. When the tester rheostat is separate from the applicator tip, an assistant is needed.
2. Review health history.	Use of the electric pulp tester is contraindicated for a client with a pacemaker or any electronic life-support device because it can interfere with the device's function and pose a serious health threat.
3. Describe the test's purpose and methods.	This familiarizes the client with the procedure. For some pulp testers, the client lightly holds the handle with the gloved clinician to complete the circuit.
4. Explain that the client may feel a tingling or a warm sensation.	
5. Identify the suspected tooth and a "control" tooth (preferably an adjacent tooth or the same tooth on the opposite side of the arch) to be tested, then dry these teeth and isolate them with cotton rolls (Figure 14-1).	Drying the teeth prevents the current from passing to the gingiva.

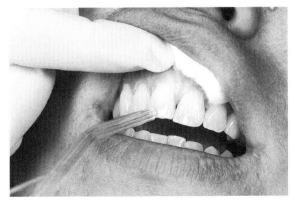

Figure 14-1. (From Bird DL, Robinson DS: *Torres and Ehrlich modern dental assisting,* ed 9, St Louis, 2009, Saunders.)

STEPS	RATIONALES
6. Instruct client to raise a hand or make a sound on feeling a sensation.	This promotes communication to enhance testing effectiveness.
7. Set the dial (current level) on the tester to zero.	
8. Place a thin layer of toothpaste on the tip of the tester.	Toothpaste acts as a conductor, and its consistency allows it to remain in place.

(Continued)

Copyright © 2010 by Saunders, an imprint of Elsevier Inc. All rights reserved.

Procedure 14-1   USE OF AN ELECTRIC PULP TESTER TO DETERMINE PULP VITALITY—*cont'd*

STEPS—*cont'd*	RATIONALES—*cont'd*
9. Test the control tooth first.	This approach determines a normal response for the client and familiarizes him or her with the procedure.
10. Apply moistened tip, without pressure but with definite contact, first to the control tooth (Figure 14-2).	

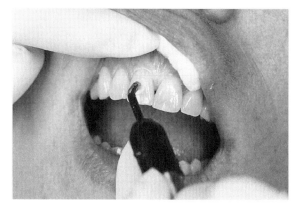

Figure 14-2.   (From Bird DL, Robinson DS: *Torres and Ehrlich modern dental assisting,* ed 9, St Louis, 2009, Saunders.)

11. Place tip on sound tooth structure on the middle third of the crown of a single-rooted tooth and the middle third of each cusp of a multirooted tooth.	These locations allow the tester to detect the presence of vital pulp tissue.
12. Avoid contact with gingival or other soft tissue.	A low-resistance circuit can be formed to bypass the tooth.
13. Avoid contact with metallic restorations.	The metal forms a more rapid conductor than does tooth structure.
14. Insert a nonconductive plastic matrix strip to separate two metallic restorations.	When approximal restorations are in contact, the circuit can be transmitted to the adjacent tooth and prevent a reading from being obtained from the tooth in question.
15. Start with the rheostat at zero and advance slowly but steadily, stopping only momentarily after each number.	This approach allows time for the client to discriminate response to a specific reading of current flow.
16. Test each tooth at lease twice. Average the readings.	Responses may vary with each test.
17. Repeat the procedure on the tooth in question.	Establishes reliability.
18. Record in client's chart the pulp tester used and the lowest number (average) at which a minimal stimulus induced a response for all teeth tested.	The same pulp tester should be used for a specific client at continuing comparative tests to obtain consistent readings. This also provides a legal record.

Please refer to the Evolve website (http://evolve.elsevier.com/Darby/hygiene) for competency forms to help evaluate your mastery of each procedure in this chapter.

Copyright © 2010 by Saunders, an imprint of Elsevier Inc. All rights reserved.

Oral Hygiene Assessment: Soft and Hard Deposits

Procedure 15-1	ORAL DEPOSIT ASSESSMENT

EQUIPMENT

Personal protective equipment
Antimicrobial mouth rinse
Mouth mirror
Periodontal explorer
Gauze
Disclosing solution
Cotton tip applicators
Compressed air
Intraoral light source
Client hand mirror
Oral hygiene assessment form (including a dental index)

STEPS	RATIONALES
1. Place client in supine position; position light source to illuminate client's mouth.	Allows visualization of both arches.
2. Using compressed air, dry the supragingival tooth surfaces a sextant at a time; using mouth mirror and direct and indirect vision, examine for supragingival calculus deposit.	Makes deposits more visible; deposits will appear chalky against tooth surface. Using both direct and indirect vision allows clinician to maintain proper ergonomic positioning.
3. Identify tooth surfaces and soft tissues with supragingival calculus and surfaces with stain; record these areas on assessment form.	Allows for assessment of change over time and illustrates areas requiring additional oral hygiene.
4. Apply disclosing agent, rinse, and dry with compressed air.	Makes supragingival oral biofilm easy to identify for both clinician and client; rinsing removes excess agent; drying improves visibility.
5. Examine tooth surfaces and soft tissues with mouth mirror for areas of stained plaque; have client watch with a hand mirror.	Engages client in assessment and educational process.
6. Record plaque-covered tooth areas on assessment form using red ink. Comment about oral biofilm on soft tissues and appliances.	Facilitates assessment of change over time; illustrates areas requiring additional oral hygiene. Recording in red ink will correlate with red disclosing agent to assist clients in making the connection between what they see in their mouths and documentation on form.
7. Using periodontal explorer and mouth mirror, explore subgingival tooth surfaces for calculus deposits.	Accesses the root surfaces; transmits tactile information because of the finer gauge of the tip, allowing the clinician to discriminate root deposits.
8. Record subgingival calculus deposits on assessment form.	Assists clinician in removing deposits during instrumentation.
9. Communicate findings to client.	Encourages client to participate in decision making regarding oral health.
10. Record service in "services rendered" section of client record (e.g., "Computed plaque-free score of 75%.")	Allows for ongoing high-quality care; reduces risk of malpractice.

Please refer to the Evolve website (http://evolve.elsevier.com/Darby/hygiene) for competency forms to help evaluate your mastery of each procedure in this chapter.

Copyright © 2010 by Saunders, an imprint of Elsevier Inc. All rights reserved.

Dental Caries Management by Risk Assessment

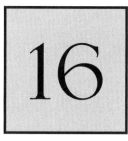

| Procedure **16-1** | USE OF THE CARIES RISK ASSESSMENT FORM |

STEPS	**RATIONALES**
1. Based on data obtained from the health histories and clinical examination, circle the *Yes* categories in the three columns on the form presented in Figure 16-1.	The three columns on the form include a hierarchy of disease indicators, risk factors, and protective factors that are based on the best scientific evidence available at this writing.
2. Make notations regarding the number of carious lesions present, the oral hygiene status, the brand of fluorides used, the type of snacks eaten, and the names of medications or drugs causing dry mouth.	Assesses the client's caries disease indicators, risk factors, and protective factors.
3. If the answer is *Yes* to any one of the four disease indicators in the first column, then take a bacterial culture using the Caries Risk Test (see Procedure 16-2) (Vivadent, Amherst, New York) or an equivalent test.	Allows a bacterial culture to be made from collected saliva and is sensitive enough to determine a level of low, medium, or high cariogenic bacterial challenge. The level of bacterial challenge has implications for caries risk and caries management. Results of this test also can be used to motivate client compliance with recommended antibacterial regimens.
4. Make an overall judgment as to whether the client is at low, moderate, high, or extreme risk depending on the balance between the disease indicators or risk factors and the protective factors using the caries balance concept. (Clients who have a current caries lesion or had one in the recent past are at high risk for future caries. Clients who are at high risk and have severe salivary gland hypofunction or special needs are at extreme risk and require very intensive therapy. If the client is not at high or low risk, then he or she by default is at moderate risk.)	The goal of caries risk assessment for clients 6 years of age or older is to assign a client to a risk level for development of future caries as the first step in managing the disease process. This assessment occurs in two phases. First, the clinician assesses an individual's caries disease indicators, risk factors, and protective factors. Second, the clinician determines the level of caries risk (low, moderate, high, or extreme) based on the presence of caries disease indicators and the balance between pathologic and protective factors.

Copyright © 2010 by Saunders, an imprint of Elsevier Inc. All rights reserved.

| Procedure **16-1** | USE OF THE CARIES RISK ASSESSMENT FORM—*cont'd* |

Patient Name: _____ CHART #: _____ DATE: _____

Assessment Date: _____ Is This (please circle) Baseline or Recall

	YES = CIRCLE	YES = CIRCLE	YES = CIRCLE
Disease Indicators (any one YES signifies likely "High Risk" and to do a bacteria test**)			
Cavities/radiograph to dentin	YES		
Approximal enamel lesions (by radiograph)	YES		
White spots on smooth surface	YES		
Restorations past 3 years	YES		
Risk Factors (biological predisposing factors)		YES	
MS and LB both medium or high (**by culture**)		YES	
Visible heavy plaque on teeth		YES	
Frequent snack (>3 times daily between meals)		YES	
Deep pits and fissures		YES	
Recreational drug use		YES	
Inadequate saliva flow by observation or measurement (**if measured, note the flow rate below)		YES	
Saliva-reducing factors (medications/radiation/systemic)		YES	
Exposed roots		YES	
Orthodontic appliances		YES	
Protective Factors			
Lives/work/school fluoridated community			YES
Fluoride toothpaste at least once daily			YES
Fluoride toothpaste at least 2 times daily			YES
Fluoride mouth rinse (0.05% NaF) daily			YES
5000 ppm F fluoride toothpaste daily			YES
Fluoride varnish in past 6 months			YES
Office F topical in past 6 months			YES
Chlorihexidine prescribed/used 1 week each of past 6 months			YES
Xylitol gum/lozenges 4 times daily past 6 months			YES
Ca and PO_4 supplement paste during past 6 months			YES
Adequate saliva flow (>1 mL/min stimulated)			YES
Bacteria/Saliva Test Results: MS: LB: Flow Rate: mL/min. Date:			

VISUALIZE CARIES BALANCE
(Use circled indicators/factors above)

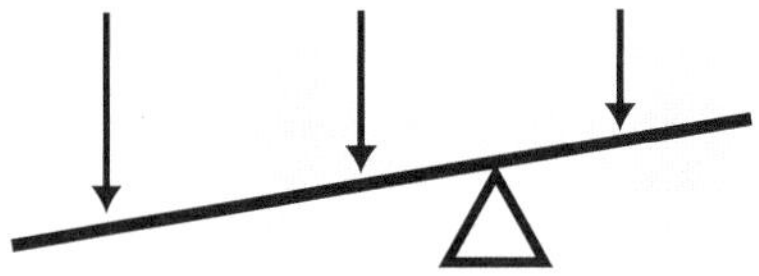

CARIES RISK ASSESSMENT (CIRCLE): EXTREME HIGH MODERATE LOW

(EXTREME RISK = HIGH RISK + SEVERE XEROSTOMIA)
Doctor signature/#: _____ Date: _____

Figure 16-1. Caries risk assessment form—children age 6 through adults. (Redrawn from Featherstone JDB, Domejean-Orliaquet S, Jenson L, et al: Caries assessment in practice for age 6 through adult, *J Calif Dent Assoc* 35:704, 2007.)

Copyright © 2010 by Saunders, an imprint of Elsevier Inc. All rights reserved.

Procedure 16-2   TESTING SALIVARY FLOW RATE AND LEVEL OF CARIES BACTERIAL CHALLENGE

EQUIPMENT
Paraffin pellets
Measuring cup
Commercially available caries bacterial test kit, such as the Caries Risk Test (Vivadent, Amherst, New York) or an
    equivalent test
Incubator
Personal protective barriers

STEPS	RATIONALES
1. Determine salivary flow rate.	Saliva neutralizes acids and provides minerals and proteins that protect the teeth from dental caries. If saliva flow appears inadequate or if the client reports having a dry mouth, then a saliva flow rate test should be conducted.
• Have the client chew a paraffin pellet for 3 to 5 minutes (timed) and spit all saliva generated into a measuring cup.	Chewing paraffin stimulates salivary flow and bacterial loading for both *Streptococcus mutans* and lactobacilli. Stimulated saliva provides an easy means to sample the oral biofilm from the whole mouth and reflects the cariogenic bacteria in the biofilm on the teeth. Depositing stimulated saliva in a measuring cup allows the amount of saliva generated to be measured.
• At the end of the 3 to 5 minutes, measure the amount of saliva in milliliters (mL) and divide that amount by time to determine the mL/min of stimulated salivary flow.	This procedure allows flow rate calculation.
• A flow rate of 1 mL/min or higher is considered normal; a level of 0.7 mL/min is low; and anything at 0.5 mL/min or less is dry, indicating severe salivary gland hypofunction.	These parameters guide the clinician in determining salivary flow rate for the client. Low salivary flow rate contributes to the level of risk for having new carious lesions in the future or for having the existing lesions progress.
• Investigate the reason for the flow rate if it is 0.7 mL/min or less (medication, radiation, systemic condition).	Allows identification of the cause of low salivary flow rate. Allows for planning protective factors in caries management.
2. Initiate bacterial testing.	Currently there are several commercially available kits for use at chairside for caries bacterial testing.
• The kit comes with a two-sided selective media stick that assesses mutans streptococci (MS) on the blue side and lactobacilli (LB) on the green side.	This test allows a bacterial culture to be made from collected saliva. Bacterial testing is needed to determine whether cariogenic pathogens are present both before and after dental caries treatment and at what level these bacteria are present in the mouth. Dental caries is caused by mutans streptococci (MS) (a group that includes the *Streptococcus mutans* and *Streptococcus sobrinus* species) and lactobacilli (LB) that live in the oral biofilm that attach to teeth.
• Remove the selective media stick from the culture tube. Peel off the plastic cover sheet from each side of the stick.	The media stick provides a selective environment that will promote MS and LB bacterial growth.
• Pour (do not streak) the collected saliva over the media on each side until it is entirely wet.	Allows for the growth of bacteria present in the saliva sample.
• Place one of the sodium bicarbonate tablets included in the kit in the bottom of the tube.	Creates a favorable condition for bacterial growth.
• Replace the media stick in the culture tube, screw the lid on, and label the tube with the client's name, registration number, and date.	Labeling the tube ensures a correct match among bacterial test, client, and when test occurred.

Copyright © 2010 by Saunders, an imprint of Elsevier Inc. All rights reserved.

Procedure 16-2   TESTING SALIVARY FLOW RATE AND LEVEL OF CARIES BACTERIAL CHALLENGE—*cont'd*

STEPS—*cont'd*

- Place the tube in the incubator at 37° C for 72 hours (Figure 16-2).* (Incubators suitable for a dental office are also sold by the company.)

RATIONALES—*cont'd*

Incubation promotes growth of cariogenic bacteria present in the collected saliva.

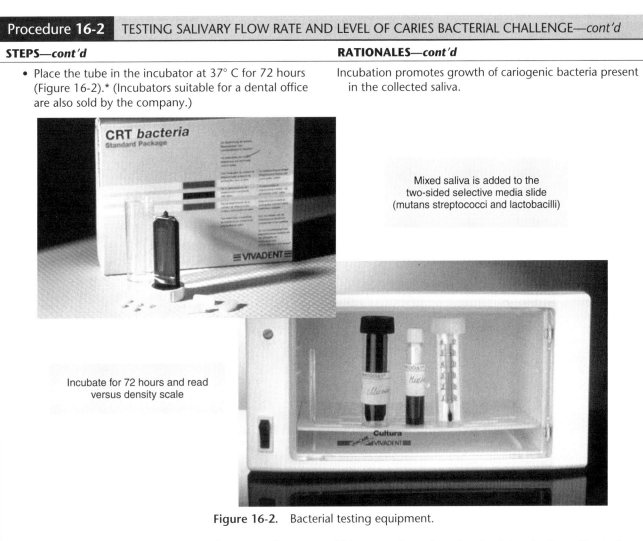

Mixed saliva is added to the two-sided selective media slide (mutans streptococci and lactobacilli)

Incubate for 72 hours and read versus density scale

Figure 16-2. Bacterial testing equipment.

- Collect the tube after 72 hours, and compare the densities of bacterial colonies with the pictures provided in the kit indicating relative bacterial levels. The dark blue agar is selective for MS, and the light green agar is selective for LB.
- Record the level of bacterial challenge in the client's chart as low, medium, or high, and inform client of results.

This comparison allows for the determination of level of cariogenic bacterial challenge: low, medium, or high. A 72-hour incubation period is required to obtain reliable results.

Documents results in client record. It is important to inform the client of the implications of the results for caries risk and caries management.

*Tests have shown that 72 hours' incubation produces more reliable results than the 48 hours recommended by the manufacturer.

Please refer to the Evolve website (http://evolve.elsevier.com/Darby/hygiene) for competency forms to help evaluate your mastery of each procedure in this chapter.

Copyright © 2010 by Saunders, an imprint of Elsevier Inc. All rights reserved.

Periodontal and Risk Assessment

17

| Procedure 17-1 | PERIODONTAL CHARTING AND ASSESSMENT |

EQUIPMENT
Personal protective equipment
Periodontal probe
Nabers probe
Mouth mirror
Dental light
Red and blue pencils
Compressed air

STEPS	**RATIONALES**
1. Use direct and indirect lighting, mouth mirror, and compressed air to determine findings.	For visualizing subtle changes in color, consistency, surface texture, contour, size of the gingiva; for reading periodontal and Nabers probes.
2. Use proper client and operator body mechanics.	Improves visualization and comfort; prevents repetitive strain injuries.
3. Question client about existing conditions.	Determines client risk status and association with systemic health.
4. Hold probe with modified pen grasp; establish appropriate fulcrum.	Provides instrument control and stability.
5. Gingival recession: Use periodontal probe to determine location of the gingival margin in relation to the cementoenamel junction (CEJ). Recession of ≥1 mm is recorded; draw gingival margin in blue on chart (Figure 17-1).	Necessary to later determine clinical attachment levels.

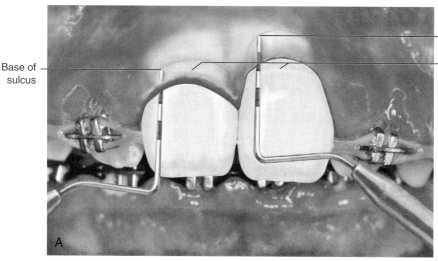

Base of sulcus

Base of periodontal pocket
Cementoenamel junction

Figure 17-1. Measuring clinical attachment levels. **A,** On the maxillary right central incisor, the inflamed gingival margin hides the cementoenamel junction (CEJ), resulting in a 4-mm psuedopocket (gingival pocket). There is no clinical attachment loss and no bone loss. The base of the sulcus is in a normal relationship to the CEJ and alveolar bone. On the maxillary left central incisor, the gingival margin has receded 2 to 3 mm, exposing the CEJ, and bone loss is evident. There is clinical attachment loss of 6 mm and a 5-mm periodontal pocket. (**A,** Adapted from Newman MG, Takei HH, Klokkevold PR, Carranza FA, eds: *Carranza's clinical periodontology*, ed 10, St Louis, 2006, Saunders.)

Copyright © 2010 by Saunders, an imprint of Elsevier Inc. All rights reserved.

Procedure **17-1**	PERIODONTAL CHARTING AND ASSESSMENT—*cont'd*

STEPS—*cont'd*	**RATIONALES**—*cont'd*

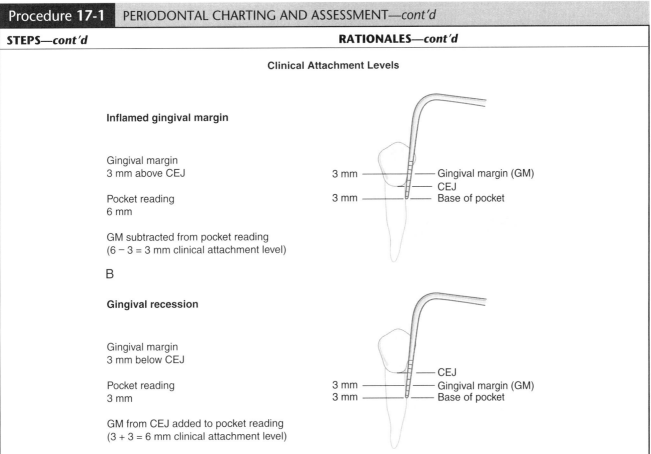

Clinical Attachment Levels

Inflamed gingival margin

Gingival margin
3 mm above CEJ

Pocket reading
6 mm

GM subtracted from pocket reading
(6 − 3 = 3 mm clinical attachment level)

B

3 mm ———— Gingival margin (GM)
———— CEJ
3 mm ———— Base of pocket

Gingival recession

Gingival margin
3 mm below CEJ

Pocket reading
3 mm

GM from CEJ added to pocket reading
(3 + 3 = 6 mm clinical attachment level)

C

———— CEJ
3 mm ———— Gingival margin (GM)
3 mm ———— Base of pocket

Figure 17-1. cont'd.   B, Gingival margin 3 mm above CEJ. **C,** Gingival margin 3 mm below CEJ (gingival recession).

6. Frenal involvement: Determine abnormal muscle pull on gingiva and/or short frenum; draw a right angle in blue pencil with the apex occlusally oriented in area of involvement.

Muscle pull contributes to recession, inadequate attached gingiva, and risk of disease progression.

7. Measure periodontal pockets with periodontal probe.
   a. Insert tip to junctional epithelium (JE); maintain tip against tooth structure.

Ensures accurate periodontal probe depth measurement.

   b. Angle probe slightly on proximal surfaces to reach directly apical to the contact point (Figures 17-2 and 17-3).

Ensures that the disease susceptible col area is measured correctly.

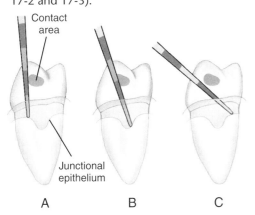

Contact area

Junctional epithelium

A   B   C

Figure 17-2.   A, Incorrect technique for probing the interproximal area. **B,** Correct technique. **C,** Incorrect technique. (Adapted from Perry D, Beemsterboer P, Carranza FA: *Techniques and theory of periodontal instrumentation,* Philadelphia, 1990, Saunders.)

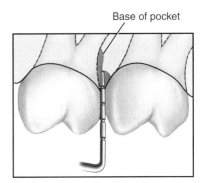

Base of pocket

Figure 17-3. Failure to tilt the probe far enough to keep its end in contact with the tooth surface. Probe is resting on the pocket wall, resulting in an inaccurate probing depth measurement. (Adapted from Newman MG, Takei HH, Klokkevold PR, Carranza FA, eds: *Carranza's clinical periodontology,* ed 10, St Louis, 2006, Saunders.)

Copyright © 2010 by Saunders, an imprint of Elsevier Inc. All rights reserved.   *(Continued)*

STEPS—*cont'd*	**RATIONALES**—*cont'd*
c. "Walk" tip along JE in 1-mm increments (Figure 17-4).	Ensures that the entire sulcus or pocket area is assessed and periodontal pockets and loss of attachment are not overlooked.

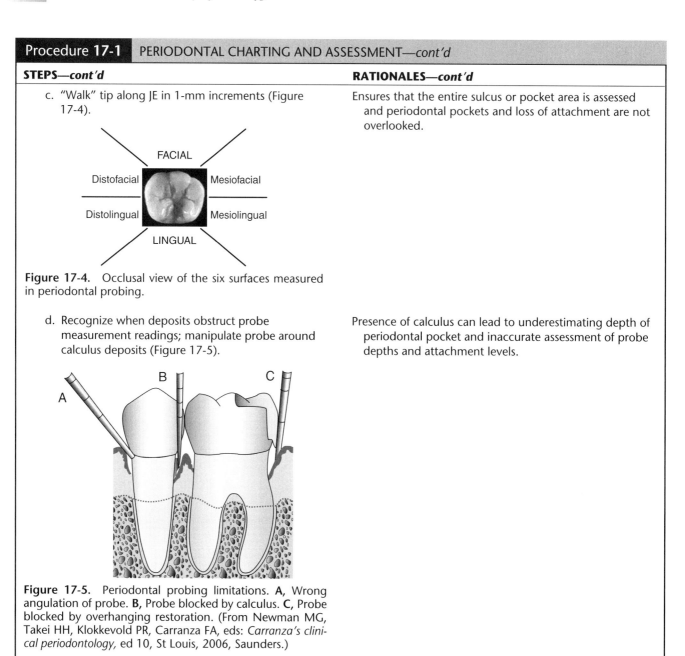

Figure 17-4.   Occlusal view of the six surfaces measured in periodontal probing.

d. Recognize when deposits obstruct probe measurement readings; manipulate probe around calculus deposits (Figure 17-5).	Presence of calculus can lead to underestimating depth of periodontal pocket and inaccurate assessment of probe depths and attachment levels.

Figure 17-5.   Periodontal probing limitations. **A,** Wrong angulation of probe. **B,** Probe blocked by calculus. **C,** Probe blocked by overhanging restoration. (From Newman MG, Takei HH, Klokkevold PR, Carranza FA, eds: *Carranza's clinical periodontology,* ed 10, St Louis, 2006, Saunders.)

8. Record proximal, facial, and lingual readings >3 mm (±1 mm) where there is no recession. Where recession is present, record all measurements to reflect clinical attachment level (CAL).	Ensures that abnormal CALs around each tooth are identified and recorded.
a. Record measurements in blue pencil; circle bleeding points in red.	Facilitates differentiation between healthy and diseased sites.
9. Draw clinical attachment level in red throughout dentition.	Displays location and topography of base of periodontal pockets; guides instrumentation and client instructions.
10. Furcation involvement: Use Nabers probe to determine classification of involvement present (Table 17-1).	Avoids overlooking a furcation; guides instrumentation and client instructions.
11. Mobility: Use handles of two instruments to rock the tooth; classify amount of movement obtained (Table 17-2).	Important for determining long-term prognosis of tooth.
12. Evaluate drifting, extrusion, and malalignment.	Tooth movement often associated with periodontitis and mobility.
13. Evaluate areas of food impaction.	Serves as a guide to contributory factors and client instruction.
14. Evaluate open contacts with dental floss.	Identify areas at risk for periodontal disease.

Copyright © 2010 by Saunders, an imprint of Elsevier Inc. All rights reserved.

Procedure **17-1** PERIODONTAL CHARTING AND ASSESSMENT—*cont'd*

STEPS—*cont'd*	**RATIONALES**—*cont'd*
15. Assess fremitus, occlusal disharmonies, and wear facets (Table 17-3 and Figure 17-6).	Facilitates identification of occlusal trauma that may be contributing to periodontal disease.

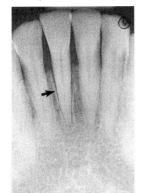

Figure 17-6. Radiograph showing widening of the periodontal ligament associated with occlusal trauma *(arrow).*

16. Gingival examination on periodontal chart:
  a. Record gingival disease entity, severity, and location (Table 17-4).
  b. Use correct dental terminology when describing severity and location (see Table 17-4).
17. Amount of attached gingiva: Subtract the depth of the pocket from the distance from the gingival margin to the mucogingival line (Figure 17-7); difference is the amount of attached gingiva.
	Ensures comprehensive gingival evaluation in terms of color, contour, consistency, and surface texture.
	Ensures that gingival condition is accurately described and documented.
	Inadequately attached gingiva must be identified and treated, or else disease progression is likely.

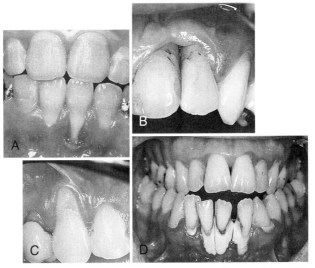

Figure 17-7. Mucogingival defects. **A,** Irregular gingival contours and recession with severe gingival inflammation. **B,** Gingival recession, crater formation, and chronic inflammation with fibrotic tissue. Bottom of the pocket is beyond mucogingival junction. **C,** Recession on maxillary canine with presence of shallow pocket and absence of attached gingiva. **D,** Advanced gingival recession and inflammation caused by heavy plaque and calculus accumulation. (Courtesy Dr. Kenneth Marinak, Adjunct Clinical Instructor, Gene W. Hirschfeld School of Dental Hygiene, Old Dominion University, Norfolk, Virginia.)

(Continued)

Copyright © 2010 by Saunders, an imprint of Elsevier Inc. All rights reserved.

Procedure **17-1** PERIODONTAL CHARTING AND ASSESSMENT—*cont'd*	
STEPS—*cont'd*	**RATIONALES**—*cont'd*
a. <2 mm should be noted as IAG (inadequately attached gingiva).	
b. <1 mm should be noted as NAG (no attached gingiva) in apical area of the facial aspect of tooth in red pencil.	
18. Periodontal examination on periodontal chart:	Necessary for care planning and referral to periodontist.
a. Record severity of periodontitis.	
b. Record location of periodontitis.	
19. Record disease (gingivitis and/or periodontitis).	Necessary for care planning and referral to a periodontist.
20. Assign appropriate periodontal classification number according to the American Academy of Periodontology (AAP) Guidelines and record.	Necessary for filing dental insurance forms (see the discussion of insurance codes in Chapter 20 of the textbook).
21. Use appropriate charting symbols (Figure 17-8).	Ensures accurate documentation, interpretable over time and by other professionals.

Copyright © 2010 by Saunders, an imprint of Elsevier Inc. All rights reserved.

Procedure 17-1 | PERIODONTAL CHARTING AND ASSESSMENT—*cont'd*

PERIODONTAL CHARTING CODE

Tooth Number	Description of symbols	Tooth Number	Description of symbols
1	5-mm pocketing with bleeding (fac.)	19	3-mm periodontal pocket on mesial facial (due to gingival enlargement)
2	Class I furcation		
3	2-mm gingival enlargement	20	4-mm pocketing with bleeding (ling.)
4	Gingival margin at CEJ	21	Gingival margin at CEJ
5	Class II mobility	22	2-mm gingival enlargement (fac.)
6	6-mm pocketing with 2-mm of recession equals 8-mm of CAL	23	3-mm probe reading due to gingival enlargement
7	5-mm pocket with 2-mm of gingival hyperplasia equals 3-mm CAL	24	Gingival margin at CEJ
		25	Healthy area on facial
8	2-mm of recession	26	Class III mobility and insufficient attached gingiva
9	Class I mobility		
10	8-mm of recession	27	Healthy area; 2-mm pocketing with no bleeding (ling.)
11	Insufficient attached gingival		
12	4-mm periodontal pocket (fac.)	28	2-mm of recession (fac.)
13	Gingival margin at CEJ	29	5-mm of CAL (mes. fac.)
14	2-mm of recession	30	Class II furcation involvement
15	Class III furcation involvement	31	6-mm periodontal pocket and 6-mm CAL on mes. fac.
16	1-mm of gingival enlargement (fac.)		
17	2-mm of gingival enlargement (ling.)	32	4-mm periodontal pocket (ling.)
A 18	Class I furcation involvement		

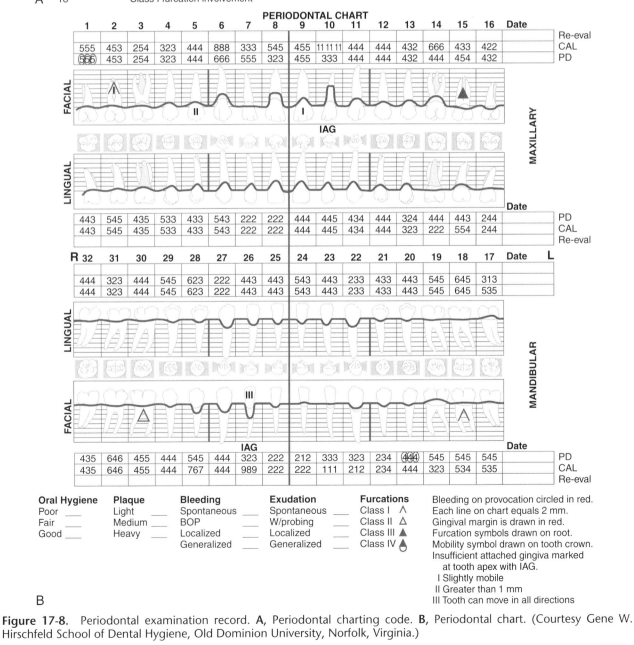

PERIODONTAL CHART

Figure 17-8. Periodontal examination record. **A,** Periodontal charting code. **B,** Periodontal chart. (Courtesy Gene W. Hirschfeld School of Dental Hygiene, Old Dominion University, Norfolk, Virginia.)

Copyright © 2010 by Saunders, an imprint of Elsevier Inc. All rights reserved. *(Continued)*

Procedure 17-1   PERIODONTAL CHARTING AND ASSESSMENT—*cont'd*

STEPS—*cont'd*	RATIONALES—*cont'd*
22. Correlate radiographic and clinical readings (Table 17-5).	Assists in disease diagnosis and documentation.
23. Use appropriate infection control protocols.	Protects client and others from disease transmission.
24. Record service in client chart under "Services Rendered"—e.g., 9/19/09: periodontal and risk assessment complete. Communicated signs of periodontitis to client. Recommended referral to periodontist.	Provides legal evidence that standard of care was provided and client was informed of findings.

Adapted from the process evaluation form used at the Gene W. Hirschfeld School of Dental Hygiene, Old Dominion University, Norfolk, Virginia.

TABLE 17-1 Classifications of Furcations

Class	Description
Class I	Beginning involvement. Concavity of furcation can be detected with an explorer or probe, but it cannot be entered. Cannot be detected radiographically.
Class II	The clinician can enter the furcation from one aspect with a probe or explorer but cannot penetrate through to the opposite side.
Class III	Through-and-through involvement, but the furcation is still covered by soft tissue. A definite radiolucency in the furcation area on a radiograph is visible.
Class IV	A through-and-through furcation involvement that is not covered by soft tissue. Clinically it is open and exposed.

TABLE 17-2 Classification of Mobility

Class	Description
Class I	Tooth can be moved up to 1 mm in any direction.
Class II	Tooth can be moved >1 mm in any direction but is not depressible in socket.
Class III	Tooth can be moved in a buccolingual direction and is depressible in socket.

TABLE 17-3 Classification of Fremitus

Class	Description
Class I	Mild vibration or movement detected
Class II	Easily palpable vibration but no visible movement
Class III	Movement is clearly visible

Copyright © 2010 by Saunders, an imprint of Elsevier Inc. All rights reserved.

TABLE 17-4 Terminology Used to Describe Observations Associated with Clinical Assessment of Gingiva

Characteristic	Terminology	Description	Example
Gingival color	Location Distribution Severity Quality	Generalized or localized Diffuse, marginal, or papillary Slight, moderate, severe Red, bright red, pink, cyanotic	Localized slight marginal redness lingual aspects of teeth 18, 19, 30, 31; all other areas coral pink, uniform in color
Gingival contour	Location Distribution Severity Quality	Generalized or localized Diffuse, marginal, or papillary Slight, moderate, severe Bulbous, flattened, punched-out, cratered	Localized moderately cratered papilla teeth 6-11, 22-27; all other areas within normal limits
Consistency of gingiva	Location Distribution Severity Quality	Generalized or localized Diffuse, marginal, or papillary Slight, moderate, severe Firm (fibrotic), spongy (edematous)	Generalized moderate marginal sponginess more severe on facial aspect teeth 8, 9; all other areas firm
Surface texture of gingiva	Location Distribution Quality	Generalized or localized Diffuse, marginal, or papillary Smooth, shiny, eroded, stippling	Localized smooth gingiva on facial aspect teeth 7, 8; all other areas with generalized stippling

TABLE 17-5 Relationship between Periodontal Disease Severity and Radiographic Findings

Disease	Radiographic Evidence
Gingivitis	No bone loss
Slight periodontitis	Less than 30% bone loss
Moderate periodontitis	30%-50% bone loss
Severe periodontitis	More than 50% bone loss

Please refer to the Evolve website (http://evolve.elsevier.com/Darby/hygiene) for competency forms to help evaluate your mastery of each procedure in this chapter.

Copyright © 2010 by Saunders, an imprint of Elsevier Inc. All rights reserved.

Dental Hygiene Care Plan and Evaluation

20

CHAPTER

Procedure 20-1	DENTAL HYGIENE CARE PLANNING
STEPS	**RATIONALES**
1. Link care plan to dental hygiene diagnoses.	The dental hygiene diagnosis is the foundation of the dental hygiene care plan.
2. Establish priorities of need.	Client's unmet human needs are ranked.
3. Set client-centered goals.	Addresses signs and symptoms supporting the dental hygiene diagnosis and client's desired outcome of care; also specifies the time and method of evaluation.
4. Select dental hygiene interventions.	Selected to address the contributing factors of the dental hygiene diagnosis; means to achieving the desired outcome of care.
5. Establish an appointment schedule.	Schedules the interventions that will most likely achieve the desired outcome of care.
6. Present the dental hygiene care plan.	Enables client to make informed decisions and consent to the plan.
7. Document in ink the completion of this service in the client's record under "Services Rendered" and date the entry (e.g., "Care plan was developed to address the client's unmet human need, care plan was presented and discussed with the client. Client asked clarifying questions before acceptance of care plan.").	Ensures integrity of client's record for both the client's health and legal protection of practitioner.

Copyright © 2010 by Saunders, an imprint of Elsevier Inc. All rights reserved.

Procedure 20-2   EVALUATION OF CARE

STEPS	RATIONALES
1. Identify evaluative criteria and expected outcomes of care.	Clarifies the desired outcome of the care.
2. Collect evidence to determine whether goals are being are met.	Ensures that practitioner and client are aware of the client's oral health status and prevents supervised neglect of the client.
3. Interpret and summarize the findings.	Compare new findings to baseline findings; determines factors that may be contributing to the client's success or failure.
4. Write an evaluative statement.	Provides a judgment of care plan success and recommendations for future care.
5. Propose continued care options.	Ensures that practitioner and client are aware of the client's oral health status; for example: *Goal Met*: Terminate care and recommend recare schedule; *Goal Partially Met*: Continue with care plan—client is progressing toward goal attainment; *Goal Not Met*: Modify plan—client is not progressing toward goal attainment.
6. Document in ink the completion of this service in the client's record under "Services Rendered" and date the entry; for example, "Updated client health history, reassessed client for changes in oral health status and oral health skills. *Goals Met:* Gingival and periodontal assessment indicated that the gingival tissue is pinker and firmer, no bleeding upon probing. Reassessed client's flossing technique and client is completent. Client reports adherence to oral self-care recommendations. Continued-care interval: 6 months."	Ensures the integrity of the client's record for both the client's health and the legal protection of the practitioner.

Please refer to the Evolve website (http://evolve.elsevier.com/Darby/hygiene) for competency forms to help evaluate your mastery of each procedure in this chapter.

Copyright © 2010 by Saunders, an imprint of Elsevier Inc. All rights reserved.

Mechanical Oral Biofilm Control: Interdental and Supplemental Self-Care Devices

22

CHAPTER

Procedure **22-1**	SPOOL FLOSSING METHOD: ADULTS

STEPS	RATIONALES
1. Break off a piece of floss 12 to 18 inches long from the spool.	As a rule of thumb, the appropriate length of floss should be as long as your forearm. This length ensures enough floss to cover the entire mouth, advancing to a new area after completing each interproximal space.
2. Wrap floss around middle fingers; wrap floss around right middle finger two to three times; wrap remaining floss around left middle finger (or vice versa) (Figure 22-1, *A*).	Wrapping dental floss around the middle fingers allows for increased control because the index fingers and thumbs are then free to control the floss. Be careful to wrap the floss somewhat loosely to avoid cutting off circulation to the middle fingers.

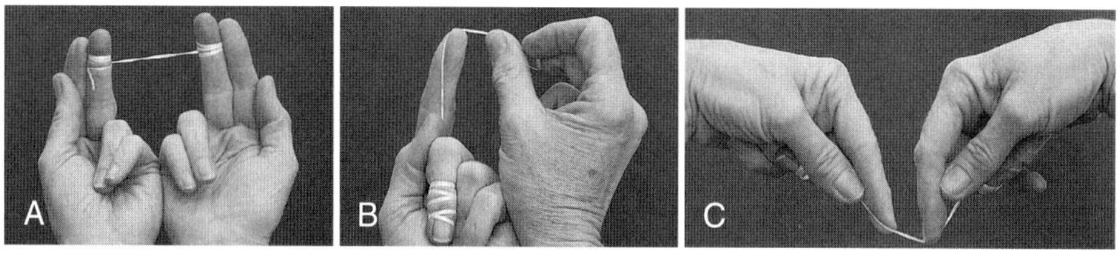

Figure 22-1.

| 3. For maxillary insertion, grasp floss firmly with thumb and index finger of each hand, using ½ inch of floss between fingertips (Figure 22-1, *B*). For mandibular insertion, direct the floss down with the index fingers (Figure 22-1, *C*). | Grasping the floss with two fingers on both hands improves control. Using only ½ inch of floss between fingers reduces the chance of floss cuts on facial or lingual surfaces adjacent to or across papillae (Figure 22-2). |

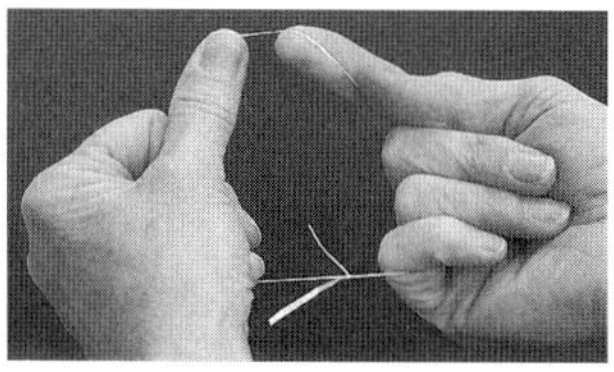

Figure 22-2.

(Continued)

Copyright © 2010 by Saunders, an imprint of Elsevier Inc. All rights reserved.

Procedure 22-1   SPOOL FLOSSING METHOD: ADULTS—*cont'd*

STEPS—*cont'd*	**RATIONALES—*cont'd***
4. Select area to begin flossing, and establish a pattern to progress throughout the mouth.	Establishing a pattern for completing flossing avoids missing areas of the mouth. Many people like to start at the midline and progress posteriorly in one quadrant and then the other in the same arch, then switch arches and progress in a similar manner. Others like to start with tooth 1 and continue in order to tooth 32. Each patient should establish a pattern that is comfortable for him or her.
5. Set a fulcrum on the cheek or in the mouth.	Setting a fulcrum increases stability and reduces the chance of popping through a contact area, possibly causing a floss cut or cleft.
6. Use gentle seesaw motion to pass through contact area.	This motion reduces the chance of popping through a contact, possibly causing a floss cut.
7. Wrap tightly in C shape around tooth (Figure 22-3).	Wrapping the floss in a C shape and keeping it tight to the tooth prevents floss cuts and increases the surface area covered by the floss, thereby disrupting more plaque biofilm.

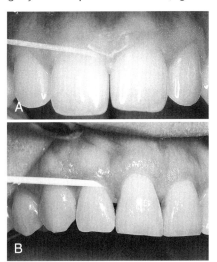

Figure 22-3.   A, Dental floss. **B,** Dental tape. (**A,** From Perry DA, Beemsterboer PL: *Periodontology for the dental hygienist,* St Louis, 2007, Saunders. **B,** From Newman MG, Takei HH, Klokkevold PR, Carranza FA: *Carranza's clinical periodontology,* ed 10, St Louis, 2006, Saunders.)

8. Move floss up and down on mesial of tooth three to four strokes, then move above papilla (just below contact); wrap in C shape on distal surface of adjacent tooth, moving floss up and down three to four strokes (Figure 22-4).	An up-and-down motion covers the entire length of the interproximal area, rather than a single area accomplished by a shoeshine motion. Moving the floss above the papilla before wrapping the C shape on the opposite surface avoids a floss cut in the papilla.

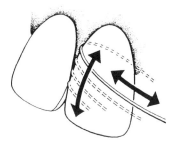

Figure 22-4. Floss wrapped around dental surface. (From Hoag PM, Pawlak EA: *Essentials of periodontics,* ed 4, St Louis, 1990, Mosby.)

(Continued)

Copyright © 2010 by Saunders, an imprint of Elsevier Inc. All rights reserved.

| Procedure 22-1 | SPOOL FLOSSING METHOD: ADULTS—*cont'd* |

STEPS—*cont'd*	RATIONALES—*cont'd*
9. Use a seesaw motion to remove floss through contact.	A seesaw motion back out of the contact allows for more gentle removal of the floss.
10. Advance floss to a new area by unwrapping floss from left-hand middle finger and wrapping onto right-hand middle finger (or vice versa; see step 2).	Floss is advanced to a new area after each interproximal space to maximize cleaning efficacy.
11. Repeat steps 5 to 11 until all teeth have been completed, continuing to grasp the floss with the thumb and index fingers.	The entire mouth should be flossed, including the distal area of the most posterior tooth in each quadrant.
12. Dispose of floss in waste receptacle.	Floss is meant for one-time use.

| Procedure 22-2 | LOOP FLOSSING METHOD: CHILDREN AND CLIENTS WITH LIMITED MANUAL DEXTERITY |

STEPS	RATIONALES
1. Break off a piece of floss 8 to 10 inches long from the spool.	Less floss is needed to loop than to wrap around the middle fingers. A midsize piece of floss is still needed, however, to advance the floss to new areas in the mouth.
2. Tie the two ends together in a knot (Figure 22-5). **Figure 22-5.**	Tying the two ends together puts the floss into a complete circle. With this method the floss does not need to be wrapped around the middle finger of each hand, which often causes the blood flow to be reduced in the fingers. A loop is also easier to control.
3-10. Follow steps listed for spool flossing method (see Procedure 22-1).	Steps 3 to 10 use the same techniques for both methods of flossing.
11. Advance floss to new area by sliding floss away from the knot.	Floss is advanced to a new area after each interproximal space to maximize cleaning efficacy.
12. Repeat steps 5 to 11 until all teeth have been completed, continuing to grasp the floss with the thumb and index fingers.	The entire mouth should be flossed, including the distal area of the most terminal teeth in each quadrant.
13. Dispose of floss in waste receptacle.	Floss is meant for one-time use.

Copyright © 2010 by Saunders, an imprint of Elsevier Inc. All rights reserved.

Procedure 22-3 | USE OF A FLOSS HOLDER

STEPS	**RATIONALES**
1. Tightly string floss on holder following the manufacturer's recommendations (Figure 22-6).	Each manufacturer will specify the directions for winding the floss on the floss holder in the directions for use. The floss must be taut in order for the floss to be seesawed through the contact area. If it is not taut, it will fall off the holder and must be restrung.

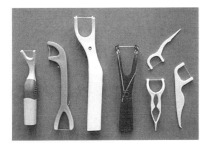

Figure 22-6. Disposable floss devices are convenient for some clients and may enhance plaque biofilm control.

STEPS	**RATIONALES**
2. Follow steps 4 to 10 for spool method of flossing.	The method for flossing with a floss holder does not differ from the spool method of flossing other than the fact that only one hand is needed.
3. To direct floss in a C shape toward mesial and distal in step 8, use push or pull motion with floss holder (Figure 22-7).	The floss should still adapt to the tooth in a C shape. In the spool method, the index fingers and thumb adapt the floss to the teeth. With the floss holder a push or pull motion adapts the floss to the tooth.

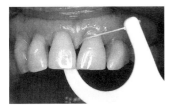

Figure 22-7. Placement of floss holder in mouth. (From Perry DA, Beemsterboer PL: *Periodontology for the dental hygienist,* St Louis, 2007, Saunders.)

STEPS	**RATIONALES**
4. To move to a new area of floss (step 11 of the spool method), the holder must be unwrapped, the floss advanced, and the holder rewrapped.	The only way to advance floss to a new area with most floss holders is to unwrap the holder and rewrap it, ensuring that a clean area of floss is placed between the prongs.
5. Continue until all teeth are completed.	The entire mouth should be flossed, including the distal area of the most terminal teeth in each quadrant.
6. Dispose of the floss in waste receptacle.	Floss is meant for one-time use.
7. Wash off floss holder with warm water and soap, dry, and store in clean, dry area until next use.	The floss holder may be reused and is normally made of plastic, a material that is durable, lightweight, and able to be cleaned. As the holder shows signs of wear or becomes difficult to clean, it should be replaced. Another recommendation is to replace the holder every 3 months, just as you would a toothbrush.

Copyright © 2010 by Saunders, an imprint of Elsevier Inc. All rights reserved.

Procedure 22-4 · USE OF A FLOSS THREADER

STEPS	RATIONALES
1. Determine the need to use a floss threader and appropriate areas for use.	See list of indications for use in Table 22-1 (see p. 93).
2. Break off a piece of floss 4 to 6 inches long from the spool.	A smaller piece of floss can be used because only one or two areas are normally flossed using a floss threader.
3. Thread floss through eye of floss threader, overlapping floss 1 to 2 inches.	Threading the floss threader is similar to threading a needle. Once it is threaded, the floss is pulled through so that 1 to 2 inches overlap (double-stranded). Overlapping the floss prevents unthreading of the floss once resistance is met; however, if the entire piece of floss is left double-stranded, it is more difficult to remove the floss threader in step 6.
4. Grasp threader with thumb and index finger of one hand.	A stable grasp prevents dropping the threader.
5. Insert tip of threader from the facial surface through an open interproximal area or area between a pontic and an abutment tooth (Figure 22-8, *A*).	Inserting the threader from a facial aspect allows better visualization of insertion and less chance of tissue trauma at the insertion point.
6. Pull floss threader toward the lingual side until threader has passed completely through the interproximal space or under a pontic (only floss is now in the space) (Figure 22-8, *B*).	For flossing to be performed correctly, the floss needs to wrap around the mesial or distal side of the tooth. Therefore the floss must pass all the way from facial to lingual for maximum coverage of surface area.

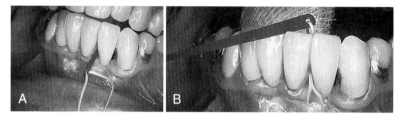

Figure 22-8.   **A,** Facial insertion of the threader tip. **B,** Threader pulled lingually through the interproximal space.

7. Slide the floss threader off the floss and remove from mouth.	Taking the floss threader off the floss and removing it from the mouth prevent loss or swallowing of the threader.
8. Move floss back and forth several times under the pontic. Then follow steps 8 and 9 of the spool method of flossing (Figure 22-9).	Once the floss is inserted into the space, the flossing method is the same. Sliding floss back and forth under the pontic removes oral biofilm and food debris from the gingival surface of the pontic.

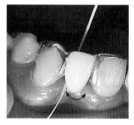

Figure 22-9.

9. Remove floss by letting go with hand that is on the lingual side and pulling floss toward the buccal side.	Because the contact area was blocked (requiring use of a floss threader), the floss will not be able to be removed by seesawing it through the contact area. Instead, letting go with the hand that is on the lingual side allows for removal from the buccal side.
10. Dispose of floss and threader in waste receptacle.	Floss and floss threader are meant for one-time use. Some patients will reuse the floss threader for the sake of cost containment. If the threader is reusable, it should be cleaned with soap and warm water, dried, and stored in a clean, dry place. If the threader becomes bent, splayed, or unusable, it should be replaced.

Copyright © 2010 by Saunders, an imprint of Elsevier Inc. All rights reserved.

Procedure 22-5   USE OF A TOOTHPICK IN A TOOTHPICK HOLDER

STEPS	RATIONALES
1. Insert a round tapered toothpick into the end of an angled plastic holder. Twist toothpick securely into holder, and break off longer end of toothpick (see Figure 22-10).	See a list of indications for use in Table 22-1 (see p. 93). Once the toothpick is inserted into the holder, it is tightened in place to avoid loosening the toothpick. Breaking off the longer end prevents the toothpick from damaging tissue in the lips or cheek during use and allows for better access to posterior areas.

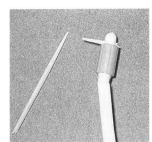

Figure 22-10.   Example of toothpick holder.

STEPS	RATIONALES
2. Moisten the end of the toothpick with saliva.	Moistening the toothpick with saliva softens the wood to prevent tissue trauma and reduce splintering.
3. Place the toothpick tip at the gingival margin with the tip pointing at a 45-degree angle to the long axis of the tooth. Trace the gingival margin around the tooth (Figure 22-11, A).	Tracing the gingival margin with the toothpick creates mechanical friction to disturb and remove oral biofilm.
4. Some clients may be dexterous enough to point the tip at less than a 45-degree angle into the sulcus or pocket and trace around the tooth surfaces and root concavities. The tip should maintain contact with the tooth at all times. Insertion should stop once the toothpick meets a slight resistance in the space without the teeth being forced apart interproximally or the tissue being impinged. Keeping the tip at the tooth, use a gentle up-and-down motion to clean concave proximal surfaces (Figure 22-11, B).	Applying the toothpick in this manner disturbs and removes plaque biofilm just below the gingival margin and from root concavities. This step is not recommended for clients with limited dexterity. The toothpick should be inserted interproximally only until the space between the teeth is filled. If the teeth are forced apart or tissue is impinged, permanent damage could result; teeth may be abraded or tissue worn away.

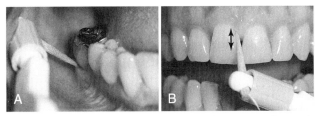

Figure 22-11.   **A,** Toothpick tip placed at gingival margin. **B,** Gentle up-and-down motion keeping tip on tooth. (From Newman MG, Takei HH, Klokkevold PR, Carranza FA: *Carranza's clinical periodontology,* ed 10, St Louis, 2006, Saunders.)

STEPS	RATIONALES
5. For exposed furcation areas, trace the furcation and use an in-and-out motion to clean the furcation. The tip should maintain contact with the tooth at all times.	Keeping the tip in contact with the tooth prevents tissue trauma.
6. If debris accumulates on toothpick, rinse under running water.	Loose debris should be rinsed away and not introduced into a new interproximal area or sulcus.
7. Once all areas of the mouth are completed, dispose of toothpick in waste receptacle.	Toothpicks made of wood will absorb blood, saliva, and bacteria and should be thrown away after one use.
8. Holder may be washed with soap and warm water and stored in a clean, dry place for reuse.	

Copyright © 2010 by Saunders, an imprint of Elsevier Inc. All rights reserved.

Procedure 22-6 USE OF A WOODEN WEDGE

STEPS	RATIONALES
1. Determine the need to use a wooden wedge and appropriate areas for use.	See a list of indications for use in Table 22-1 (see p. 93).
2. If wedge is made of wood, moisten the end of the wedge or toothpick with saliva. Establish a rest by placing the hand on the cheek or chin or by placing a finger on the gingiva convenient to the place where the tip will be applied.	Moistening the wooden wedge with saliva softens the wood to prevent tissue trauma and reduce splintering. Establishing a rest will help prevent inserting the wedge or toothpick with too much pressure.
3. Place wedge against the proximal surface of a tooth with the base of the wedge triangle toward gingival border and the tip pointing occlusally or incisally at approximately a 45-degree angle (Figure 22-12).	The base of the triangular wedge is flat instead of pointed, which reduces the possibility of damaging interdental tissue. Pointing the wedge or toothpick occlusally reduces the chance of flattening or wearing away papillae or damaging the gingival border.

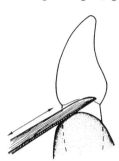

Figure 22-12. Proper placement of the Balsa wooden wedge against the proximal surface of a tooth. (From Hoag PM, Pawlak EA: *Essentials of periodontics,* ed 4, St Louis, 1990, Mosby.)

4. Use an in-and-out motion interproximally from the facial area only. Apply a burnishing stroke with moderate pressure first to the proximal surface of one tooth and then to the other, about four strokes each. Stop once wedge meets a slight resistance in the space (Figure 22-13).	Inserting the wedge interproximally should be done only until the space between the teeth is filled. If the teeth are forced apart or tissue is impinged, permanent damage could result; teeth may be abraded or tissue worn away.

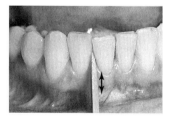

Figure 22-13. Wooden wedge placement. The tip is moved in and out to remove plaque biofilm. (From Newman MG, Takei HH, Klokkevold PR, Carranza FA: *Carranza's clinical periodontology,* ed 10, St Louis, 2006, Saunders.)

5. Trace margin of tissue to remove marginal debris, again with tip pointing occlusally (away from tissue).	Pointing the tip occlusally prevents tissue trauma.
6. If debris accumulates on wedge, rinse under running water.	Loose debris should be rinsed away and not introduced into a new interproximal area or sulcus.
7. Once all areas of mouth are completed, dispose of wedge in waste receptacle.	Wedges made of wood will absorb blood, saliva, and bacteria and should be thrown away after one use. If the wedge is plastic, it can be reused if washed with soap and warm water, then stored in a clean, dry place.

Copyright © 2010 by Saunders, an imprint of Elsevier Inc. All rights reserved.

Procedure 22-7   USE OF A RUBBER TIP STIMULATOR

STEPS	RATIONALES
1. Determine the need to use a rubber tip stimulator and appropriate areas for use.	See a list of indications for use in Table 22-2 (see p. 94).
2. Place side of rubber tip interdentally and slightly pointing coronally (45-degree angle) (Figure 22-14).	Using the side of the rubber tip allows for more surface area to be covered and reduces the chance for tissue trauma to occur. Pointing the tip coronally also decreases the risk of tissue trauma.

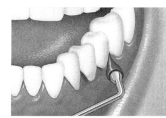

Figure 22-14.   Proper placement of a rubber tip stimulator. (Courtesy Sunstar Americas, Inc, Chicago, Illinois.)

STEPS	RATIONALES
3. Move in and out with a slow stroke, rubbing the tip against the teeth and under the contact area.	Movement into and out of the proximal space removes plaque and massages the interdental tissue. The tip should not be forced into the space, however, to prevent trauma.
4. Remove from the interproximal space and trace the gingival margin, with the tip positioned just below the margin, following the contour of the gingiva.	When the margins are traced, the marginal tissue is stimulated.
5. Once all appropriate areas are completed, rinse stimulator with soap and warm water, then store in a clean, dry place.	The stimulator is meant to be reused after cleaning. Storage is similar to that of a toothbrush.
6. Replace rubber tip as it becomes worn, cracked, or splayed.	The handle may still be kept and reused, but a worn rubber tip should be replaced to improve efficacy and reduce the possibility of tissue trauma.

Copyright © 2010 by Saunders, an imprint of Elsevier Inc. All rights reserved.

Procedure **22-8**	USE OF AN INTERDENTAL BRUSH

STEPS	**RATIONALES**
1. Determine the need to use an interdental brush and appropriate areas for use.	See a list of indications for use in Table 22-2 (see p. 94).
2. Insert bristles into embrasure at a 90-degree angle to tooth surface (long axis of the tooth) (Figure 22-15, *A*).	Inserting the bristles at a 90-degree angle prevents trauma to the sulcus or interdental papilla yet provides maximum coverage of surface area.
3. Move brush using in-and-out motion from facial and/or lingual surfaces of appropriate areas (Figure 22-15, *B*).	Because of the handle design, the interdental brush may be used from either the facial or lingual aspects. Some handles are double-ended, with one end angled for the facial surfaces and the opposite end angled for the distal surfaces.

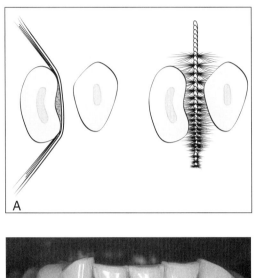

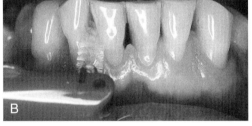

Figure 22-15. **A,** Cleaning of concave or irregular proximal tooth surfaces. Dental floss may be less effective than an interdental brush on long root surfaces with concavities. **B,** Proper placement of inderdental brush. (**A,** From Newman MG, Takei HH, Klokkevold PR, Carranza FA: *Carranza's clinical periodontology,* ed 10, St Louis, 2006, Saunders. **B,** From Perry DA, Beemsterboer PL: *Periodontology for the dental hygienist,* St Louis, 2007, Saunders.)

4. Rinse bristles under running water as necessary to remove debris.	Debris that accumulates on the bristles should be rinsed off to avoid contaminating other areas that require use of the brush.
5. On completion of use, rinse entire handle and bristles with soap and warm water.	The interdental brush is designed to be reused, just as a toothbrush is reused.
6. Store in a clean, dry place.	Storage is similar to that of a toothbrush. The interdental brush should be kept clean and dry to prevent bacterial growth.
7. Replace bristles as they become worn or splayed.	Bristles and handle should be replaced as needed to ensure cleanliness.

Copyright © 2010 by Saunders, an imprint of Elsevier Inc. All rights reserved.

Procedure 22-9 | USE OF A TONGUE CLEANER

STEPS	RATIONALES
1. Determine the need to use a tongue cleaner.	Coated tongue and/or oral malodor.
2. Hold the handle of the tongue cleaner, or if it is a strip tongue cleaner, wrap in a U shape by holding both ends of the cleaner.	The grasp on the tongue cleaner should be stable, with light pressure.
3. Start at the posterior part of the tongue, and drag the tongue cleaner to the tip of the tongue. If gag reflex is triggered, drag from the lateral border of the tongue to the opposite lateral border (Figures 22-16 and 22-17).	Drag the tongue cleaner with a light stroke to avoid tissue trauma, especially trauma to the papillae.

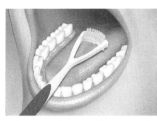

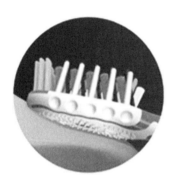

Figure 22-16. Tongue cleaner. (Courtesy Sunstar Americas, Inc, Chicago, Illinois.)

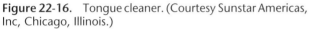

Figure 22-17. Oral-B CrossAction Pro-Health with tongue cleaner on head of brush. (Courtesy Procter & Gamble, Professional and Scientific Relations, Cincinnati, Ohio.)

STEPS	RATIONALES
4. Rinse tongue scraper with water.	Rinse the tongue cleaner to remove bacteria and debris.
5. Repeat step 3 until tongue cleaner is clean on removal, being sure to cover all aspects of the tongue with overlapping strokes.	Overlapping strokes on the surface of the tongue will prevent missing any area.
6. Rinse tongue cleaner with soap and warm water to clean. Store in a clean, dry place.	Tongue cleaners are reusable but should be replaced if they cannot be cleaned adequately or show signs of wear.

Copyright © 2010 by Saunders, an imprint of Elsevier Inc. All rights reserved.

Procedure 22-10 | USE OF A DENTAL WATER JET: JET TIP

STEPS	RATIONALES
1. Fill the reservoir with lukewarm water or an antimicrobial agent.	Reservoir is filled with about 20 oz or 500 mL of solution for full mouth irrigation. Some smaller portable units may need to be refilled to irrigate the entire mouth. An antimicrobial agent may be used and in some cases can be diluted (see Chapter 29 in the textbook).
2. Select the appropriate tip and insert into the handle, pressing firmly until it is fully engaged.	Standard jet tips are designed for full-mouth irrigation. Specially designed subgingival tips, orthodontic tips, toothbrush tips, and tongue cleaners are available with some units. Tip direction can be controlled by rotating the tip on the handle. Some units also have a pause button to stop the flow while the tips are repositioned in the mouth.
3. Adjust the pressure gauge to the lowest setting when using for the first time. Increase as needed or dicated by client comfort.	Pressure ranges vary between manufactures. It is recommended to start on the lowest pressure setting until the client is used to the device. The client may increase the setting as he or she becomes comfortable or as recommended by the dental hygienist.
4. Place the tip in the mouth, then turn the unit on. Lean over the sink and close the lips enough to prevent splashing while still allowing the water to flow from mouth into the sink.	It may take a few seconds for the flow to begin when the device is first used. Always turn the unit off or pause the flow before removing the tip from the mouth, to avoid splashing.
5. Aim the tip at a 90-degree angle to the long axis of the tooth (Figure 22-18). Starting in the posterior, follow the gingival margin, pausing between the teeth for a few seconds before continuing to the next tooth. Be sure to irrigate from the buccal and lingual aspects of all teeth.	Instructing the client to aim the tip right where the gums meet the tooth is an easy way to explain the placement. Fluid hits the tooth surface and flushes subgingivally.

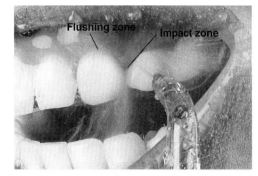

Figure 22-18. Proper placement of a standard jet tip. (From Daniel SJ, Harfst SA, Wilder RS: *Mosby's dental hygiene*, ed 2, St Louis, 2008, Mosby.)

STEPS	RATIONALES
6. Read manufacturer's instructions for each model of dental water jet before demonstration.	Not all models are designed the same, and operating instructions will vary based on the manufacturer.

Copyright © 2010 by Saunders, an imprint of Elsevier Inc. All rights reserved.

TABLE 22-1 Powered Interdental and Supplemental Self-Care Devices

Powered Interdental and Supplemental Self-Care Devices	Description and Types	Indications	Contraindications and Limitations	Common Problems That May Be Experienced during Use or Misuse
Flossing devices	Single nylon filament or a bow-shaped tip attached to a power handle Special attachment for a power toothbrush that resembles a floss holder Power floss holder with replaceable floss heads	Class I embrasures Clients with physical challenges Clients who cannot master string flossing Client preference	Class II and III embrasures Tight contacts or crowned dentition May not be able to access all proximal spaces	Floss cuts or clefts with floss holder designs Unable to maintain tension or wrap floss completely around proximal area
End- or single-tufted brush	Special attachment for power toothbrush	Type II or III embrasure depending on design (tapered or flat) Fixed dental prosthesis (e.g., orthodontic appliances, implants, pontics, maxillofacial surgery client with jaw wired shut) Difficult-to-reach areas (e.g., lingual surface of mandibular molars, abutment teeth, distal surface of terminal teeth, crowded teeth, third molars)	Type I embrasure	Tissue trauma Similar to problems associated with improper brushing technique
Interdental brushes and tips	Attached to a power handle Design similar to nonpower brushes	Type II and III embrasures Exposed root furcations Orthodontic and fixed appliances Maxillofacial surgery client with jaw wired shut Difficult-to-access areas	Class I embrasures	Clients may have difficulty controlling the tip once device is turned on
Dental water jet	Motor driven pulsating or nonpulsating device with a reservoir and specially designed tips to deliver the irrigant Nonpulsating devices attach to a faucet or showerhead	Indicated for all patient types	Children need to have the ability and dexterity to use the product	Directing the stream of water under the tongue may damage the soft tissue

Copyright © 2010 by Saunders, an imprint of Elsevier Inc. All rights reserved.

TABLE 22-2 Nonpowered Interdental Self-Care Devices

Interdental Nonpowered Self-care Products	Description and Types	Indications	Contraindications and Limitations	Common Problems That May Be Experienced during Use or Misuse
Floss	Unwaxed vs. waxed Dental tape polytetrafluoroethylene (PTFE) Braided Plain vs. flavored Therapeutic agents added (fluoride)	Type I embrasures Floss cleans between papilla and tooth Braided floss is for implants	Type II and III embrasures	Floss cuts Floss clefts Circulation to fingers cut off from wrapping too tight Inability to reach posterior teeth due to dexterity problems
Tufted dental floss	Regular diameter floss, wider tufted portion looks like yarn, and threader combination	Type II and III embrasures Mesial and distal surfaces of abutment teeth Under pontics of fixed partial dentures	Type I embrasures	Trauma from forcing threader into tissues Yarnlike portion may catch on appliances or dental work
Floss holder	Flossing aid Handle with two prongs in Y or C shape	Type I embrasures Clients lacking manual dexterity, who are physically challenged, or who have a strong gag reflex Caregivers	Type II and III embrasures	Unable to maintain tension of floss against tooth and fully wrap around proximal area Need to unwrap and rewrap floss to move to new area of floss after each tooth Need to set fulcrum to avoid floss cuts
Floss threader	Different designs that resemble a needle with a large opening to thread the floss Floss is pulled through the interproximal space to allow cleaning of the proximal surface	Type I embrasures Insert floss under tight contacts Floss between and under abutment teeth and pontics of fixed prosthesis Floss under orthodontic appliances (e.g., wires, lingual bar) Floss under bars for implants	Type II and III embrasures	Trauma from forcing threader into tissues
Toothpick (wooden or plastic)	Round Triangular	Type II and III embrasures from facial aspect only Trace gingival margin Accessible furcations Small root concavities	Type I embrasures Healthy tissue	Wearing down of papilla and marginal tissues from incorrect usage Splaying of wood ends may cause tissue trauma, cuts, or abrasions Enamel abrasion from incorrect use

Copyright © 2010 by Saunders, an imprint of Elsevier Inc. All rights reserved.

TABLE 22-2 Nonpowered Interdental Self-Care Devices—*cont'd*

Interdental Nonpowered Self-care Products	Description and Types	Indications	Contraindications and Limitations	Common Problems That May Be Experienced during Use or Misuse
Toothpick holder	Plastic handle with opening at the tip to place a toothpick	Type II and III embrasures from facial or lingual aspect Accessible furcations Concave surfaces in interproximal areas Fixed prosthetic and orthodontic appliances Sulcular cleansing in areas of shallow pocketing	Type I embrasures Healthy tissue	Wearing down of papilla and tissues from incorrect use Splaying of wood ends may cause tissue trauma, cuts, or abrasions Possible damage of epithelial attachment if used incorrectly subgingivally
Wooden wedge	Triangular wooden wedge	Type II and III embrasures from facial aspect Accessible furcations	Type I embrasures Healthy tissue	Wearing down of papilla and marginal tissues from incorrect use Splaying of wood ends may cause tissue trauma, cuts, or abrasions
Interproximal brush	Bristle inserts: tapered (conical) or straight Variety of sizes Attached to reusable handle or single disposable units	Type II and III embrasures Exposed root furcations Orthodontic and fixed appliances Difficult access areas	Type I embrasures Healthy tissue	Trauma to tooth surface or gingiva from sharp wire center of some designs
Interdental tip	Handle with soft absorbent tip or plastic filament	Type II and III embrasures Root concavities Furcations Orthodontic appliances Fixed dental appliances Application of fluoride, antimicrobial agent, or desensitizing agent	Type I embrasures Healthy tissue	Trauma caused by forcing into too small a space

Please refer to the Evolve website (http://evolve.elsevier.com/Darby/hygiene) for competency forms to help evaluate your mastery of each procedure in this chapter.

Copyright © 2010 by Saunders, an imprint of Elsevier Inc. All rights reserved.

Hand-Activated Instruments

24

Procedure 24-1   BASIC POSITIONING FOR ASSESSMENT AND TREATMENT

EQUIPMENT
Ergonomically designed dental chair and operator chair
Personal protective equipment
Protective eyewear for client
Assessment and treatment instruments (as needed)
Air-water syringe and evacuation equipment

STEPS	RATIONALES
CLIENT POSITIONING	
1a. Mandibular occlusal plane positioned parallel to floor.	Maximizes accuracy of observation and measurement.
1b. Maxillary occlusal plane positioned nearly perpendicular to floor.	Optimal accessibility for assessment and instrumentation.
1c. Client's head turned for maximum direct view of instrumentation when possible.	Enhanced client comfort.
OPERATOR POSITIONING	
2a. Right-handed operator: 8 to 10 o'clock for healthy client. The 10- to 4-o'clock positions are recommended for instrumentation of mandibular posterior teeth with moderate to severe periodontal pocket depth and sides of anterior teeth facing away from the operator. These positions usually require use of extraoral fulcrums. Occasionally, the operator may be in a standing position for very challenging deep pockets.	Accessibility to all surfaces is generally optimal from a comfortable, seated operator position next to the client. Moderate to advanced mandibular posterior depth may require an extended operator position using a maxillary reach-down extraoral fulcrum with operator in standing position for optimal instrument adaptation and insertion to base of pocket. Extended operator positioning usually allows direct vision and better control of instrument.
2b. Left-handed operator: 2 to 4 o'clock for healthy client. The 8- to 2-o'clock positions are recommended for instrumentation of mandibular posterior teeth with moderate to severe periodontal pocket depth and sides of anterior teeth facing away from the operator. These positions usually require use of extraoral fulcrums. Occasionally, the operator may be in a standing position for very challenging deep pockets.	Accessibility to all surfaces is generally optimal from a comfortable, seated operator position next to the client. Moderate to advanced mandibular posterior depth may require an extended operator position using a maxillary reach-down extraoral fulcrum with operator in standing position for optimal instrument adaptation and insertion to base of pocket. Extended operator positioning usually allows direct vision and better instrument control.
LIGHT, AIR, AND WATER AND EVACUATION	
3. Central beam illuminates working area.	Aids in comfortable instrument insertion, reducing client anxiety and stress.
4. Maintain good, unobstructed lighting; use water-air syringe and saliva evacuation when necessary. Depending on procedure, evacuation may include use of saliva ejector or high-volume evacuation by a dental assistant.	Allows operator to visualize instrument-to-tooth relationships, aiding in complete tooth surface assessment and instrumentation; improves efficiency and quality of care.

Copyright © 2010 by Saunders, an imprint of Elsevier Inc. All rights reserved.

Procedure **24-2**   USE OF THE PERIODONTAL PROBE

EQUIPMENT

Periodontal probe (Figures 24-1, *B,* and 24-2)
Mouth mirror

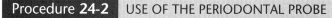

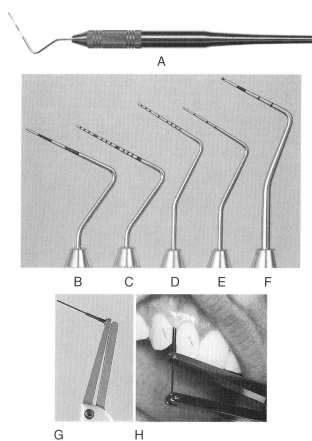

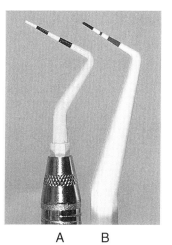

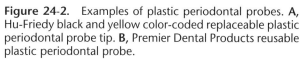

Figure 24-2. Examples of plastic periodontal probes. **A,** Hu-Friedy black and yellow color-coded replaceable plastic periodontal probe tip. **B,** Premier Dental Products reusable plastic periodontal probe.

Figure 24-1. Examples of periodontal probes. Note the differences in markings. **A,** AEP12Y/GX Probe with green band at 3 to 6 mm and yellow band at 9 to 12 mm. **B,** Marquis color-coded probe with markings at intervals of 3, 6, 9, and 12 mm. **C,** UNC-15 probe, a 15-mm-long probe with millimeter markings at each millimeter and color coding at the fifth, tenth, and fifteenth mm. **D,** University of Michigan O probe with Williams markings at 1, 2, 3, 5, 7, 8, 9, and 10 mm. **E,** Michigan O probe with markings at 3, 6, and 8 mm. **F,** World Health Organization probe, which has a 0.5-mm ball at the tip and millimeter markings at 3.5, 8.5, and 11.5 mm and color coding from 3.5 to 5.5 mm. **G,** Florida Probe Computerized Periodontal Probing and Patient-Education System. **H,** Florida Probe positioned in periodontal pocket. (**A,** Courtesy American Eagle Instruments, Missoula, Montana. **B** to **F,** From Newman MG, Takei HH, Klokkevold PR, Carranza FA: *Carranza's clinical periodontology,* ed 10, St Louis, 2006, Saunders. **H,** Courtesy Florida Probe Corporation, Gainesville, Florida.)

(Continued)

Copyright © 2010 by Saunders, an imprint of Elsevier Inc. All rights reserved.

Procedure 24-2 — USE OF THE PERIODONTAL PROBE—*cont'd*

STEPS	RATIONALES
1. Begin with Basic Positioning in Procedure 24-1.	Allows for ergonomic practice and prevention of repetitive stress injuries.
GRASP 2. Use a light, modified pen grasp.	Allows clinician to carefully insert and walk tip of instrument along junctional epithelium with minimal client discomfort. Increases maneuverability of the instrument around the tooth.
FULCRUM AND FULCRUM PRESSURE 3. Use relatively light fulcrum pressure and flexible fulcrum placement: Intraoral near the tooth being probed (Figure 24-3)	Allows movement with good adaptation of tip and first few millimeters of probe to reach base of deep periodontal pockets. Allows probe to be positioned with working end parallel to long axis of tooth.

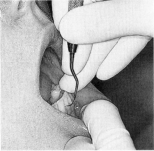

Figure 24-3. Same arch fulcrum positioned near area being scaled.

Cross-arch (Figure 24-4, *A*) Opposite arch (Figure 24-4, *B*)	Fulcrum position may be raised, lowered, tilted, and/or rotated in response to surface being measured. Because probing is an assessment function, fulcrum pressure on tooth or extraorally is light compared with a calculus removal or debridement stroke.

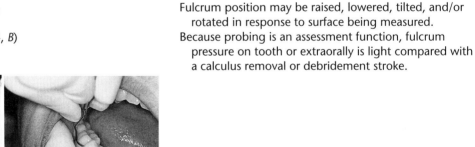

Figure 24-4. A, Cross-arch fulcrum is positioned on the same arch but across from area being scaled; fulcrum on opposite quadrant. **B,** Opposite arch fulcrum from the arch being scaled.*

*Note: Photos are included here to exemplify types of fulcrums, even though they show the fulcrums with curets and not explorers.

Copyright © 2010 by Saunders, an imprint of Elsevier Inc. All rights reserved.

Procedure 24-2 USE OF THE PERIODONTAL PROBE—*cont'd*

STEPS—*cont'd*   **RATIONALES—*cont'd***

Extraoral (Figure 24-5, *A* and *B*)

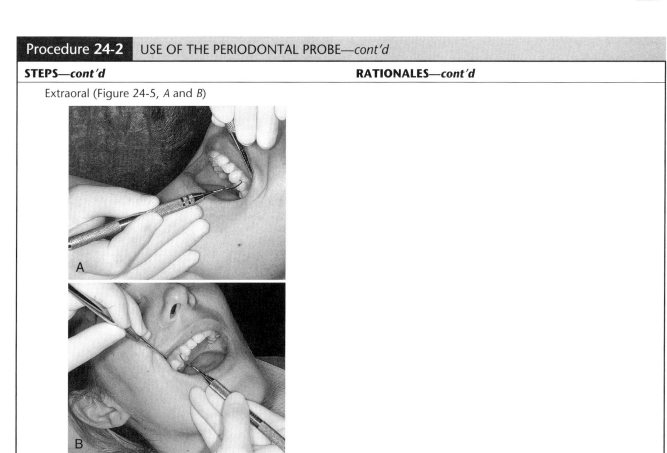

Figure 24-5. External fulcrums. **A,** Extraoral palm-down fulcrum. The front surfaces of the fingers rest on the left lateral aspect of the mandible while the maxillary left posterior teeth are instrumented. **B,** Extraoral palm-up fulcrum. The backs of the fingers rest on the right lateral aspect of the mandible while the maxillary right posterior teeth are instrumented. (From Newman MG, Takei HH, Klokkevold PR, Carranza FA: *Carranza's clinical periodontology,* ed 10, St Louis, 2006, Saunders.)

INSERTION AND ADAPTATION

4a. All periodontal probes: Insert with the lower 1 to 3 mm of the probe adapted against the tooth structure until the junctional epithelium is found. Insertion is parallel to the long axis of the tooth (see Figure 24-1).

Avoids injury and penetration of junctional epithelium, leading to client comfort and accurate readings. Parallel insertion to base of pocket leads to accurate pocket depth measurement.

4b. When the probe reaches the contact area, slant tip to the area directly under the contact (col), and with the shank touching the contact, record measurement (Figure 24-6).

Provides information to accurately diagnose furcation involvement, as treatment options, planning, and prognosis depend on assessment accuracy.

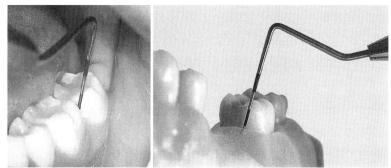

Figure 24-6. For proximal readings, periodontal probe is slightly angled under the col and positioned vertically to touch contact area between adjacent teeth.

Copyright © 2010 by Saunders, an imprint of Elsevier Inc. All rights reserved.   *(Continued)*

Procedure 24-2	USE OF THE PERIODONTAL PROBE—*cont'd*

STEPS—*cont'd*	**RATIONALES**—*cont'd*

4c. Carefully negotiate tip of probe around ledges of calculus when possible.

4d. If significant ledges of calculus prevent insertion or comfortable adaptation, remove calculus first then take readings for baseline assessment.

Ledges of calculus oftentimes interfere with periodontal probe reaching base of pocket.

5a. Nabers furcation probe (Figure 24-7, *A*): Using radiographs, previously recorded probe depths, and knowledge of root anatomy as a guide, wrap and insert the furcation probe into the furcation; note extent of penetration and classification of involvement (Figure 24-7, *B*).

Because the furcation is a tooth surface concavity, the curved furcation probe is ideal for identifying mesial and distal furcations of maxillary molars.

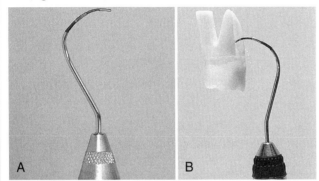

Figure 24-7.   **A,** The No. 2 Nabers probe for detection of furcation areas, with color-coded markings at 3, 6, 9, and 12 mm. **B,** Probe positioned in a furca for furcation classification. (**A,** From Newman MG, Takei HH, Klokkevold PR, Carranza FA: *Carranza's clinical periodontology,* ed 10, St Louis, 2006, Saunders.)

5b. Plastic probe (see Figure 24-2, *A*): Insert plastic probe adapted to the implant surface until resistance is met with very light pressure.

Avoid trauma and distention of soft tissue around implants.

Prevents scratching of metal surfaces.

ACTIVATION AND DIRECTION OF STROKE

6a. Move probe in small increments along base of sulcus or pocket. Under gentle pressure the junctional epithelium feels soft and resilient.

Careful and accurate activation of periodontal probe is important because this procedure is usually done without benefit of local anesthesia.

6b. Move distally in small increments until center (no contact) or col area (under contact) of tooth is reached. One side of probe must be touching tooth surface.

Avoids penetrating tissue or measuring too shallowly.

6c. Note deepest reading on distal surface.

Deepest readings offer the most accurate picture of periodontal status.

6d. Lift probe and reinsert at distal line angle; walk forward until mesial col area is reached. Probe is straightened until upper portion touches contact area.

Ensures that complete pocket area is assessed.

6e. Continue throughout mouth buccally and lingually.

Ensures that complete pocket area is assessed.

RECORDING PROBE READINGS

7a. Record deepest buccal and lingual readings from distal, buccal or lingual, and mesial surfaces. Six readings are recorded per tooth.

Deepest readings offer the most accurate picture of periodontal status and guide dentist in formulating the dental diagnosis and care plan.

7b. Stop to record in periodontal assessment section of client record after several surfaces are complete.

Enhances efficiency when clinician can remember probe readings for several teeth and chart them all at once or when a dental assistant can be used to record. Participation of a dental assistant can improve infection control and more easily avoid the contamination of charts.

Copyright © 2010 by Saunders, an imprint of Elsevier Inc. All rights reserved.

Procedure 24-3 | USE OF THE PERIODONTAL EXPLORER

EQUIPMENT
Periodontal explorer (3-A explorer or ODU 11/12 explorer) (Figure 24-8)
Mouth mirror

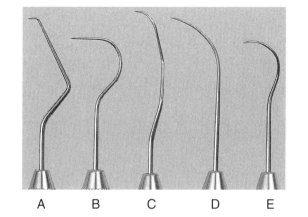

Figure 24-8. Five typical explorers. **A,** No. 17. **B,** No. 23 Shepherd's hook explorer. **C,** EXD 11/12. **D,** No. 3. **E,** No. 3CH pigtail. (From Newman MG, Takei HH, Klokkevold PR, Carranza FA: *Carranza's clinical periodontology,* ed 10, St Louis, 2006, Saunders.)

STEPS	RATIONALES
1. Begin with Basic Positioning in Procedure 24-1.	Allows for ergonomic practice and prevention of repetitive stress injuries.
SELECTING CORRECT WORKING END	
2. The 3-A extended explorer has only one working end; 11/12 extended explorers are paired with two working ends. Use the end whose curvature adapts toward the surface to be explored (see Figure 24-8, C).	Both the 3-A and 11/12 explorers are curved explorers. When curve is adapted toward tooth surface, the tip is also adapted, minimizing tissue discomfort to client.
GRASP	
3a. Use a light to moderate modified pen grasp.	Enhances tactile sensitivity, allowing operator to feel slight vibrations conducted through shank and handle with pads of tripod of fingers. Increases maneuverability of instrument around tooth. Reduces muscle fatigue in operator's hands and fingers. Grasp strength is increased when more pressure is necessary to interpret density and topography of harder structures such as burnished calculus, irregular cementum, or restorative materials.
3b. Grasp pressure is slightly increased when explorer pressure against the tooth must be increased to distinguish between tooth structure, restorative material(s), and/or calculus.	
3c. Move grasp further away from working end as you go from anterior to posterior teeth. When fulcrum moves cross-arch, opposite arch, or extraorally, move grasp away from working end of explorer.	Accessibility to posterior pockets improves with extension of fulcrum away from tooth being explored. This extension requires movement of grasp away from working end.
FULCRUM AND FULCRUM PRESSURE	
4. Use relatively light fulcrum pressure and flexible fulcrum placement:	Allows extended movement with good adaptation to base of deep periodontal pockets.

(Continued)

Copyright © 2010 by Saunders, an imprint of Elsevier Inc. All rights reserved.

Procedure 24-3   USE OF THE PERIODONTAL EXPLORER—*cont'd*

STEPS—*cont'd*	RATIONALES—*cont'd*
Intraoral near the tooth being explored (Figure 24-9) 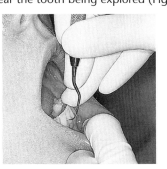 **Figure 24-9.** Same arch fulcrum positioned near area being scaled.	Allows movement of explorer in a variety of directions (vertical, horizontal, oblique). Fulcrum position may be raised, lowered, tilted, and/ or rotated in response to changing tooth surface topography. Because exploring is an assessment function, fulcrum pressure on tooth or extraorally is light compared with a calculus removal or debridement stroke.
Cross-arch (Figure 24-10, *A*) Opposite arch (Figure 24-10, *B*)	

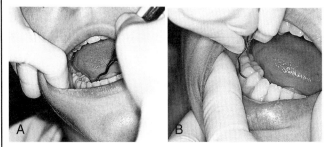

Figure 24-10.   **A,** Cross-arch fulcrum is positioned on the same arch but across sfrom area being scaled; fulcrum on opposite quadrant. **B,** Opposite arch fulcrum from the arch being scaled.*

Copyright © 2010 by Saunders, an imprint of Elsevier Inc. All rights reserved.

Procedure **24-3**   USE OF THE PERIODONTAL EXPLORER—*cont'd*

STEPS—*cont'd*	RATIONALES—*cont'd*

Extraoral (Figure 24-11)

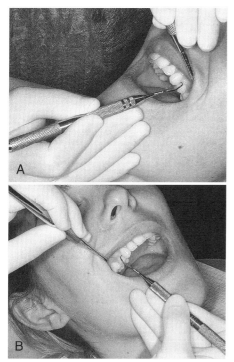

Figure 24-11.   External fulcrums. **A,** Extraoral palm-down fulcrum. The front surfaces of the fingers rest on the left lateral aspect of the mandible while the maxillary left posterior teeth are instrumented. **B,** Extraoral palm-up fulcrum. The backs of the fingers rest on the right lateral aspect of the mandible while the maxillary right posterior teeth are instrumented. (From Newman MG, Takei HH, Klokkevold PR, Carranza FA: *Carranza's clinical periodontology,* ed 10, St Louis, 2006, Saunders.)*

INSERTION AND ADAPTATION

5a. Insert with lower 1 to 3 mm of explorer adapted or curved toward tooth structure until junctional epithelium is found.

5b. Adapt explorer tip to root surface.

5c. In anesthetized clients or after clinician understands pocket topography, reinsert tip of explorer pointed downward like a periodontal probe. Adaptation of explorer curves toward tooth surface. Insert tip in a downward direction (first 1 to 2 mm must be adapted to root).

3-A and 11/12 extended explorers: Tactile evaluation of irregularities on root surface and subgingival calculus exploration begins with explorer insertion.

Reduces possibility of soft-tissue injury.

Enhances clinician's ability to reach the base of moderate to deep pocket depth and maneuver around line angles and curvatures.

11/12 extended explorer:

Anterior teeth: 11/12 Explorer is more effective when clinician uses opposite end of instrument to explore the surface sides away from the clinician on anterior teeth. It is easier for curvature of the instrument to adapt to the root surface.

Posterior teeth: Using the same end of the 11/12 explorer on the distal, buccal, and mesial surfaces on posterior teeth allows tip to remain in contact with root surface and access base of pocket.

(Continued)

Copyright © 2010 by Saunders, an imprint of Elsevier Inc. All rights reserved.

Procedure 24-3   USE OF THE PERIODONTAL EXPLORER—*cont'd*

STEPS—*cont'd*	RATIONALES—*cont'd*
ACTIVATION, DIRECTION OF STROKE, AND EFFICIENCY	
6a. Begin activation with insertion stroke (vertical direction). Stroke activation is both a push and pull stroke.	Push or downward action is important in identifying roughness that may be detectable only from the upper edge of a calculus deposit.
6b. Assess root surfaces in multiple directions (vertical, horizontal, oblique):	Burnished calculus is usually smoothest at base and may not easily be detected from bottom. Therefore, multidirection exploration is important.
Use sweeping strokes to initially determine surface irregularities.	Results in accurate identification of size and location of calculus.
Strokes are short and restricted around pieces of calculus or surface irregularities.	Long, sweeping exploratory strokes allow clinician to evaluate shape of tooth surface and effectively compare surfaces.
Strokes are long and sweeping to evaluate root smoothness.	
Use many stroke directions to assess calculus, burnished calculus, root caries, or restorative margins.	
Use fewer strokes when surface is smooth during final evaluation phase of care.	
PRESSURE	
7a. Use light pressure when assessing light calculus, little pocket depth, and friable soft tissue.	Easier to feel calculus and irregularities when lightly exploring tooth surface.
7b. Increase pressure with moderate to heavy calculus to detect burnished calculus and root irregularities.	Easier to feel heavy, tenacious calculus with either light or moderate pressure strokes.
	Moderate pressure strokes allow the clinician to assess the hardness for appropriate care planning and instrument selection for removal.
7c. Use light pressure to assess root planing outcomes.	Evaluation of scaling and root planing requires light, long, fluid strokes that do not hang up or inadvertently catch on root anatomy. It is important to assess overall smoothness over large areas.

*Note: Photos are included here to exemplify types of fulcrums, even though they show the fulcrums with curets and not explorers.

Copyright © 2010 by Saunders, an imprint of Elsevier Inc. All rights reserved.

Procedure 24-4   USE OF ANTERIOR SICKLE SCALER

EQUIPMENT
Anterior sickle scaler (Figure 24-12, *A-C*)
Subgingival explorer
Mouth mirror

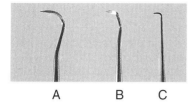

Figure 24-12. Comparison of various sickle scalers. **A,** Curved anterior sickle. **B,** Jacquette (double-ended) sickle. **C,** Morse anterior sickle.

STEPS	RATIONALES
1. Begin with Basic Positioning in Procedure 24-1.	Allows for ergonomic practice and prevention of repetitive stress injuries.
SELECTING CORRECT WORKING END	
2a. Select correct adaptation and working end based on the amount of calculus present and tissue tone.	Selection of correct end reduces possible injury from sharp point and allows better adaptation to tooth surfaces.
2b. Use straight end of the SH 5/33 on anterior interproximal surfaces (Table 24-1 on p. 107).	
2c. Use the slight contra-angle design of the SH 6/7 in anterior and premolar areas.	
GRASP	
3. Use a moderate modified pen grasp.	Allows clinician to carefully engage tip of sickle scaler under calculus and remove it with light to firm force, depending on tenacity.
FULCRUM AND FULCRUM PRESSURE	
4. Use stable, moderate fulcrum pressure during working stroke. Fulcrum placement: Intraoral near tooth being scaled (Figure 24-13)	Allows cutting edge and tip to be well adapted to tooth surface. Fulcrum position may be raised, lowered, tilted during calculus removal. Maximizes stability.

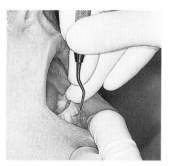

Figure 24-13. Same arch fulcrum positioned near area being scaled.*

(Continued)

Copyright © 2010 by Saunders, an imprint of Elsevier Inc. All rights reserved.

Procedure 24-4   USE OF ANTERIOR SICKLE SCALER—*cont'd*

STEPS—*cont'd*	RATIONALES—*cont'd*
Opposite arch	
INSERTION AND ADAPTATION	
5a. Engage lower edge of interproximal supragingival ledge of calculus. Engagement may extend, when soft tissue permits, 1 to 2 mm subgingivally.	Enhances probability of popping off pieces of calculus rather than relying on multiple shaving motions, which may burnish calculus.
5b. Adapt cutting edge of sickle to tooth surface.	Proper adaptation of a large-pointed instrument prevents possible injury from slippage.
	Slightly offset position of the lower shank allows access interproximally and subgingivally.
	The long blade with large, rounded back does not permit comfortable and atraumatic adaptation and insertion deeper than 1 to 2 mm.
ACTIVATION, DIRECTION OF STROKE, AND PRESSURE	
Supragingival Use	
6a. Engage large calculus deposit with a vertical to oblique stroke direction.	Allows clinician to use safest method of calculus removal without injuring soft tissue.
6b. Use a pull stroke with moderate pressure.	An oblique stroke directed toward contact area prevents losing control of instrument beyond immediate area and injuring client's soft tissues.
Subgingival Use	
7. Activate with a pull stroke in a vertical direction with moderate pressure.	Because toe of sickle scaler is a sharp point, the vertical stroke avoids injury to soft tissue or cementum.

*Note: Photo is included here to exemplify type of fulcrum, even though it shows the fulcrum with a curet and not an anterior sickle scaler.

Copyright © 2010 by Saunders, an imprint of Elsevier Inc. All rights reserved.

TABLE 24-1 Anterior Sickle Scaler Design and Selection

Common Design Specifications of All Anterior Sickle Scalers
Single-ended straight shank.
Double-ended, paired design when the shank is slightly bent.
Blade, shank, and handle are in the same plane.
Two cutting edges on a straight blade that end in a point or two cutting edges on a curved blade that end in a sharp point.
Cross-sectional view is triangular.
Back is a sharp edge of the meeting of the two sides or flattened depending on manufacturer.

Instrument Examples	Design, Function, and Recommendation
SH 6/7 Design	Paired, contra-angle, curved sickle design. Short lower shank with slight angulation for accessibility; however, blades, shank, and handle should be considered to be within the same plane and therefore are anterior sickles. Blade is long, relatively thin, with a large rounded back.
Function	Use for anterior and premolar supragingival and subgingival (1-2 mm) calculus removal. Contra-angle design allows easier access interproximally than with a straight shank. With good adaptation, this instrument could be used to remove heavy ledges of calculus on lingual surfaces of posterior teeth in a horizontal direction.
Recommendation	Not recommended for subgingival calculus removal ≥3 mm or root planing.
SH 5/33 Design	Double-ended with a straight sickle on one end and a curved sickle on other end. Both blades are within the same plane as the shank and handle. Both blades are relatively thin.
Function	Use both ends for anterior supragingival and subgingival (1-2 mm) calculus removal.
Recommendation	Not recommended for subgingival calculus removal ≥3 mm or root planing.

Copyright © 2010 by Saunders, an imprint of Elsevier Inc. All rights reserved.

Procedure 24-5 | USE OF THE POSTERIOR SICKLE SCALER

EQUIPMENT
Posterior sickle scaler (Figure 24-14)
Subgingival explorer
Mouth mirror

Figure 24-14. Posterior sickle.

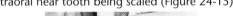

STEPS	RATIONALES
1. Begin with Basic Positioning in Procedure 24-1.	Allows for ergonomic practice and prevention of repetitive stress injuries.
SELECTING CORRECT WORKING END 2a. Select correct adaptation and working end based on amount of calculus present, tissue tone, and pocket depth. 2b. Use the SCNEVI2 rather than the S204SD for more periodontally involved clients (Table 24-2 on p. 110).	Selection of correct end of the sickle scaler reduces possible injury from sharp point and enhances clinician effectiveness.
GRASP 3. Use a moderate modified pen grasp.	Allows clinician to carefully engage tip of sickle scaler under calculus and remove it with light to firm force, depending on tenacity.
FULCRUM AND FULCRUM PRESSURE 4. Use stable, moderate fulcrum pressure during working stroke. Fulcrum placement: Intraoral near tooth being scaled (Figure 24-15)	Bends in posterior sickles allow for fulcrum placement away from area being scaled. Allows cutting edge and tip to be well adapted to tooth surface. Fulcrum position may be raised, lowered, tilted during calculus removal. Maximizes stability.

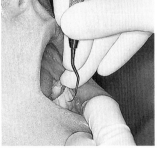

Figure 24-15. Same arch fulcrum positioned near area being scaled.

Cross-arch (Figure 24-16, *A*)

Opposite arch (Figure 24-16, *B*)

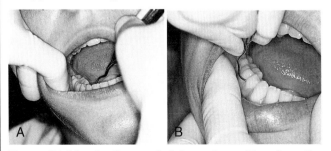

Figure 24-16. A, Cross-arch fulcrum is positioned on the same arch but across from area being scaled; fulcrum on opposite quadrant. **B,** Opposite arch fulcrum from the arch being scaled.*

Copyright © 2010 by Saunders, an imprint of Elsevier Inc. All rights reserved.

Procedure 24-5   USE OF THE POSTERIOR SICKLE SCALER—cont'd

STEPS—cont'd	RATIONALES—cont'd
INSERTION AND ADAPTATION	
5a. Insert to greatest depth tissue allows. Side of tip remains well adapted to root surface.	Proper adaptation and engagement of calculus are critical to safe subgingival instrumentation with a sickle scaler. Avoid possible injury to soft tissue and cementum.
5b. Engage lower edge of supragingival ledge of calculus.	Inserting subgingivally to find deepest part of calculus ledge is a safer stroke than attempting to fracture calculus simply to stay supragingival.
5c. Tilt tip slightly downward.	Enhances probability of popping off pieces of calculus rather than relying on multiple shaving motions, which may burnish calculus.
5d. Engage ledge of subgingival calculus. (Use opposite end for alternate sides of tooth.)	In loose, deep periodontal pockets, the curved, thin sickle blade inserts subgingivally and the curvature allows proper adaptation to root surfaces.
ACTIVATION, DIRECTION OF STROKE, AND PRESSURE	
Supragingival Use	
6a. Engage large pieces of calculus with a vertical to oblique stroke direction.	Allows clinician to use safest method of calculus removal without injuring soft tissue.
6b. Use pull stroke with moderate pressure, moving across tooth surface until all gross calculus is removed.	Prevents losing control of instrument beyond immediate area and injuring client's soft tissues.
Subgingival Use	
7a. Activate stroke with a pull stroke in a vertical direction using moderate pressure.	Because toe of sickle scaler is a sharp point, the vertical stroke avoids injury to soft tissue or cementum.
7b. Move across subgingival area until all gross calculus is removed.	

*Note: Photos are included here to exemplify types of fulcrums, even though they show the fulcrums with curets and not explorers.

Copyright © 2010 by Saunders, an imprint of Elsevier Inc. All rights reserved.

TABLE 24-2 Posterior Sickle Scaler Design and Selection

Common Design Specifications of All Posterior Sickle Scalers
Double-ended, paired design with a bent shank for posterior interproximal access.
Two straight or curved cutting edges that end in a sharp point.
Cross-sectional view is triangular.
Back is a sharp edge of the meeting of the two sides or flattened depending on manufacturer.

Instrument Examples	Design, Function, and Recommendation	
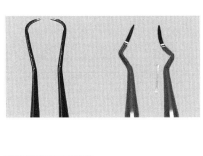	*S204SD*	
	Design	Paired, contra-angle, curved sickle design.
		Shank is bent in two places.
		Blade is small, about half the width and length of the anterior SH 6/7 sickle scaler.
	Function	Bent lower shank allows access interproximally in anterior and posterior areas.
		Short narrow blade allows access subgingivally.
	Recommendation	Use for supragingival and subgingival calculus removal (where tissue permits).
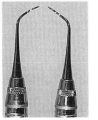	*SJ 34/35*	
	Design	Paired, contra-angle, straight sickle design (Jacquette scaler).
		Shank is bent in two places.
		The 34/35 is a miniature sickle scaler.
	Function	Bent lower shank allows access interproximally and subgingivally in anterior and posterior areas.
	Recommendation	Access may be limited owing to size of blade.
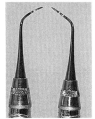	*SCNEVI2*	
	Design	Paired, contra-angle, curved sickle design.
		Shank is acutely bent.
		The blade is long and thin.
	Function	Bent lower shank allows ideal access interproximally in anterior and particularly in posterior areas.
	Recommendation	Use for supragingival and subgingival calculus removal (where tissue permits).

Copyright © 2010 by Saunders, an imprint of Elsevier Inc. All rights reserved.

Procedure 24-6   USE OF UNIVERSAL CURET

EQUIPMENT
Universal curet (Figure 24-17)
Subgingival explorer
Mouth mirror

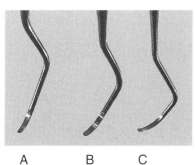

A   B   C

Figure 24-17. Universal curets. **A,** Columbia 2R/2L. **B,** Columbia 4R/4L. **C,** Columbia 13/14.

STEPS	RATIONALES
1. Begin with Basic Positioning in Procedure 24-1.	Allows for ergonomic practice and prevention of repetitive stress injuries.
SELECTING CORRECT WORKING END	
2a. See Table 24-3 (p. 113) to determine anterior versus posterior instrument usage.	
2b. Posterior instrument end selection is simple if the clinician first positions blade against buccal surface. Choose end that offers a more closed adaptation to tooth. This same end is used on mesial and distal surface from the buccal aspect.	Correct blade selection avoids excessive hard- and soft-tissue trauma and allows instrument to reach base of periodontal pocket.
2c. Follow this same rule for the lingual aspect.	
2d. For anterior instrument end selection, select either end of the universal curet.	Blade selection of anterior areas is based on thickness of instrument blade, tightness of tissue, pocket depth, and amount of calculus present.
GRASP	
3a. Use a moderate modified pen grasp. Grasp should be secure but responsive to changes during calculus removal and root topography such as line angles and concavities.	Maximizes tactile sensitivity.
3b. Roll handle of instrument around convexities and into concavities with fluid motion.	A moderate grasp (versus a heavy grasp) responds better to the anatomy of calculus and root structure(s), which is important for skillful scaling and root planing.
FULCRUM AND FULCRUM PRESSURE	
4. Use stable, moderate fulcrum pressure during working stroke. Fulcrum placement:	Allows cutting edge and tip to be well adapted to tooth surface.
Intraoral near tooth being scaled	Maximizes stability.
Cross-arch	Fulcrum position may be raised, lowered, tilted during calculus removal.
Opposite arch	
Extraoral	

(Continued)

Copyright © 2010 by Saunders, an imprint of Elsevier Inc. All rights reserved.

Procedure **24-6**	USE OF UNIVERSAL CURET—*cont'd*

STEPS—*cont'd*	**RATIONALES**—*cont'd*

INSERTION, ADAPTATION, AND ANGULATION

5a. Insert blade in a relatively closed position to base of pocket (Figure 24-18).

Correct blade selection and subsequent insertion avoid excessive soft-tissue trauma.

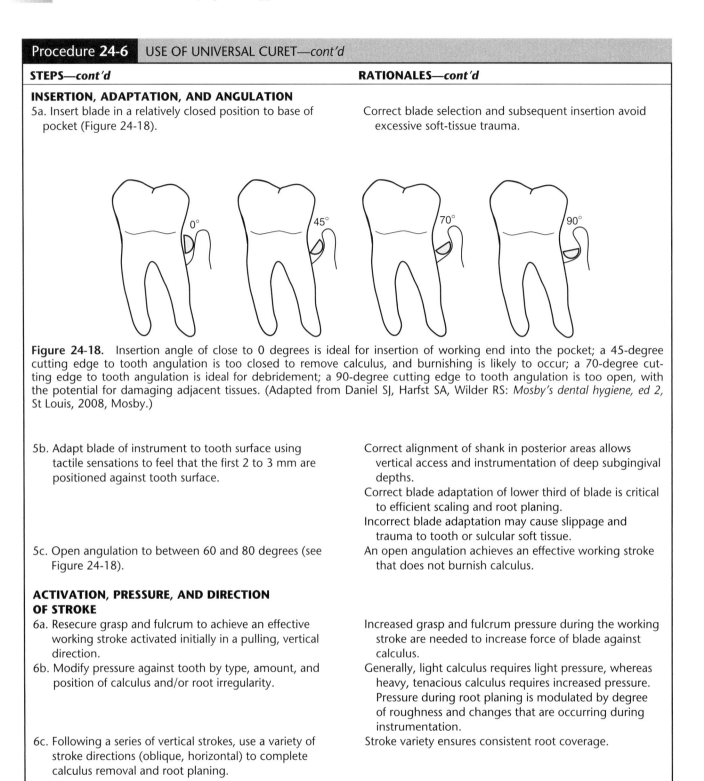

Figure 24-18. Insertion angle of close to 0 degrees is ideal for insertion of working end into the pocket; a 45-degree cutting edge to tooth angulation is too closed to remove calculus, and burnishing is likely to occur; a 70-degree cutting edge to tooth angulation is ideal for debridement; a 90-degree cutting edge to tooth angulation is too open, with the potential for damaging adjacent tissues. (Adapted from Daniel SJ, Harfst SA, Wilder RS: *Mosby's dental hygiene, ed 2,* St Louis, 2008, Mosby.)

5b. Adapt blade of instrument to tooth surface using tactile sensations to feel that the first 2 to 3 mm are positioned against tooth surface.

Correct alignment of shank in posterior areas allows vertical access and instrumentation of deep subgingival depths.

Correct blade adaptation of lower third of blade is critical to efficient scaling and root planing.

Incorrect blade adaptation may cause slippage and trauma to tooth or sulcular soft tissue.

5c. Open angulation to between 60 and 80 degrees (see Figure 24-18).

An open angulation achieves an effective working stroke that does not burnish calculus.

ACTIVATION, PRESSURE, AND DIRECTION OF STROKE

6a. Resecure grasp and fulcrum to achieve an effective working stroke activated initially in a pulling, vertical direction.

Increased grasp and fulcrum pressure during the working stroke are needed to increase force of blade against calculus.

6b. Modify pressure against tooth by type, amount, and position of calculus and/or root irregularity.

Generally, light calculus requires light pressure, whereas heavy, tenacious calculus requires increased pressure. Pressure during root planing is modulated by degree of roughness and changes that are occurring during instrumentation.

6c. Following a series of vertical strokes, use a variety of stroke directions (oblique, horizontal) to complete calculus removal and root planing.

Stroke variety ensures consistent root coverage.

Copyright © 2010 by Saunders, an imprint of Elsevier Inc. All rights reserved.

TABLE 24-3 Universal Curet Design and Selection

Common Design Specifications of All Universal Curets
Double-ended, mirror image working ends.
Two curved cutting edges that end in a rounded toe.
Face is at 90 degrees or perpendicular to lower shank.
Cross-sectional view is semicircular.
Back is round.
Differences in shank length, design, and blade size affect use.
One curet can be used throughout the healthy mouth of a child, adolescent, or adult.

Instrument	Design, Function, and Recommendation	
Posterior and Anterior Application		
(A) Columbia 13/14	Design	Short lower shank.
(B) Barnhardt 5/6		Rigid or regular flexibility in shank.
(C) Younger Good 7/8	Function	Scaling and root planing of supragingival and subgingival biofilm and calculus.
		Use on all anterior tooth surfaces.
	Recommendation	May be useful in posterior areas of the healthy mouth.
A B C		
Posterior Application		
(A) Columbia 4R/4L	Design	Long lower shank.
(B) Columbia 2R/2L		Rigid or regular flexibility in shank.
(C) Barnhardt 1/2	Function	Scaling and root planing of supragingival and subgingival biofilm and calculus.
		Use on all posterior tooth surfaces in clients with moderate to deep pocket depth.
	Recommendation	The more bent the shank, the easier it is to reach interproximally (A and C). The straighter the shank, the easier it is to reach buccally and lingually (B).
A B C		May be useful on anterior teeth where there are deep pockets and or recession.

Copyright © 2010 by Saunders, an imprint of Elsevier Inc. All rights reserved.

Procedure 24-7 | USE OF AREA-SPECIFIC CURETS

EQUIPMENT
Area-specific curets, e.g., Gracey curets (Figures 24-19 and 24-20)
Subgingival explorer
Mouth mirror

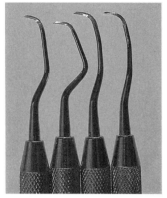

Figure 24-19. Gracey curets 5/6, 7/8, 11/12, and 13/14.

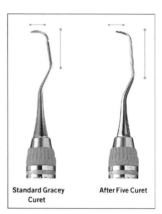

Standard Gracey Curet   After Five Curet

Figure 24-20. Gracey curet tip comparisons.

STEPS	RATIONALES
1. Begin with Basic Positioning in Procedure 24-1.	Allows for ergonomic practice and prevention of repetitive stress injuries.
SELECTING CORRECT WORKING END 2. See Table 24-4 on p. 117 for area-specific curet variations. See Table 24-5 on p. 118 for design and selection criteria of area-specific curets.	Uniquely designed for deep periodontal scaling and root planing. Offset blade, one cutting edge design, and shank angulation require knowledge of specific usage and strengths of each instrument in set. Gracey 5/6, 7/8, 11/12, and 13/14 are used as a basic set.
GRASP 3a. Use a moderate modified pen grasp. Grasp should be secure but responsive to changes during calculus removal and root topography, such as line angles and concavities.	Maximizes tactile sensitivity.
3b. Grasp allows handle (and hence blade) to roll around convexities and into concavities with fluid motion.	A moderate grasp (versus a heavy grasp) responds better to calculus and root structure(s), which is important for skillful scaling and root planing.

Copyright © 2010 by Saunders, an imprint of Elsevier Inc. All rights reserved.

Procedure 24-7 USE OF AREA-SPECIFIC CURETS—*cont'd*

STEPS—*cont'd*	RATIONALES—*cont'd*
FULCRUM AND FULCRUM PRESSURE 4. Use stable, moderate fulcrum pressure during working stroke. Fulcrum placement: Intraoral near tooth being scaled (Figure 24-21)	Allows cutting edge and tip to be well adapted to tooth surface. Maximizes stability. Fulcrum position may be raised, lowered, tilted during calculus removal.

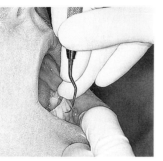

Figure 24-21. Same arch fulcrum positioned near area being scaled.

Cross-arch (Figure 24-22, *A*)

Opposite arch (Figure 24-22, *B*)

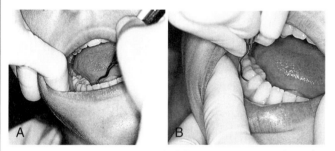

Figure 24-22. A, Cross-arch fulcrum is positioned on the same arch but across from area being scaled; fulcrum on opposite quadrant. **B,** Opposite arch fulcrum from the arch being scaled.*

(Continued)

Copyright © 2010 by Saunders, an imprint of Elsevier Inc. All rights reserved.

Procedure 24-7   USE OF AREA-SPECIFIC CURETS—*cont'd*

STEPS—*cont'd*	**RATIONALES**—*cont'd*

Extraoral (Figure 24-23)

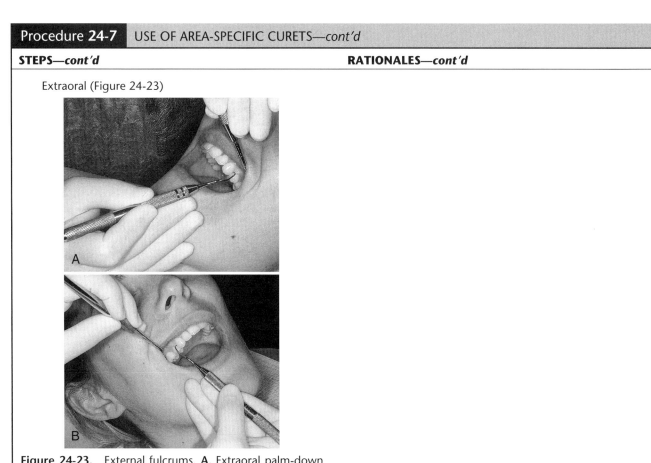

Figure 24-23.   External fulcrums. **A,** Extraoral palm-down fulcrum. The front surfaces of the fingers rest on the left lateral aspect of the mandible while the maxillary left posterior teeth are instrumented. **B,** Extraoral palm-up fulcrum. The backs of the fingers rest on the right lateral aspect of the mandible while the maxillary right posterior teeth are instrumented. (From Newman MG, Takei HH, Klokkevold PR, Carranza FA: *Carranza's clinical periodontology,* ed 10, St Louis, 2006, Saunders.)

INSERTION, ADAPTATION, AND ANGULATION

5a. Select correct end of curet by positioning longer, lower cutting edge of blade against tooth. (The correct end positions face of blade toward the root surface; with a vertical stroke, the lower shank should be parallel to the long axis of the tooth.)

Correct blade selection, alignment, and subsequent insertion.

5b. Insert blade in a relatively closed position to base of pocket.

Avoids excessive soft-tissue trauma and allows vertical access and instrumentation of deep subgingival depths.

5c. Adapt blade of instrument to tooth surface using tactile sensations to feel that the first 2 to 3 mm are positioned against tooth surface.

Correct blade adaptation of lower third of blade is critical to efficient scaling and root planing. Incorrect blade adaptation may cause slippage on and trauma to tooth or sulcular soft tissue.

5d. Open angulation to between 60 and 80 degrees.

Angulation must be opened to achieve an effective working stroke that does not burnish calculus.

Copyright © 2010 by Saunders, an imprint of Elsevier Inc. All rights reserved.

Procedure 24-7	USE OF AREA-SPECIFIC CURETS—*cont'd*

STEPS—*cont'd*	**RATIONALES**—*cont'd*
ACTIVATION, PRESSURE, AND DIRECTION OF STROKE	
6a. Resecure grasp and fulcrum to achieve an effective working stroke activated initially in a pulling, vertical direction.	Increased grasp and fulcrum pressure during working stroke are needed to increase force of blade against calculus.
6b. Modify pressure against tooth by type, amount, and position of calculus and/or root irregularity.	Generally, light calculus requires light pressure; heavy, tenacious calculus requires increased pressure. Pressure during root planing is modulated by degree of roughness and changes that are occurring during instrumentation.
6c. Following a series of vertical strokes, use a variety of stroke directions (oblique, horizontal) to complete calculus removal and root planing.	Stroke variety ensures consistent root coverage.

*Note: Photos are included here to exemplify types of fulcrums, even though they show the fulcrums with curets and not explorers.

TABLE 24-4 Area-Specific Curet Design Variations (see Figure 24-20)

Common Design Specifications of All Area-Specific Curets

Double-ended, mirror-image working ends.

Each blade has two curved cutting edges that end in a rounded toe; however, only one cutting edge per working end is used.

When the lower shank is held vertically, only lower edge of blade is identified as the cutting edge.

Face is offset or tilted at approximately 60 to 70 degrees to the lower shank for perfect working angulation.

Cross-sectional view is semicircular.

Back is round.

Shank design varies with each instrument, making them specific to areas and tooth surfaces where they are used.

All Gracey curets may be used for supragingival and subgingival biofilm and calculus removal and root planing.

Variations	**Options**	**Comparisons**	**Application**
Shank strength	Standard	Slight flexion with moderate to heavy instrumentation pressure	Healthy or maintenance clients
	Rigid and extra rigid	Larger, stronger, less-flexible shank	Moderate to heavy tenacious calculus removal
Shank length	Standard	Area specificity allows for deep scaling, root planing, and periodontal debridement	Healthy or maintenance clients
	Examples by manufacturer: After-Five (Hu-Friedy); Extended Gracey (G. Hartzell & Son)	Terminal shank elongated by 3 mm Deep periodontal pockets	
Blade size	Standard	Offset blade relative to the lower shank, curved upward with a curved blade producing an elongated cutting edge	Healthy to periodontally involved clients
	Examples by manufacturer: Mini-Five (Hu-Friedy); Mini-Extended Gracey (G. Hartzell & Son); Micro-Mini Five (Hu-Friedy)	Terminal shank elongated by 3 mm and blade length reduced by half standard blade 20% thinner blade than the Mini-Five Gracey curets, shank rigidity greater than the Mini-Five Gracey curets	Deep, narrow periodontal pockets and furcations Precise debridement of root and tooth surfaces in challenging periodontal pockets

Copyright © 2010 by Saunders, an imprint of Elsevier Inc. All rights reserved.

TABLE 24-5 Area-Specific Curet Design and Selection

Instrument	Design and Selection	
 A B	*Gracey 1/2* Design Function	Straight shank in the Gracey 1/2 (**A**) similar to that of a Gracey 5/6 (**B**), but shorter. Maxillary and mandibular anterior incisors and canines. Shorter shank length limits this instrument to shallower depth than the Gracey 5/6.
 A B	*Gracey 3/4* Design Function	Bent shank in the Gracey 3/4 (**A**) similar to that of a Gracey 7/8 (**B**), but shorter. Maxillary and mandibular anterior incisors and canines. Shorter shank length limits this instrument to shallower depth than the Gracey 7/8.
(See comparison above with Gracey 1/2)	*Gracey 5/6* Design Function	Similar straight shank to that of a Gracey 1/2, but longer. Maxillary and mandibular anterior incisors, canines, and premolars.
(See comparison above with Gracey 3/4)	*Gracey 7/8* Design Function	Similar shank bend to that of a Gracey 3/4, but longer. Maxillary and mandibular anterior incisors, canines, premolars, and molars. Limitations on distal surfaces of molars.
	Gracey 9/10 Design Function	Shank bend is more pronounced than on a Gracey 7/8. Maxillary and mandibular molar buccal and lingual surfaces.
	Gracey 11/12 Design Function	Shank is slightly angulated at two points for adaptation to mesial surfaces. Maxillary and mandibular molar and premolar mesial surfaces.
	Gracey 13/14 Design Function	Shank is angulated for adaptation to distal surfaces. Maxillary and mandibular molar and premolar distal surfaces. Using extraoral fulcrums and a variety of operator positions around the client, the clinician also may be able to use the 13/14 in nontraditional areas such as lingual surfaces.

Copyright © 2010 by Saunders, an imprint of Elsevier Inc. All rights reserved.

TABLE 24-5 Area-Specific Curet Design and Selection—*cont'd*

Instrument	Design and Selection	
	Gracey 15/16 Design Function	Same shank angulation as the Gracey 13/14, but nonworking blade is now the cutting edge, thereby positioned to reach mesial posterior surfaces. Maxillary and mandibular molar and premolar mesial surfaces.
	Gracey 17/18 Design Function	Accentuated shank angles for access to distal posterior surfaces. Smaller blade and slightly longer terminal shank. Maxillary and mandibular molar distal surfaces.

Copyright © 2010 by Saunders, an imprint of Elsevier Inc. All rights reserved.

Procedure 24-8 | BASIC OPERATOR POSITIONING STRATEGIES FOR PROTECTIVE SCALING

EQUIPMENT
Ergonomically designed dental chair, equipment, and operator chair

STEPS	RATIONALES
1. Position self comfortably in chair with weight distributed evenly on seat (Figure 24-24). 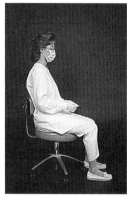 **Figure 24-24.**	Operator chairs are small and tip over or move if operator's weight is unevenly distributed over seat. Safe, effective periodontal instrumentation requires a balanced body.
2. Lower back should be straight but need not be against backrest. At times, when speaking with client or if a moment of relaxation is required, backrest may be used for support. Maintain a straight lower back for much of the time during the appointment.	It is impossible to keep lower back against the backrest during scaling. It is necessary to lean over the client to distribute body weight over the scaling arm to transfer some workload to upper arm and shoulder. A straight lower back reinforces good postural habits and minimizes possible back injury.
3. Knees should be bent in a sitting position, not crossed or straight. From this position, lean over client, concentrating more total body effort to control scaling actions.	It is easier to control the movable operator's stool when knees are bent; lessens chance that chair will flip out from under operator. Bent knees are more balanced and allow changes in upper body position at a moment's notice.
4. Legs do not have to be kept together (i.e., they may straddle the chair). Pant dressing is essential (Figure 24-25). 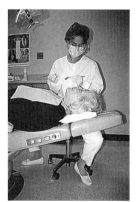 **Figure 24-25.**	Straddling the client's chair provides better stability when it is necessary to lean over the client.
5. Both feet do not have to be positioned squarely on floor. Either knee or both knees may be dropped, which changes foot position to a side or toe placement instead of feet flat on floor (Figure 24-26).	A right-angle knee position limits the ability to position client's chair in a low supine position. A variety of foot positions allows clinician to stretch and maintain agility, thereby improving balance throughout the day.

Copyright © 2010 by Saunders, an imprint of Elsevier Inc. All rights reserved.

| Procedure **24-8** | BASIC OPERATOR POSITIONING STRATEGIES FOR PROTECTIVE SCALING—*cont'd* |

STEPS—*cont'd*   **RATIONALES**—*cont'd*

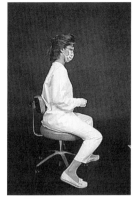

Figure 24-26.

6. Right-handed or left-handed operator may move anywhere from an 8-o'clock to a 4-o'clock seated position around client.

7. Standing approach is useful in all positions from 8 o'clock to 4 o'clock (Figure 24-27).

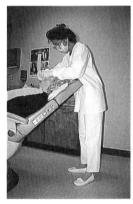

Figure 24-27.

8. Standing position is useful when vision becomes difficult (e.g., in situations where client is seated slightly upright, the mouth is small, or the client's chair does not drop low enough).

Allows clinician to move to positions that are ergonomically sound and safe for both clinician and client.
Some areas of the mouth are easier to reach from different angles.
Standing position is easier in some areas of the mouth (e.g., mandibular posterior mesial surfaces) because it allows traction and versatility to move over a client.
Clinician may need to perform instrumentation without risk or need to control a movable stool.

Allows the clinician to reach down and use a pull stroke while keeping wrist and arm in line with shoulder.

(Continued)

Copyright © 2010 by Saunders, an imprint of Elsevier Inc. All rights reserved.

Procedure 24-8   BASIC OPERATOR POSITIONING STRATEGIES FOR PROTECTIVE SCALING—*cont'd*

STEPS—*cont'd*	**RATIONALES**—*cont'd*
9. In standing position, feet may be positioned squarely on floor but may lift off onto ball of left foot (right-handed clinician) with the right hip leaning against client's chair (Figure 24-28).	By lifting slightly up on the toes and bracing the lower body against the client's chair, the clinician may lean across the client and work with maximal control.

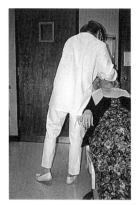

Figure 24-28.

Please refer to the Evolve website (http://evolve.elsevier.com/Darby/hygiene) for competency forms to help evaluate your mastery of each procedure in this chapter.

Copyright © 2010 by Saunders, an imprint of Elsevier Inc. All rights reserved.

Ultrasonic and Sonic Instrumentation

25

Procedure 25-1	INSTRUMENTATION WITH THE MAGNETOSTRICTIVE ULTRASONIC UNIT

EQUIPMENT

Personal protective equipment, including face shield
Ultrasonic unit (manual or autotuned) tuned appropriately
Inserts (standard and/or precision thin)
Subgingival explorer
Mouth mirror
Files
Curets
High-speed evacuation
Preprocedural mouth rinse of 0.12% chlorhexidine gluconate
Protective eyewear and drape for client

STEPS	RATIONALES
PREPARATION	
1. Connect ultrasonic unit to water source on dental unit and electrical power source.	Provides power source to operate equipment.
2. Turn ultrasonic unit on, and allow water to flow through handpiece for 2 to 5 minutes (30 seconds between clients).	Allows stagnant water and trapped air to flush through handpiece. Decreases biofilm in water line.
3. Select a straight-angled tip and insert into water-filled handpiece of ultrasonic unit.	
4. Holding handpiece over a water receptacle, adjust water and power to desired setting. Tip emits mist of water without excessive dripping.	The higher the power setting, the more water is needed to keep tip properly cooled.
POSITIONING	
5. Place client in appropriate supine position: Have client tilt head toward right or left depending on area being treated and place suction appropriately. Provide protective eyewear, plastic drape, and paper towels.	Prevents lavage from pooling in client's throat and directs fluid to the suction. Protective barrier protects client's eyes and clothing.
GRASP	
6. Use light pen or modified pen grasp.	Minimizes lateral pressure.
FULCRUM	
7. Employ conventional, opposite arch, cross-arch, or other fulcrum.	Enhances control and access.
8. Use intraoral fulcrum for standard designs and extraoral fulcrum for precision thin designs.	Both are needed for periodontal debridement with mechanized instrument.
MIRROR USE	
9. Prepare mirror to allow water to pool on its surface.	Enhances care, retraction, and client comfort.
ADAPTATION	
10. Explore or visually locate deposit. Position side of insert tip on deposit (standard) or at epithelial attachment (precision thin).	Point of working end causes tooth structure damage and must be avoided.

(Continued)

Copyright © 2010 by Saunders, an imprint of Elsevier Inc. All rights reserved.

Procedure 25-1	INSTRUMENTATION WITH THE MAGNETOSTRICTIVE ULTRASONIC UNIT—*cont'd*
STEPS—*cont'd*	**RATIONALES**—*cont'd*
11. Apply insert tip at no more than a 15-degree angle to tooth surface.	Use of active tip and appropriate surfaces is essential for successful debridement.
12. Adapt back or lateral surfaces of insert tip parallel to long axis of tooth.	Allows access to larger surface area.
13. Adapt insert tip diagonally (bisecting the long axis) on proximal surface. Back of precision thin insert might be adapted in pocket on proximal surfaces or in furcation invasions.	Allows access to larger surface area.
14. Roll insert within handpiece to adapt to various tooth surfaces. (Hu-Friedy Satin Swivel is designed to facilitate adaptation in an ergonomic manner.)	Facilitates adaptation to variable tooth surfaces.
15. Extend insert tip to midline of proximal surfaces.	Facilitates comprehensive instrumentation.
ACTIVATION	
16. Keep insert in motion at all times.	Prevents unnecessary loss of tooth structure.
17. Use quick, controlled, eraser-like motions with standard inserts. Speed of movement is slower with precision thin inserts, except where smoothing is indicated (vibrato stroke).	Speed of movement is adjusted depending on the purpose of the debridement and insert used.
18. Use overlapping, multidirectional strokes.	Varying stroke direction is essential for complete debridement.
19. Do not apply excessive lateral pressure.	Allows the tip of the instrument to work.
20. Stop periodically to allow complete evacuation.	Assists in visibility.
21. Evaluate progress and product with light, air, and explorer. Retreat areas as necessary with manual or mechanized instruments.	Maximizes efficiency; allows clinician to modify technique as necessary.
DOCUMENTATION	
22. Record services rendered in client record (e.g., oral debridement of mandibular left quadrant using universal tip insert).	Maintains accurate record for legal purposes and monitoring of care.
23. Follow current infection control protocol.	Aerosolization of contaminants requires strict infection control.

Please refer to the Evolve website (http://evolve.elsevier.com/Darby/hygiene) for competency forms to help evaluate your mastery of each procedure in this chapter.

Copyright © 2010 by Saunders, an imprint of Elsevier Inc. All rights reserved.

Root Morphology and Instrumentation Applications

26

Procedure 26-1 ROOT MORPHOLOGY AND IMPLICATIONS FOR ROOT INSTRUMENTATION

ASSUMPTION

The clinician has mastered instrumentation procedures from textbook Chapter 17, Periodontal and Risk Assessment; Chapter 24, Hand-Activated Instruments; and Chapter 25, Ultrasonic and Sonic Instrumentation.

Select ultrasonic insert and universal and area-specific curets for use on cementum and root surfaces.

STEPS	RATIONALES
1. Make a mental image of the unseen portion of the tooth to be instrumented and the width and height of the adjacent alveolar bone.	Provides information on the anatomy of the tooth and alveolar bone.
2. Review periodontal parameters recorded on the periodontal assessment form.	Free gingival margin and attachment level demarcate the subgingival area to be instrumented.
3. Observe clinical and radiographic alignment of the tooth and adjacent teeth.	Identifies where instrument placement may be difficult, e.g., narrow space normally on the lower anterior teeth, or interferences created by crowding.
GENERAL CHARACTERISTICS OF ROOTS AND THEIR IMPLICATIONS FOR INSTRUMENTATION	
4. Adapt instrument so that it follows the long axis of the root and the taper or convergence of root surfaces apically. For curets, use the terminal shank of the instrument as the guide to maintain parallelism. For periodontal probe and universal ultrasonic inserts, use working end to maintain parallelism.	Ensures instrument adaptation to the tooth surface and movement apically to reach the junctional epithelium; instrument must be in line with the inclination of the long axis of the root being instrumented.
5. Adapt instrument to the taper or convergence of the proximal surfaces toward the lingual surface. If the convergence of the proximal surfaces is pronounced as in maxillary anterior teeth and maxillary molars, approach more of the proximal surfaces from the lingual surface.	Maxillary incisors, canines, and sometimes mandibular premolars have roots with proximal surfaces that converge toward the lingual surface. For these teeth, there is more room to access the proximal surface from the lingual.
6. Adapt instrument so that it also accounts for the position of the tooth in the alveolar bone and the client's position in the chair.	Teeth are positioned in the alveolar bone so that maxillary teeth overlap mandibular teeth in centric occlusion. In a facial or lingual plane, crowns of all anterior and maxillary posterior teeth are positioned more facial than their roots, except crowns of mandibular molars, which are positioned more lingual than their roots. Mesiodistally, crowns of canines and posterior teeth are also positioned more mesially than their roots. Tooth position is also influenced by client and operator positioning.
7. Use multidirectional strokes, alternating horizontal, vertical, and oblique stroke directions.	Ensures complete coverage of all surfaces.
8. Adapt instrument to the lingual inclination of mandibular posterior teeth by slightly angling instrument shank toward the lingual surface.	Crowns of mandibular teeth are tilted slightly toward the lingual surface.
9. Use alternative instrument placement or an alternative instrument for very narrow spaces, e.g., posterior curet or scaler on an anterior tooth.	Mandibular incisors have very narrow facial and lingual surfaces and broad mesial and distal surfaces and are frequently crowded. They are positioned closest of all teeth because their crowns are narrow and their proximal crests only slightly convex.

(Continued)

Copyright © 2010 by Saunders, an imprint of Elsevier Inc. All rights reserved.

| Procedure **26-1** | ROOT MORPHOLOGY AND IMPLICATIONS FOR ROOT INSTRUMENTATION—*cont'd* |

STEPS—*cont'd* | **RATIONALES**—*cont'd*

ROOT MORPHOLOGY INSTRUMENTATION

Specific Characteristics of Roots and Their Implications for Instrumentation (Table 26-1)

10. Adapt instrument to curvature of the cementoenamel junction (CEJ) on the proximal surface of anterior teeth by turning toe end of a curet or ultrasonic insert into the most incisal portion of it, which may be very narrow. The end of a scaler may be needed to access this area.

On proximal mesial surfaces of anterior teeth, the CEJ is curved sharply toward the incisal surface, especially on maxillary central incisors. Curvature of the CEJ on proximal surfaces of posterior teeth is not sharply pointed toward the occlusal surface.

11. Adapt toe end of instrument's cutting edge to proximal root concavities with small overlapping strokes that are gradually channeled into the concave area from both facial and lingual approaches. If tooth has more than one root, adapt instrument similarly to the slight concave area approaching the furcation.

Most roots have longitudinal concavities on proximal surfaces and concave areas on root trunks before a furcation begins.

12. Adapt instrument into furcations.

12a. If there are (anatomic) concavities cervical to or with Class I furcation involvement, scale area with very small strokes and turn toe into concave area that marks the very initial stages of division.

Concavities may appear as normal anatomic variants on root trunks just apical to the CEJ, especially on buccal surfaces of maxillary or mandibular first molars. Expect furcations on mesial and distal surfaces of maxillary first premolars; on mesial, facial, and distal surfaces of maxillary molars, and on the facial and lingual surfaces of mandibular molars.

12b. With Class II, III, or IV furcation involvement, instrument furcation area as if there were two or three distinct roots. If access is very limited, furcation or ultrasonic instruments can be used. Refer to the dentist of record when Class II or higher furcation involvement is found.

Proximal surface furcations are much more difficult to instrument because of access.

In Class III and IV furcation involvement, roots of the tooth must be treated as individual roots, e.g., the mandibular molars have two roots, one mesial and one distal each, with mesial, facial, distal, and lingual surfaces.

VARIATIONS

13. For concrescence, use toe end of curet to instrument area of junction of the roots.

Occurs after formation, when roots of two adjacent teeth become joined by cementum.

14. For palatogingival groove, use toe end of a micro-, mini-, or extended-shank curet to access the groove.

Sometimes occurs on the maxillary lateral incisor; has potential for creating a long thin pocket.

15. Document in ink the completion of the services in the client's record under "Services Rendered," and date the entry. For example:

Ensures integrity of the client's record for both the client's health and the protection of the practitioner from legal risks.

08-24-10: No. 30 facial, Class II furcation present; ultrasonics and 11-14 Gracey used for full instrumentation of furcation; spoke with client at length regarding prognosis and need for follow-up treatment; no anesthesia; client tolerated well; reinforced OHI in area; referred to dentist of record.

Provides guidance on instrument selection at future appointments. Furcation files can also be used after the Gracey curets.

or

06-14-10: No. 3 Class II mesial furcation present, used ultrasonics and curets for full furcation instrumentation; access easiest from lingual aspect; reinforced OHI in area; advised on need for periodontal evaluation; referred to dentist of record.

Copyright © 2010 by Saunders, an imprint of Elsevier Inc. All rights reserved.

TABLE 26-1 Characteristics of Roots

Maxillary Arch

Central Incisor

One cone-shaped root
Does not have prominent root concavities
Most prominent cementoenamel junction (CEJ)
    curvature toward incisal on mesial surface
Lingual surface is smaller than facial
    because proximal surface tapers
    toward the lingual surface
Cervical cross-section is a "rounded" triangle in shape
Flat mesial surface
Root is approximately one and one third times the length
    of the crown*

See Figure 26-15, *A* (p. 131)

Tooth No. 8

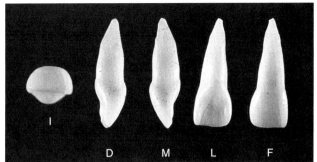

Figure 26-1. (Courtesy former Department of Dental Hygiene, Marquette University.)

Lateral Incisor

One cone-shaped root
May have a palatogingival groove
Lateral root is rounder
Lateral root longer than central root*

Tooth No. 7

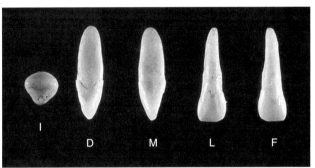

Figure 26-2. (Courtesy former Department of Dental Hygiene, Marquette University.)

Canine

One long cone-shaped root
Generally has proximal root concavities
Distal crest of curvature in the crown may hinder
    access to the mesial surface of the first premolar
Root length is one and a half times the length
    of the very long crown*

Tooth No. 6

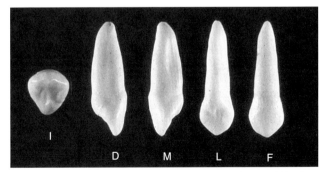

Figure 26-3. (Courtesy former Department of Dental Hygiene, Marquette University.)

(Continued)

Copyright © 2010 by Saunders, an imprint of Elsevier Inc. All rights reserved.

TABLE 26-1 Characteristics of Roots—*cont'd*

Maxillary Arch

First Premolar

Two roots, F and L (may have only one)
Prominent mesial root concavity that extends apically
  from the mesial contact on the crown
Bifurcated in cervical third to half
Elliptic in shape in cervical cross-section; narrow facial
  and lingual root surfaces, broad proximal surfaces
Root is approximately one and three fourths times
  the length of the crown*

Second Premolar

One root
Mesial concavity not as pronounced as in first
  premolar (may be prominent)
Elliptic in cross-section; broad proximal surfaces
Root is approximately one and one third times the length
  of the crown*

First Molar

Three roots, mesiobuccal, distobuccal, and palatal
Palatal root is longest and extends out
  beyond the lingual surface of the crown (lingual root
  concavity on its palatal surface)
Root concavities may be present on the
  mesiobuccal and palatal roots and also
  on furcal surfaces
Mesiobuccal and distobuccal roots may appear as a "pair"
  with their apices curved toward each
  other; look like pliers
Mesiobuccal root has a mesial concavity
Furcations are an the facial, mesial, and
  distal aspects and begin gradually before
  the entrance, which is located near the
  junction of the cervical and middle third
  of the root
The root trunk on the mesial surface is the shortest and on
  the distal surface is the longest
Mesial furcation is located more toward the lingual asepect
Roots are one and three fourths the length
  of the crown*

See Figure 26-15, *A* (p. 131)

Tooth No. 5

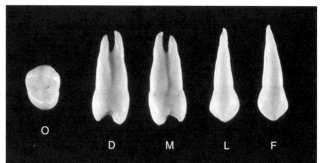

Figure 26-4. (Courtesy former Department of Dental Hygiene, Marquette University.)

Tooth No. 4

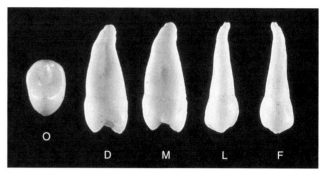

Figure 26-5. (Courtesy former Department of Dental Hygiene, Marquette University.)

Tooth No. 3

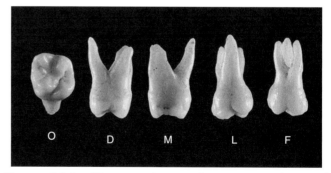

Figure 26-6. (Courtesy former Department of Dental Hygiene, Marquette University.)

Copyright © 2010 by Saunders, an imprint of Elsevier Inc. All rights reserved.

TABLE 26-1 Characteristics of Roots—*cont'd*

Maxillary Arch

Second Molar
Three roots: mesiobuccal, distobuccal, and
   palatal
Longer root trunk than first molar
Roots are closer together with more distal
   orientation
Less interradicular bone than on first
   molar

See Figure 26-15, *B* (p. 131)

Tooth No. 2

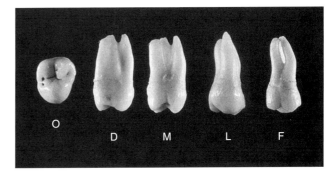

Figure 26-7. (Courtesy former Department of Dental Hygiene, Marquette University.)

Third Molar
Root morphology varies greatly; may be three rooted, roots
   may be fused and may have accessory roots

Mandibular Arch

Central and Lateral Incisor
Very similar
One cone-shaped root
Cervical cross-section is elliptic in shape with very narrow
   facial and lingual surfaces and broader proximal surfaces
Frequently have very shallow root concavities on proximal
   surfaces
Root is one and a half times the length of
   the crown*

See Figure 26-15, *B* (p. 131)

Tooth No. 25

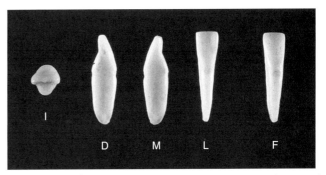

Figure 26-8. (Courtesy former Department of Dental Hygiene, Marquette University.)

Tooth No. 26

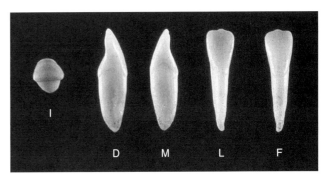

Figure 26-9. (Courtesy former Department of Dental Hygiene, Marquette University.)

(Continued)

Copyright © 2010 by Saunders, an imprint of Elsevier Inc. All rights reserved.

TABLE 26-1   Characteristics of Roots—*cont'd*

Mandibular Arch

See Figure 26-15, *B* (p. 131)

Canine

One cone-shaped root

Cervical cross-section is ovoid in shape with small lingual surface

Proximal root concavities are present

Root length is about one and a half times the length of the crown[*]

Occasionally the root apex is bifurcated into a facial and a lingual root

Tooth No. 27

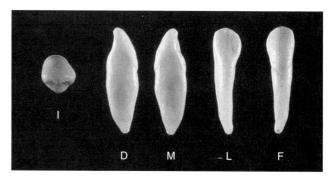

Figure 26-10. (Courtesy former Department of Dental Hygiene, Marquette University.)

First Premolar[†]

One cone-shaped root

Cervical cross-section may be elliptic or ovoid in shape

Facial and lingual root surfaces converge markedly toward the apex

May have root concavities deep on distal surface

Root length is one and two thirds the length of the crown[*]

Tooth No. 28

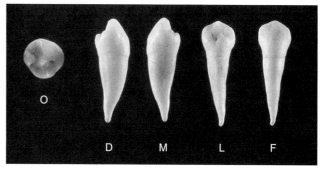

Figure 26-11. (Courtesy former Department of Dental Hygiene, Marquette University.)

Second Premolar[†]

One cone-shaped root

Cervical cross-section may be elliptic or ovoid in shape

Mandibular premolars may have proximal root concavities

Root length is one and two thirds the length of the crown[*]

Tooth No. 29

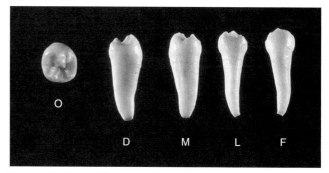

Figure 26-12. (Courtesy former Department of Dental Hygiene, Marquette University.)

Copyright © 2010 by Saunders, an imprint of Elsevier Inc. All rights reserved.

TABLE 26-1 Characteristics of Roots—*cont'd*

Mandibular Arch

First Molar†
Two roots: mesial and distal, which is narrower
Furcations on facial and lingual surface, facial concavity before the furcation begins just apical to the CEJ
Short root trunk, about 3 mm on the facial surface, one fourth the length of root trunk; longer on lingual surface
Large interradicular area
Proximal and furcal concavities on mesial root, furcal concavity on distal root
Roots are one and three fourths times the length of the crown
Cervical enamel projections may be present

Second Molar†
Two roots: mesial and distal
Roots are likely to be closer together with a longer root trunk than first molar
Mesial root concavities are not as prominent as in first molar
Roots are one and three fourths times the length of the crown
Cervical enamel projections may be present

Third Molar†
Root structure varies greatly
Typically has two roots
Roots are frequently shorter, fused, and dilacerated

See Figure 26-15, *B*

Tooth No. 30

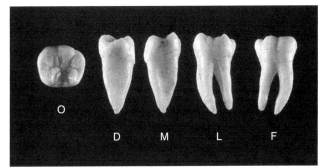

Figure 26-13. (Courtesy former Department of Dental Hygiene, Marquette University.)

Tooth No. 31

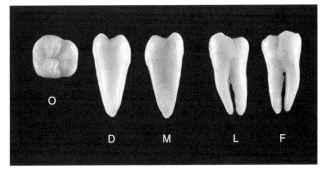

Figure 26-14. (Courtesy former Department of Dental Hygiene, Marquette University.)

I, Incisal; *D,* distal; *M,* mesial; *L,* lingual; *F,* facial; *O,* occlusal.
*Knowing the length of the crown of a tooth is helpful in assessing the length of its root and the amount of attachment:
- Maxillary central and lateral incisor crowns are the longest in the dentition, being approximately ½ inch in length.
- Anterior crowns are approximately 2 to 3 mm longer than posterior crowns. Roots range from approximately 12 to 17 mm in length; incisor roots are the shortest, and canines are the longest.
- Proportionally, when the length of roots is compared with the length of crowns, molars have the longest roots (because of their short crowns), and maxillary incisors have the shortest.
†Crowns of all mandibular posterior teeth are lingually inclined and make instrument placement more difficult.

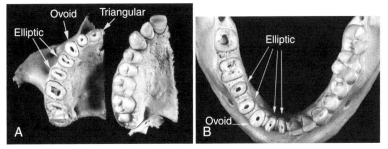

Figure 26-15. Root shapes in cervical cross-section. **A,** Maxillary teeth: triangular, elliptic, and ovoid. **B,** Mandibular teeth: elliptic and ovoid. (Courtesy former Department of Dental Hygiene, Marquette University.)

Please refer to the Evolve website (http://evolve.elsevier.com/Darby/hygiene) for competency forms to help evaluate your mastery of each procedure in this chapter.

Copyright © 2010 by Saunders, an imprint of Elsevier Inc. All rights reserved.

Management of Extrinsic and Intrinsic Stains

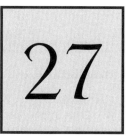

27

Procedure 27-1 RUBBER-CUP POLISHING

EQUIPMENT

Polishing paste, esthetic restoration polishing paste, and low-abrasive toothpaste
Prophylaxis angle and toothbrush
Dental floss or tape
Floss threader (if needed)
Rubber cups and pointed bristle brushes
Low-speed handpiece
Gauze squares
Mouth mirror, air-water syringe
Disclosing solution
Preprocedural antimicrobial mouth rinse
Saliva ejector or high-volume evacuation (HVE) tip
Safety glasses for client
Personal protective equipment (PPE)

STEPS	RATIONALES
PREPARATION AND POSITIONING	
1. Evaluate client's health and pharmacologic history to determine need for antibiotic premedication.	Ensures protection from health risks.
2. Identify tooth surfaces indicated and contraindicated for polishing. Always polish esthetic restorations first, then polish teeth.	Prevents unnecessary removal of tooth structure; maintains esthetic dental material by using specially designed nonabrasive polishing parts; ensures protection from health risks.
3. Educate client about selective polishing procedure.	Facilitates client acceptance.
4. Select polishing abrasive based on type of stain and oral restorations and assemble basic setup (Figure 27-1).	Prevents unnecessary removal of tooth structure.

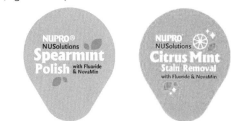

Figure 27-1. Examples of commercial prophylaxis pastes in unit doses. (Courtesy DENTSPLY Preventive Care Division, York, Pennsylvania.)

5. Wear appropriate PPE and provide protective eyewear for client.	Prevents cross-contamination; protects client's eyes from spatter.
6. Provide client with a preprocedural antimicrobial rinse polishing.	Reduces aerosol microorganisms; minimizes occurrence of bacteremia in at-risk clients.
7. Have client tilt head up and turn slightly away when polishing maxillary and mandibular right buccal surfaces of posterior teeth (left buccal if left-handed practitioner) and maxillary and mandibular left lingual surfaces of posterior teeth (right lingual if left-handed practitioner).	Enhances access and visibility; prevents occupational injury.

132

Copyright © 2010 by Saunders, an imprint of Elsevier Inc. All rights reserved.

Procedure 27-1   RUBBER-CUP POLISHING—*cont'd*

STEPS—*cont'd*	RATIONALES—*cont'd*

GRASP

8. Use modified pen grasp (Figure 27-2).   Facilitates movement of handpiece.

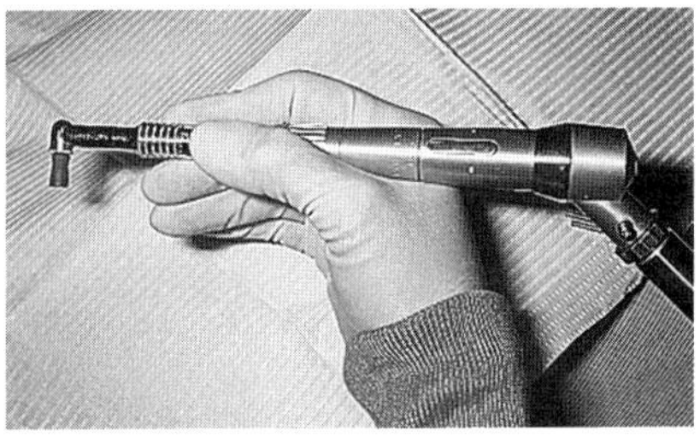

Figure 27-2. Handpiece grasp.

9. Rest handpiece in V of hand.   Transfers handpiece weight from fingers to hand to decrease fatigue.
10. Have all fingers in contact as a unit.   Facilitates wrist-forearm motion.

FULCRUM

11. Establish intraoral fulcrum close to working area.   Enhances control of handpiece.
12. Fulcrum on ring finger.   Facilitates pivoting for wrist-forearm motion.
13. Use moderate fulcrum pressure.   Enhances stabilization.

ADAPTATION

14. Angle rubber cup to flare at gingival margin.   Enhances stain removal at cervical third of tooth.
15. Adapt rubber cup to reach distal, facial and lingual, or mesial surfaces.   Ensures access to all surfaces with extrinsic stain.
16. Adapt cup to tooth by rotating handpiece or pivoting on fulcrum as necessary.   Decreases tissue trauma; provides adequate tooth coverage.
17. Adapt brush to occlusal surface.   Removes extrinsic stain from pits and grooves.

STROKE

18. Fill cup with paste and evenly apply to surfaces to be polished.   Ensures adequate and even distribution of paste.
19. Place cup on tooth; activate handpiece by gently stepping on rheostat. Stroke from the gingival third to the incisal third with just enough pressure to make the cup flare while using wrist-forearm motion to polish the teeth.   Controls speed of handpiece; reduces finger fatigue.
20. Use low speed and intermittent, dabbing, overlapping strokes with light to moderate pressure in a cervical to occlusal or incisal direction (Figure 27-3).   Dissipates heat, reduces abrasion, ensures complete coverage where needed.

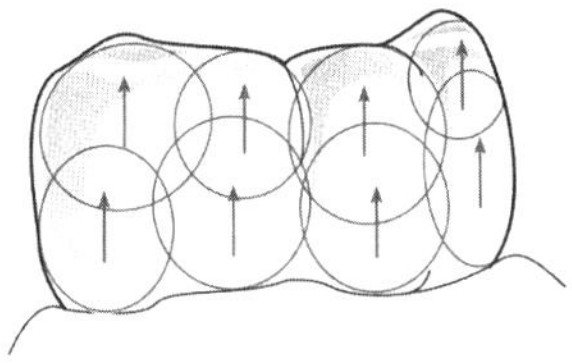

Figure 27-3. Overlapping strokes to ensure complete coverage of the tooth as needed. (From Bird DL, Robinson DS: *Torres and Ehrlich modern dental assisting,* ed 9, St Louis, 2009, Saunders.)

21. Remove rubber cup from tooth at completion of stroke; readapt cup for next stroke.   Dissipates heat.
22. Hold mirror in nondominant hand to retract buccal mucosa. Instruct client to close mouth halfway and to tilt head slightly toward the ceiling. Polish buccal surfaces of maxillary right posterior quadrant (Figure 27-4).   Mirror use facilitates access and direct observation of buccal and mesial surfaces and indirect observation of distal surfaces.

Copyright © 2010 by Saunders, an imprint of Elsevier Inc. All rights reserved.

(Continued)

Procedure 27-1 RUBBER-CUP POLISHING—*cont'd*

STEPS—*cont'd*	RATIONALES—*cont'd*

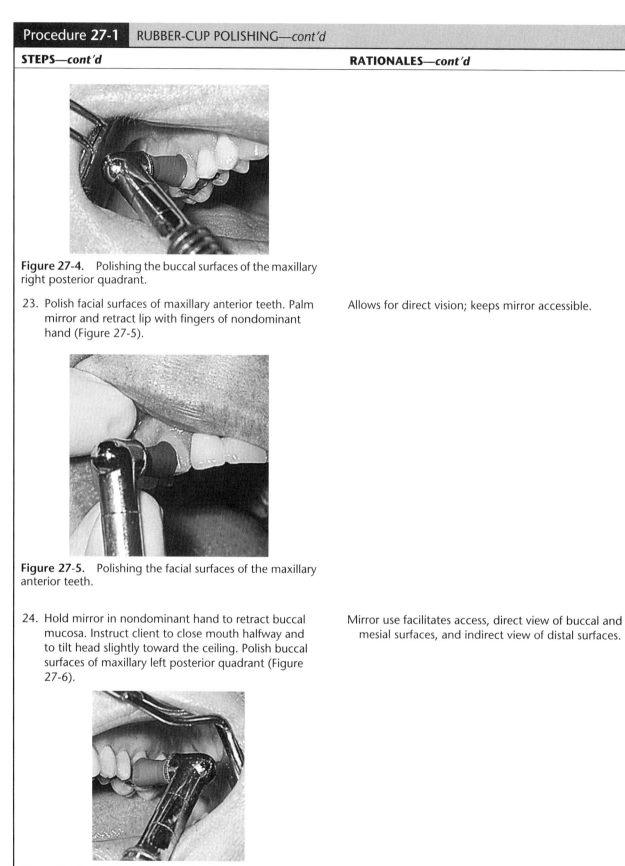

Figure 27-4. Polishing the buccal surfaces of the maxillary right posterior quadrant.

23. Polish facial surfaces of maxillary anterior teeth. Palm mirror and retract lip with fingers of nondominant hand (Figure 27-5).

Allows for direct vision; keeps mirror accessible.

Figure 27-5. Polishing the facial surfaces of the maxillary anterior teeth.

24. Hold mirror in nondominant hand to retract buccal mucosa. Instruct client to close mouth halfway and to tilt head slightly toward the ceiling. Polish buccal surfaces of maxillary left posterior quadrant (Figure 27-6).

Mirror use facilitates access, direct view of buccal and mesial surfaces, and indirect view of distal surfaces.

Figure 27-6. Polishing the buccal surfaces of the maxillary left posterior quadrant.

Copyright © 2010 by Saunders, an imprint of Elsevier Inc. All rights reserved.

Procedure 27-1 | RUBBER-CUP POLISHING—cont'd

STEPS—cont'd

25. Polish lingual surfaces of maxillary right posterior quadrant. Use mirror for indirect view and indirect lighting (Figure 27-7).

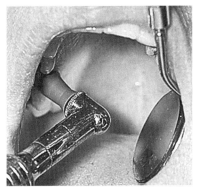

Figure 27-7. Polishing the lingual surfaces of the maxillary right posterior quadrant.

26. Polish lingual surfaces of maxillary anterior teeth. Use mirror for indirect vision (Figure 27-8).

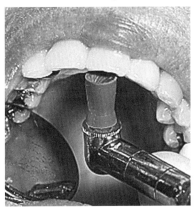

Figure 27-8. Polishing the lingual surfaces of the maxillary anterior teeth.

27. Polish lingual surfaces of maxillary left posterior quadrant. Use mirror for indirect vision (Figure 27-9).

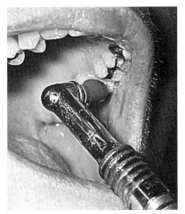

Figure 27-9. Polishing the lingual surfaces of the maxillary left posterior quadrant.

RATIONALES—cont'd

Use of indirect vision promotes good posture and visibility of lingual surfaces. Using the mirror to reflect additional light improves visibility.

Use of indirect vision promotes good posture and visibility of lingual surfaces.

Use of indirect vision promotes good posture and good visibility of lingual surfaces. Using the mirror to reflect additional light improves visibility.

Copyright © 2010 by Saunders, an imprint of Elsevier Inc. All rights reserved.   *(Continued)*

Procedure 27-1   RUBBER-CUP POLISHING—*cont'd*

STEPS—*cont'd*	RATIONALES—*cont'd*
28. Rinse client's teeth.	Removes prophylaxis paste from client's mouth.
29. Hold mirror in nondominant hand to retract right buccal mucosa. Polish buccal surfaces of mandibular right posterior quadrant (Figure 27-10).	Retracting buccal mucosa with mirror facilitates access, direct view of buccal and mesial tooth surfaces, and indirect view of distal surfaces.

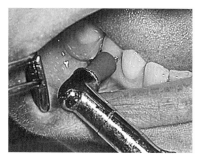

Figure 27-10. Polishing the buccal surfaces of the mandibular right posterior quadrant.

30. Palm grasp mirror and retract lip with fingers of nondominant hand. Polish facial surfaces of mandibular anterior teeth (Figure 27-11).	Allows for direct vision; palm grasp of mirror handle keeps mirror accessible.

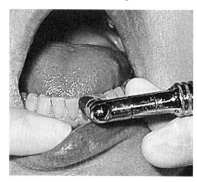

Figure 27-11. Polishing the facial surfaces of the mandibular anterior teeth.

31. Retract buccal mucosa with mirror and polish buccal surfaces of mandibular left posterior quadrant (Figure 27-12).	Allows for direct view of buccal and mesial surfaces and indirect view of distal surfaces.

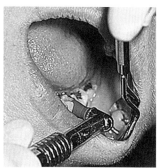

Figure 27-12. Polishing the buccal surfaces of the mandibular left posterior quadrant.

32. Polish lingual surfaces of mandibular right posterior quadrant. Use mirror to retract tongue and for indirect vision and lighting (Figure 27-13).	Retracting the tongue facilitates direct and indirect vision.

Copyright © 2010 by Saunders, an imprint of Elsevier Inc. All rights reserved.

Procedure 27-1 | RUBBER-CUP POLISHING—*cont'd*

STEPS—*cont'd*   **RATIONALES—*cont'd***

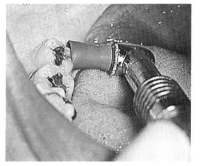

Figure 27-13. Polishing the lingual surfaces of the mandibular right posterior quadrant.

33. Polish lingual surfaces of mandibular anterior teeth (Figure 27-14). Use mirror for indirect vision and indirect lighting. Avoid resting mirror on sublingual mucosa.

Resting the mirror on sublingual mucosa is very uncomfortable for client. Rim of cup can be used to polish concave lingual surfaces of anterior teeth.

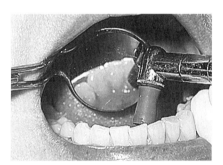

Figure 27-14. Polishing the lingual surfaces of the mandibular anterior teeth.

34. Polish lingual surfaces of mandibular left posterior quadrant (Figure 27-15). Use mirror to retract tongue and for indirect vision and lighting. Replace rubber cup with flat or pointed brush and remove occlusal stain.

Use of mirror facilitates access and visibility of lingual surfaces. Brushes adapt to pits and fissures.

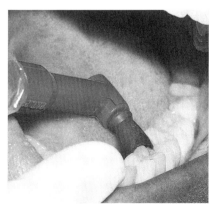

Figure 27-15. Polishing the lingual surfaces of the mandibular left posterior quadrant. (From Bird DL, Robinson DS: *Torres and Ehrlich modern dental assisting,* ed 9, St Louis, 2009, Saunders.)

Copyright © 2010 by Saunders, an imprint of Elsevier Inc. All rights reserved.

(Continued)

Procedure 27-1   RUBBER-CUP POLISHING—*cont'd*

STEPS—*cont'd*	RATIONALES—*cont'd*
35. Floss client's teeth with abrasive agent still on teeth, then rinse.	Removes prophylaxis paste from client's mouth; facilitates the removal of interproximal stain.
36. Apply topical fluoride therapy (see Chapter 31 in the textbook).	Replaces fluoride removed from the outer surfaces of enamel by selective polishing.
37. Document completion of service in client's record under "Services Rendered" and date the entry—e.g.,"Removed tobacco stain with rubber-cup polishing on No. 6-11L, 22-27L; removed client oral biofilm from remaining teeth with a soft toothbrush and fluoride gel toothpaste. Flossed all teeth. APF topical fluoride gel treatment—tray method—provided for 4 minutes. Advised client not to eat, drink, or rinse for 30 minutes."	Ensures integrity of client's record for client's health and legal protection of practitioner.

Photographs courtesy Dr. Margaret Walsh, University of California–San Francisco.

Copyright © 2010 by Saunders, an imprint of Elsevier Inc. All rights reserved.

Procedure 27-2 | AIR POLISHING TECHNIQUE

EQUIPMENT
Sodium bicarbonate powder or aluminum trihydroxide air polishing powder and low-abrasive toothpaste (Figure 27-16)
Air-polisher device (Figure 27-17) and toothbrush
Dental floss or tape
Mouth mirror, air-water syringe
Disclosing solution
Lubricant for client's lips
Saliva ejector and high-volume evacuation (HVE) tip
Safety glasses for client
Personal protective equipment (PPE)
Preprocedural antimicrobial mouth rinse

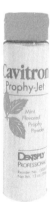

Figure 27-16.   Flavored prophy powder for use in air polishing device. (Courtesy DENTSPLY Preventive Care Division, York, Pennsylvania.)

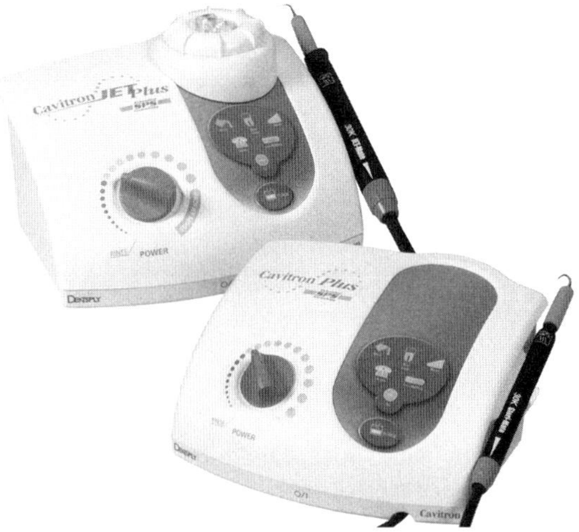

Figure 27-17.   Prophy-Jet and ultrasonic scaler combination *(top unit)*. (Courtesy DENTSPLY Preventive Care Division, York, Pennsylvania.)

STEPS	RATIONALES
PREPARATION AND POSITIONING	
1. Evaluate client's health and pharmacologic history to determine need for antibiotic premedication.	Ensures safe treatment.
2. Identify tooth surfaces and restorations indicated and contraindicated for polishing and agents to be used.	Prevents unnecessary removal of tooth structure.
3. Educate client about selective polishing procedure.	Facilitates client acceptance of procedure.
4. Assemble high-speed evacuation and saliva ejector.	Reduces amount of aerosol released into atmosphere.
5. Verify that slurry exits from device tip when held outside the mouth; adjust saliva ejector as necessary.	Ensures adequate evacuation.
6. Use appropriate PPE and provide protective eyewear for client.	Reduces risk of infection in client and practitioner.
7. Clinician, client, and equipment must be in appropriate position for each area.	Enhances access and visibility; prevents occupational injury.
GRASP	
8. Use modified pen grasp.	Facilitates movement of handpiece.
9. Rest handpiece in V of hand.	Transfers handpiece weight from fingers to hand to decrease fatigue.
10. Have all fingers in contact as a unit.	Facilitates wrist-forearm motion.
11. Tuck excess cord around pinkie finger, if desired.	Decreases pull from handpiece cord.
FULCRUM	
12. Use external soft tissue fulcrums.	Facilitates access.

(Continued)

Copyright © 2010 by Saunders, an imprint of Elsevier Inc. All rights reserved.

| Procedure **27-2** | AIR POLISHING TECHNIQUE—*cont'd* |

STEPS—*cont'd* | **RATIONALES**—*Cont'd*

ADAPTATION AND STROKE

13. Activate foot pedal by pushing halfway down for water and all the way down for combined air-water-powder spray.

Provides adequate coverage of tooth surface.

14. At about 3 to 4 mm from tooth surface and at correct angulation, use constant circular sweeping motions, from proximal to proximal; pivot nozzle to surface being polished; polish several teeth for 1 to 2 seconds each and rinse. Surfaces without stain are cleaned with a toothbrush and low-abrasive toothpaste (Figure 27-18).

Ensures adequate stain removal; provides pleasant aftertaste; ensures adequate biofilm removal.

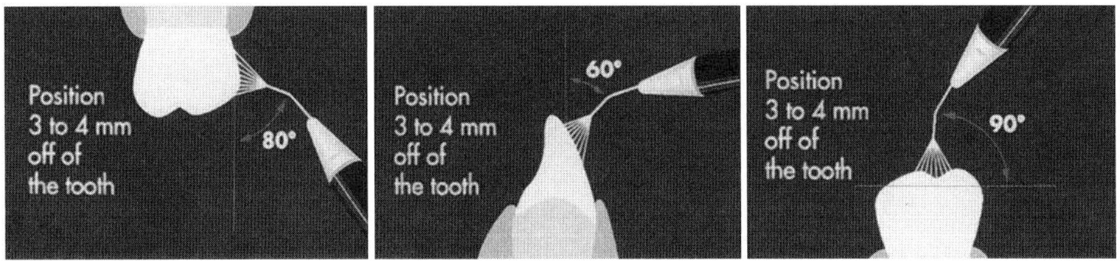

Figure 27-18. Recommended angulations of Prophy-Jet nozzle to tooth surface. (Adapted from DENTSPLY Preventive Care Division, York, Pennsylvania.)

OTHER

15. Rinse with water; floss all teeth (or have client do so and evaluate their flossing technique).

Removes any remaining polishing paste.

16. Evaluate effectiveness with disclosing solution, compressed air, and good lighting.

Ensures complete extrinsic stain removal.

17. Provide professionally applied topical fluoride treatment.

Replenishes any fluoride lost from outer fluoride-rich surface layer of enamel.

18. Dispose of single-use items according to federal, state, and local regulations.

Ensures compliance with law.

19. Properly disinfect and sterilize all other equipment.

Prevents cross-examination between clients.

20. Document completion of service in client's record under "Services Rendered" and date the entry, e.g., "Removed tobacco stain with air polishing on No. 6-11L, 22-27L; removed client oral biofilm from remaining teeth with a soft toothbrush and fluoride toothpaste. Flossed all teeth. APF topical fluoride gel treatment—tray method—provided for 4 minutes. Advised client not to eat, drink, or rinse for 30 minutes."

Ensures integrity of client's record for client's health and legal protection of practitioner.

Please refer to the Evolve website (http://evolve.elsevier.com/Darby/hygiene) for competency forms to help evaluate your mastery of each procedure in this chapter.

Copyright © 2010 by Saunders, an imprint of Elsevier Inc. All rights reserved.

Decision Making Related to Nonsurgical Periodontal Therapy

28

Procedure 28-1 | USE OF EXTENDED SHANK AND MINIBLADED CURETS

EQUIPMENT
Personal protective equipment
Subgingival periodontal explorer
Set of extended shank area-specific curets (minimum recommendations for a quadrant include an anterior curet such as the Gracey 1/2 and posterior curets 11/12 and 13/14 (or 11/14 and 12/13)
Set of minibladed area-specific curets for specific locations
Pockets >5 mm
2 × 2 gauze

STEPS	RATIONALES
1. Refer to periodontal assessment.	Identifies pocket depths >5 mm, gingival contour and tone, pocket topography.
2. Self-assess clinician and client positioning.	Improves positioning for area-specific design and pocket depth or root anatomy.
3. Use modified pen grasp with thumb and index finger across from each other near the junction of the shank and handle, or further up on the handle, depending on the fulcrum used.	Facilitates tactile sensitivity, adaptation, activation, and comfort for client and operator.
4. Select an appropriate fulcrum such as conventional or opposite arch. Vary fulcrum position when negotiating deep pockets. It is advisable to extend to the depth of pocket or underneath calculus, adapt the blade, then place the fulcrum.	Provides stability for activation. Fulcrums are modified depending on depth of pocket. Conventional fulcrums are still the most useful; opposite arch fulcrum is useful for molars, especially on maxillary arch.
5. Use dental mirror.	Needed for retraction, indirect vision, reflection, and/or transillumination.
6. Select appropriate working end and blade. Hold instrument with terminal shank perpendicular to floor. Viewing face of blade from above, the larger, convex curved lower blade is the correct blade, or adapt the cutting edge that tilts away from the terminal shank.	Only one cutting edge is appropriate to use on a specific surface.
7. Insert working end into pocket with blade as closed as possible to reach epithelial attachment or to extend 1 mm below the calculus, whichever is appropriate.	Reaches base of pocket or deposit in a nontraumatic manner.
8. Use vertical position of terminal shank as a visual cue to recognize correct working end and blade.	Terminal shank should be parallel with surface being treated.
9. Use handle position as a visual cue to recognize correct working end and blade.	Handle should be as parallel as possible with long axis of tooth in the buccolingual dimension. Handle should not cross the occlusal plane.
10. Adapt terminal 1 to 2 mm of blade to the root.	Using too much of the blade (more than the terminal one third) hinders effective channeling, can be uncomfortable for the client, and/or does not provide correct adaptation to convex and concave root surfaces.
11. Acquire correct blade-to-root angle for the procedure (from 45 to 90 degrees depending on mode of attachment of the lighter calculus).	Provides appropriate angle to meet the purpose of the stroke (exploratory, working, planing, or debridement).

(Continued)

Copyright © 2010 by Saunders, an imprint of Elsevier Inc. All rights reserved.

Procedure 28-1	USE OF EXTENDED SHANK AND MINIBLADED CURETS—*cont'd*
STEPS—*cont'd*	**RATIONALES**—*cont'd*
12. Activate with lateral pressure, length of stroke, and direction of stroke.	Lateral pressure and length of the stroke (1 to 3 mm) depend on the purpose of stroke (light calculus deposit removal or debridement). Direction of stroke depends on the purpose: oblique strokes are necessary on proximal surfaces of molars and premolars to maintain adaptation and achieve oral clearance of handle from opposite arch.
13. Use rock, roll, and pivot to maintain adaptation.	Facilitates adaptation to convex and concave surfaces.
14. View radiographs throughout procedure.	Complements tactile sensitivity.
15. Evaluate instrument sharpness throughout procedure.	Effectiveness of mechanical therapy depends on a sharp blade.
16. Evaluate root surface with periodontal explorer.	Determines relative smoothness and clinical endpoint.
17. Record in client record the curets used and where, e.g., periodontal debridement of maxillary right quadrant using Gracey 11/12 and 13/14.	Aids in instrument selection at subsequent nonsurgical periodontal therapy and/or periodontal maintenance appointments; maintains accurate documentation for legal purposes.

Please refer to the Evolve website (http://evolve.elsevier.com/Darby/hygiene) for competency forms to help evaluate your mastery of each procedure in this chapter.

Copyright © 2010 by Saunders, an imprint of Elsevier Inc. All rights reserved.

Chemotherapy for the Control of Periodontal Diseases

29

Procedure **29-1**	PLACEMENT OF CONTROLLED-RELEASE DRUG: TETRACYCLINE FIBER

EQUIPMENT

Personal protective equipment
Mouth mirror
Periodontal probe
Cotton pliers
Cord-packing instrument
Scaler(s)
Scissors
Tetracycline fiber
Water-soluble lubricant

STEPS	RATIONALES
1. Determine need for controlled-release tetracycline fiber therapy (indicated for reduction of pocket depth in sites ≥5 mm not responding to mechanical therapy alone in persons with chronic periodontitis).	Prevents indiscriminate use of antibiotics and development of antibiotic-resistant microorganisms.
2. Evaluate contraindications and precautions to treatment.	Ensures quality of care; manages legal risks.
3. Explain risks and benefits and alternative to treatment. Obtain informed consent.	Encourages active decision making by client; manages legal risks.
4. Remove fiber from package before use. Cut fiber into 2- to 3-inch segments.	Facilitates organization and placement.
5. Place fiber around the tooth; thread interproximally with a floss threader. Insert fiber subgingivally into bottom of pocket using a cord-packing instrument. Fill entire pocket by overlapping (layering) fiber over itself within 1 mm of gingival margin. For furca, pack with a small piece of fiber, then fill pocket.	Fiber must be in the pocket to produce therapeutic effect.
6. Secure fiber in pocket with cyanoacrylate tissue adhesive (verify that client is not allergic to adhesive). Isolate and dry area. Apply small amounts of adhesive quickly all around margin. Apply water-soluble lubricant to prevent sticking. Discard unused fiber. Replace any fiber lost before day 7.	Provides fiber retention. Fiber replacement ensures therapeutic effect.
7. Instruct client not to brush or floss area for 10 days, and to use 0.12% chlorhexidine gluconate oral rinse twice daily.	Brushing or flossing may prematurely dislodge fiber.
8. Remove fiber with cotton pliers after 10 to 14 days.	Fiber is nonbioresorbable. Time required for a therapeutic effect.
9. Schedule reevaluation and/or reapplication. Can coincide with periodontal maintenance visits.	Host response to therapy must be observed and documented.
10. Document in client's record under Service Rendered, and date the entry, e.g., "Tetracycline fiber placed in the sites not responding to mechanical debridement alone for the reduction of pocket depths: No. 2M, No. 3D, No. 30M, D, No. 31D. Cyanoacrylate adhesive placed for retention at each site. Client instructed not to brush or floss areas for 10 days and to call if loss of fiber occurs before day 7."	Ensures integrity of client's record for both client's health and legal protection of practitioner. Client must understand that the fiber is nonresorbable and must be removed by the dentist or dental hygienist.

Copyright © 2010 by Saunders, an imprint of Elsevier Inc. All rights reserved.

Procedure 29-2   PLACEMENT OF CONTROLLED-RELEASE DRUG: CHLORHEXIDINE CHIP

EQUIPMENT

Personal protective equipment
Mouth mirror
Periodontal probe
Cotton pliers, cotton rolls, dry angles
Scaler(s)
Chlorhexidine chips

STEPS	RATIONALES
1. Determine need for controlled-release chlorhexidine chip therapy (indicated for reduction of pocket depth in sites ≥5 mm not responding to mechanical therapy alone in persons with chronic periodontitis).	Prevents indiscriminate use of chemotherapeutic agent.
2. Evaluate contraindications to and precautions for treatment.	Ensures quality of care; manages legal risks.
3. Explain risks and benefits and alternatives to treatment. Obtain informed consent.	Encourages active decision making by client; manages legal risks.
4. Remove required number of chips from package. Note that product is stored at controlled room temperature of 59° to 77° F (15° to 25° C).	
5. Isolate and dry area to prevent wetting chip during placement. Grasp square end of chip with cotton pliers, and insert subgingivally.	Chip is bioresorbable and self-retentive in pocket.
6. Use cotton pliers or an instrument of choice to advance chip into deepest part of pocket.	Chip is difficult to place if it gets wet. Rounded end is for adaptation to subgingival anatomy.
7. Instruct client not to floss area for 10 days and that some moderate sensitivity may be experienced for about 1 week in the area of placement. Client should clean other areas of mouth as usual and call office if any pain, swelling, or problem occurs.	Flossing may prematurely dislodge the chip. Time required for therapeutic effect.
8. Schedule reevaluation and/or reapplication. Reevaluation of probe depths and clinical attachment levels can coincide with periodontal maintenance visit.	Host response must be observed and documented. Maximum benefit is attained after three consecutive administrations at 3-month intervals over a 9-month period.
9. Document in client's record under Services Rendered, and date the entry, e.g., "Chlorhexidine chip placed in sites not responding to mechanical debridement alone for the reduction of pocket depths: No. 2M, No. 3D, No. 30M, D, No. 31D. Client instructed not to brush or floss the area for 10 days and to call if loss of chip occurs."	Ensures integrity of client's record for client's health and legal protection of practitioner.

Copyright © 2010 by Saunders, an imprint of Elsevier Inc. All rights reserved.

Procedure 29-3	PLACEMENT OF CONTROLLED-RELEASE DRUG: DOXYCYCLINE GEL

EQUIPMENT
Personal protective equipment
Mouth mirror
Periodontal probe
Scaler(s) or cord packer instrument
Lubricant
Two unit-dosed syringes for coupling
Blunt-ended cannula
Doxycycline gel product

STEPS	RATIONALES
1. Determine need for controlled-release doxycycline therapy (indicated for the reduction of pocket depth and gains in clinical attachment in sites ≥5 mm not responding to mechanical therapy alone in persons with chronic periodontitis).	Prevents indiscriminate use of an antibiotic and development of antibiotic-resistant microorganisms.
2. Evaluate contraindications to and precautions for treatment.	Ensures quality of care and manages legal risks.
3. Explain risks and benefits and alternative to treatment. Obtain informed consent.	Encourages active decision making by the client and manages legal risks.
4. Remove syringes for coupling (one containing 10% doxycycline hyclate and one containing liquid polymer) from package. Contains enough material to treat three to four teeth.	Product requires storage in refrigeration at 36° to 46° F.
5. Hold uncapped syringes with the nozzles upright to avoid spilling before coupling.	Ensures a sealed container for the mix.
6. Mix by holding the coupled syringes together horizontally in both hands. Inject liquid contents of syringe with stripe into syringe with yellow powder, then push the contents back into syringe with purple stripe again. This constitutes one mixing cycle and should be repeated for 1½ to 2 minutes for 100 cycles. Finish with contents in syringe with purple stripe by holding the coupled syringes vertically with purple stripe syringe at the bottom. Pull back on purple stripe syringe plunger and allow gel to flow down barrel. Twist and lock syringes together per manufacturer's instructions. Lock open ends of both syringes together by twisting together until they lock.	Ensures adequate mixing of ingredients.
7. Uncouple syringes and attach enclosed cannula to syringe by twisting in place. Cannula can be bent at desired angle to resemble a periodontal probe. Product is now ready to use. If product is mixed in advance, refresh mixture with 10 mixing cycles before uncoupling the syringes.	Product can be prepared in advance and stored at room temperature for up to 3 days.
8. Insert tip of cannula near base of pocket; express gel into pocket while slowly withdrawing tip coronally until material can be seen at gingival margin. Gel will begin setting reaction immediately on contact with pocket. Separate tip from newly placed material by using a twisting motion, or cut material by pushing cannula tip against tooth surface or using a wet blunt instrument.	Increases likelihood of 100% coverage.
9. Wipe excess material protruding from pocket with a wet cotton swab, or pack into pocket and interproximal embrasures with back surface of a wet curet or cord packer instruments. Use water or lubricant to prevent sticking. Drip a few drops of water onto the surface of gel in the pocket to aid in coagulation.	Removal of excess material increases longevity of the material within the pocket.

(Continued)

Copyright © 2010 by Saunders, an imprint of Elsevier Inc. All rights reserved.

Procedure 29-3 | PLACEMENT OF CONTROLLED-RELEASE DRUG: DOXYCYCLINE GEL—*cont'd*

STEPS—*cont'd*	RATIONALES—*cont'd*
10. Secure gel in pocket by applying cyanoacrylate tissue adhesive or noneugenol-type periodontal dressing.	Provides retention. Gel must be present in the pocket to produce therapeutic effect.
11. Remove retention after 10 days of therapy with cotton pliers.	Removal increases client comfort. Gel is bioresorbable (30% gone in approximately 7 days; 98% gone in approximately 28 days).
12. Instruct client to avoid chewing, brushing and interdental cleaning around area for 7 days; recommend oral rinsing with an effective antimicrobial agent. Client should not be alarmed if small amounts of hardened gel become visible at gumline or are dislodged because it is harmless if swallowed.	Brushing or interdental cleaning may prematurely dislodge the gel.
13. Schedule reevaluation and/or reapplication. Reevaluation of pocket depth and clinical attachment levels can coincide with periodontal maintenance visit.	Host response to therapy must be observed and documented.
14. Document in client record under Services Rendered, and date the entry. For example, "Doxycycline gel placed in sites not responding to mechanical debridement alone for the reduction of pocket depths: No. 2M, No. 3D, No. 30M, D, No. 31D. Cyanoacrylate adhesive placed for retention at each site. Client instructed not to brush or floss the area for 10 days and to report any loss of gel to the office."	Ensures integrity of client's record for both quality care and legal protection of practitioner.

Copyright © 2010 by Saunders, an imprint of Elsevier Inc. All rights reserved.

Procedure 29-4	PLACEMENT OF CONTROLLED-RELEASE DRUG: MINOCYCLINE HYDROCHLORIDE MICROSPHERES

EQUIPMENT
Personal protective equipment
Mouth mirror
Periodontal probe
Scaler(s)
Unit-dosed cartridge of minocycline hydrochloride product
Dispensing handle

STEPS	RATIONALES
1. Determine need for controlled-release minocycline microspheres therapy (indicated for the reduction of pocket depth in sites ≥5 mm not responding to mechanical therapy alone in persons with chronic periodontitis).	Prevents indiscriminate use of an antibiotic and development of antibiotic-resistant microorganisms.
2. Evaluate contraindications to and precautions for treatment.	Ensures quality of care and manages legal risks.
3. Explain risks and benefits and alternative to treatment. Obtain informed consent.	Encourages active decision making by the client and manages legal risks.
4. Remove number of unit-dosed cartridges needed for treatment.	Store at 68° to 77° F. Avoid excessive heat.
5. Insert cartridge into sterile cartridge handle to administer product, and follow manufacturer directions.	Minimizes risk of cross-contamination.
6. Bend cartridge tip to improve access to diseased sites. Insert tip of cartridge subgingivally to base of pocket; tip should be parallel to long axis to tooth. Press thumb ring to express powder while gradually withdrawing tip from base of pocket. Do not force tip into base of pocket. Withdraw tip further if resistance is felt.	Product must be in pocket to produce therapeutic effect.
7. No dressing or adhesive is required. Microspheres activate and adhere on contact with moisture in pocket. Discard cartridge and resterilize dispensing handle.	Product is bioresorbable and self-retentive in pocket.
8. Instruct client to delay brushing for first 12 hours after treatment. For 10 days clients should abstain from interdental cleaning in area and from eating hard, crunchy, or sticky foods.	Interdental cleaning or certain foods may prematurely dislodge product.
9. Schedule reevaluation and/or reapplication. Reevaluation of pocket depths and clinical attachment levels can coincide with periodontal maintenance visits. Repeat treatment as needed.	Maximum benefit is attained after 3 consecutive administrations at 3-month intervals over a 9-month period.
10. Document in client record under Services Rendered, and date the entry. For example, "Minocycline microspheres placed in sites not responding to mechanical debridement alone for the reduction of pocket depths: No. 2M, No. 3D, No. 30M, D, No. 31D. Client instructed to delay brushing for first 12 hours after treatment and to abstain from interdental cleaning in area and from eating hard, crunchy, or sticky foods for 10 days."	Ensures integrity of client's record for both high-quality care and legal protection of practitioner.

Please refer to the Evolve website (http://evolve.elsevier.com/Darby/hygiene) for competency forms to help evaluate your mastery of each procedure in this chapter.

Copyright © 2010 by Saunders, an imprint of Elsevier Inc. All rights reserved.

Acute Gingival and Periodontal Conditions, Lesions of Endodontic Origin, and Avulsed Teeth

| Procedure **30-1** | EMERGENCY MANAGEMENT OF THE AVULSED TOOTH |

EQUIPMENT
Clean cup or other container
Transport medium

STEPS	RATIONALES
1. Calm the individual or parent.	Quick action is necessary to increase the chance of successful replantation; emotional upset can cause delays.
2. Locate tooth.	Often the child or parent will not know that the tooth can be replanted.
3. Handle only by the crown and do not dry the tooth; do not debride the tooth.	Successful tooth replantation can occur only if periodontal ligament cells are alive and intact on the tooth surface.
4. Place in transport medium (Table 30-1).	Options for keeping the surface cells viable must be thought through quickly. A child may be too young to retain the tooth either in the socket or in the mouth.
5. Contact dentist, dental office, or other emergency facility, such as a dental clinic or hospital emergency room.	Client or parent may be too upset to know where to call. Facilitate timely response to this emergency.
6. Arrange for transportation to treatment facility immediately.	If not personally taking the client to the treatment facility, make sure the parent or other driver knows where to go.
7. Record services rendered in dental chart.	Provides continuity of care and manages legal risks.

TABLE 30-1	Storage of Avulsed Teeth during Transportation for Treatment
Choice	**Transportation Medium**
First	Replace in socket
Second	Store in physiologic saline
Third	Store in cold, fresh milk
Fourth	Place in the individual's mouth, under the tongue or in the cheek
Fifth	Store in warm saltwater
Sixth	Store in tap water

Please refer to the Evolve website (http://evolve.elsevier.com/Darby/hygiene) for competency forms to help evaluate your mastery of each procedure in this chapter.

Copyright © 2010 by Saunders, an imprint of Elsevier Inc. All rights reserved.

Caries Management: Fluoride, Chlorhexidine, Xylitol, and Amorphous Calcium Phosphate Therapies

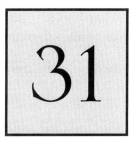

Procedure 31-1	PROFESSIONALLY APPLIED TOPICAL FLUORIDE USING THE TRAY TECHNIQUE FOR IN-OFFICE FLUORIDE TREATMENT (GEL OR FOAM)

EQUIPMENT

Mouth mirror
Cotton forceps
Fluoride tray(s)
Cotton rolls
1.23% acidulated phosphate fluoride (APF) or 2.0% sodium fluoride gel
Air syringe

Timer
Saliva ejector
2 × 2 gauze
Tissues
2-oz cup
Personal protective barriers and equipment barriers

STEPS	RATIONALES
1. Assemble equipment (Figure 31-1).	Promotes efficiency and infection control.

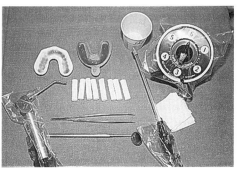

Figure 31-1.

| 2. Seat client in upright position. Reiterate benefits and obtain informed consent (Figure 31-2). | Prevents gagging and accidental ingestion of fluoride gel or foam. Manages legal risk. |

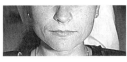
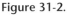

Figure 31-2.

| 3. Try tray of appropriate size. Complete dentition must be covered, including areas of recession (Figure 31-3). | Trays must be pliable, comfortable, and deep enough to cover all surfaces and must have a distal dam to keep fluoride in the tray. |

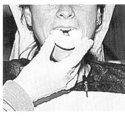

Figure 31-3.

(Continued)

Copyright © 2010 by Saunders, an imprint of Elsevier Inc. All rights reserved.

| Procedure 31-1 | PROFESSIONALLY APPLIED TOPICAL FLUORIDE USING THE TRAY TECHNIQUE FOR IN-OFFICE FLUORIDE TREATMENT (GEL OR FOAM)—*cont'd* |

STEPS—*cont'd*

RATIONALES—*cont'd*

4. Load fluoride gel into trays: 2 mL maximum per tray for small children; 4 mL maximum per tray for large children (>44 lb), 2.5 mL maximum per tray for adults (Figure 31-4).

Recommendations of the American Academy of Pediatric Dentistry; trays deliver fluoride to exposed tooth surfaces.

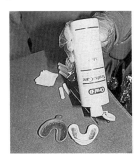
Figure 31-4.

5. Isolate teeth with cotton rolls. Dry with air syringe (Figure 31-5).

A dry field maintains fluoride concentration and maximizes fluoride uptake.

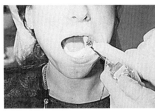
Figure 31-5.

6. Insert both trays in mouth (Figures 31-6 and 31-7).

Mandibular tray stays in place more easily than maxillary tray. Most trays connect both a mandibular and a maxillary arch into one device designed for efficiency of insertion.

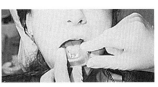
Figure 31-6.

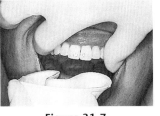
Figure 31-7.

Copyright © 2010 by Saunders, an imprint of Elsevier Inc. All rights reserved.

| Procedure **31-1** | PROFESSIONALLY APPLIED TOPICAL FLUORIDE USING THE TRAY TECHNIQUE FOR IN-OFFICE FLUORIDE TREATMENT (GEL OR FOAM)—*cont'd* |

STEPS—*cont'd* | **RATIONALES—*cont'd***

7. Press tray against teeth, and ask client to close mouth and bite gently on trays or cotton rolls (Figure 31-8).

Slight pressure from biting helps force fluoride gel around all surfaces. Ensures coverage into interproximal spaces.

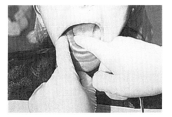

Figure 31-8.

8. Place saliva ejector over mandibular tray. Set timer for 4 minutes. Never leave client unattended during procedure (Figure 31-9).

Prevents saliva from diluting fluoride concentration. Maximum fluoride exposure requires 4 minutes. Supervision prevents accidental ingestion of fluoride response if gagging results.

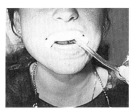

Figure 31-9.

9. Tilt chin down to remove trays (Figure 31-10).

Allows fluids to flow to anterior region of mouth for easy evacuation.

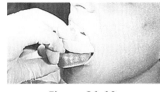

Figure 31-10.

10. Ask client to expectorate; suction excess fluoride from the mouth with saliva ejector (Figure 31-11).

Prompt removal of fluoride gel or foam from mouth minimizes swallowing of excess gel or foam and risk of acute fluoride toxicity.

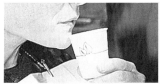

Figure 31-11.

11. Instruct client not to eat, drink, or rinse for 30 minutes.

Allows residual fluoride to remain in contact with teeth.

12. Record service in client's chart under "services rendered"; e.g., "Applied topical APF fluoride gel to existing teeth for 4 minutes. Used stock trays to apply approx. 2 to 2.5 mL of 1.23% APF (insert brand name). Client consented to procedure; no complications or adverse reactions during treatment. Client instructed not to eat, rinse, or drink for 30 minutes."

Documentation ensures continuity of high-quality care and risk management.

Copyright © 2010 by Saunders, an imprint of Elsevier Inc. All rights reserved.

Procedure **31-2**	PROFESSIONALLY APPLIED SODIUM FLUORIDE VARNISH USING THE PAINT-ON TECHNIQUE

EQUIPMENT
Mouth mirror
5% Sodium fluoride varnish (unit dosage)
Cotton-tip applicators or syringe applicator
Paper cup
Personal protective barriers and equipment barriers

STEPS	RATIONALES
1. Select unit dose fluoride varnish product; gather equipment and supplies for application.	Enhances time efficiency, ensures client comfort and safety, and promotes maintenance of infection control.
2. Provide client with information about procedure; reiterate benefits. Obtain informed consent.	Encourages client participation in care and manages risk.
3. Unless an oral prophylaxis has been performed at the same appointment, have client cleanse teeth with toothbrush.	Brushing is adequate preparation for placement of varnish.
4. Recline client for ergonomic access to oral cavity.	Ensures operator and client comfort.
5. Wipe application area with gauze or cotton rolls and insert a saliva ejector. Can be applied in the presence of saliva and without a saliva ejector.	Varnish sets in contact with intraoral moisture, so drying with compressed air is unnecessary; removal of saliva facilitates client comfort and cooperation.
6. Using a cotton-tip, brush, or syringe-style applicator, apply 0.3 to 0.5 mL of varnish (unit dose) to clinical crown of teeth: application time is 1 to 3 minutes.	Varnish is not permanent; a thin layer will promote fluoride release and absorption.
7. Dental floss may be used to draw the varnish interproximally.	This procedure is optional because it must be done quickly, as the varnish dries on contact with moisture.
8. Allow client to rinse on completion of procedure.	Varnish sets on contact; no need to avoid rinsing after application.
9. Remind client to avoid eating hard foods, drinking hot or alcoholic beverages, brushing, and flossing until the next day or at least for 4 to 6 hours after application. Drink through a straw for the first few hours after application.	Prevents premature removal of varnish and maximizes fluoride contact and release time.
10. Record service in client's record under "Services Rendered," e.g., "Applied 0.3 mL of 5% (22,600 ppm) sodium fluoride varnish (insert brand name) per tooth. Client consented to this procedure; no complications or adverse reactions during treatment. Client instructed to keep varnish on the teeth for at least 4 to 6 hours or preferably until the next day. Client told to drink through a straw and avoid hard foods, alcoholic and hot beverages, brushing, and flossing until preferably the next day to prolong the varnish treatment. Varnish can be removed the next day with toothbrushing and interdental cleaning."	Documentation is important for continuity of high-quality care and for risk management purposes.

Please refer to the Evolve website (http://evolve.elsevier.com/Darby/hygiene) for competency forms to help evaluate your mastery of each procedure in this chapter.

Copyright © 2010 by Saunders, an imprint of Elsevier Inc. All rights reserved.

Pit and Fissure Sealants

32

Procedure 32-1 | APPLYING LIGHT-CURED (PHOTOPOLYMERIZED) SEALANTS

EQUIPMENT

Mouth mirror
Explorer
Cotton forceps
Saliva ejector
Sealant kit
Cotton rolls and rubber dam
Air-water syringe tip
Dri-Angles
High-speed evacuation tube
Low-speed handpiece or air-polishing device

Bristled brush
Pumice
Floss
Light protective shield
Client protective eyewear
Personal protective equipment
Light cure unit
Round finishing burr
Articulating paper

STEPS

1. Assemble sealant armamentarium (Figure 32-1).

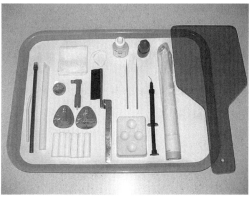

Figure 32-1.

2. Provide client with protective eyewear with filter. Wear personal protective equipment.

3. Identify tooth or teeth to be sealed.
4. Polish the intended surface with a slurry of pumice and water. Use air polishing or a bristled brush attached to a low-speed handpiece. Rinse with water (Figures 32-2 and 32-3).

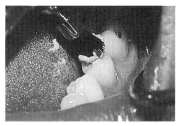

Figure 32-2.

RATIONALES

Armamentarium and procedure may differ with product. Always read manufacturer's directions.

Protect clients and clinicians from potential retinal damage from the blue curing light. Use of eyeglasses is a standard infection control procedure.

Surfaces to be sealed must be free of deposits and organic debris. Commercial pastes contain coloring and/or flavoring agents, glycerin, and/or fluoride, which may interfere with bonding. A bristled brush efficiently cleans the occlusal surface. Air polishing is preferred.

(Continued)

Copyright © 2010 by Saunders, an imprint of Elsevier Inc. All rights reserved.

Procedure 32-1   APPLYING LIGHT-CURED (PHOTOPOLYMERIZED) SEALANTS—*cont'd*

STEPS—*cont'd*	RATIONALES—*cont'd*

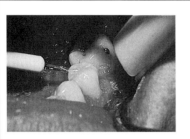

Figure 32-3.

5. Isolate teeth with a rubber dam, or place Dri-Angle over Stensen's duct and insert cotton rolls. Place saliva ejector into client's mouth.

Treatment site should be visible, accessible, and dry for proper sealant placement and retention.

6. Dry the site to be sealed with compressed air that is free of oil and moisture (Figure 32-4).

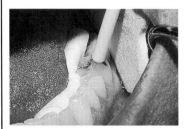

Figure 32-4.

7. Apply phosphoric acid to the clean, dry tooth surface. Etch the tooth for 10 to 20 seconds. If using a liquid etch, apply it with a brush. If using a gel etch, apply it and leave undisturbed.

Acid etches the enamel to produce micropores into which the sealant flows and hardens; it is mechanically locked into place. Successful sealant retention depends on proper etching technique. Rubbing the gel acid burnishes the enamel surface and causes it to become smooth again, which decreases the retention and adversely affects bond strength.

8. Rinse etched surfaces for 30 to 60 seconds using a water syringe and high-speed evacuation. If gel etch is used, rinse for an additional 30 seconds (Figure 32-5).

Rinsing removes the acid. If etched surface becomes contaminated with saliva, re-etch for 10 seconds.

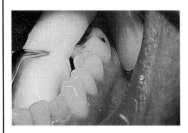

Figure 32-5.

9. Using cotton forceps, replace cotton rolls and Dri-Angles as they become wet (Figure 32-6).

Moisture interferes with bonding and retention.

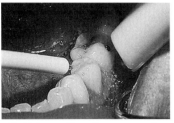

Figure 32-6.

Copyright © 2010 by Saunders, an imprint of Elsevier Inc. All rights reserved.

Procedure 32-1   APPLYING LIGHT-CURED (PHOTOPOLYMERIZED) SEALANTS—*cont'd*

STEPS—*cont'd*	RATIONALES—*cont'd*
10. Dry the treatment site with compressed air for 10 seconds. Evaluate etched surface (Figure 32-7).	A properly etched area appears white, dull, and frosty.

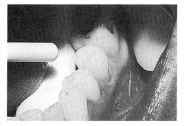

Figure 32-7.

11. Apply hydrophilic primer and dry with compressed air.	
12. Apply liquid sealant over the pits and fissures at <90 degrees. Allow the sealant to flow into the etched surfaces (Figure 32-8).	A low-viscosity sealant prevents air entrapment.

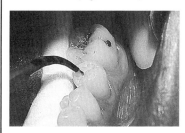

Figure 32-8.

13. Apply light-cure tip to sealant. Place tip of light source 2 mm from sealant. Check manufacturer's instructions for time before advancing the light to another area (Figure 32-9).	The curing process of the sealant is initiated by the light source. Time varies from 20 to 30 seconds.

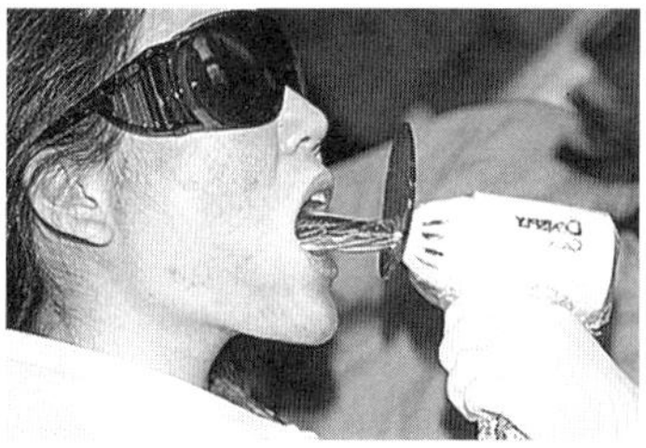

Figure 32-9.

14. After the polymerization process, evaluate the sealant with an explorer and check for hard, smooth surface and retention. Set sealant appears as a thin, polymerized film.	A successful sealant feels hard and smooth and firmly bonded to the tooth. Air bubbles should not be present.
15. If imperfections are noted (e.g., incomplete coverage: air bubbles), re-etch tooth for 10 seconds; wash and dry teeth and apply additional sealant (Figures 32-10 and 32-11).	Air bubbles or a loose sealant do not provide effective caries prevention.

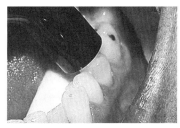

Figure 32-10.

(Continued)

Copyright © 2010 by Saunders, an imprint of Elsevier Inc. All rights reserved.

Procedure 32-1	APPLYING LIGHT-CURED (PHOTOPOLYMERIZED) SEALANTS—*cont'd*

STEPS—*cont'd*	**RATIONALES—*cont'd***

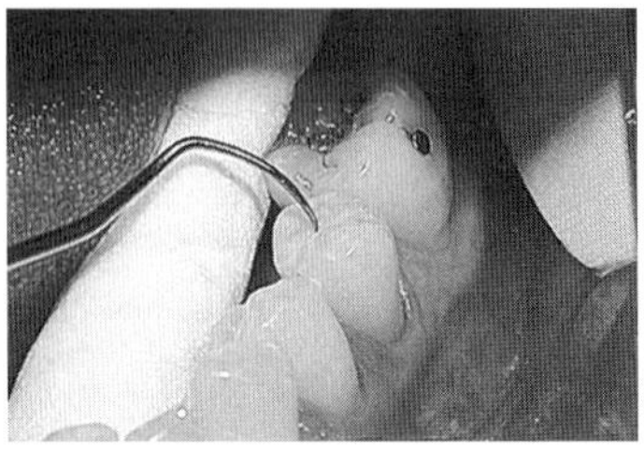

Figure 32-11.

16. Check occlusion with articulating paper to detect high spot areas. Remove excess filled sealant material with a finishing burr (Figure 32-12).

High spot areas contain excess sealant material that interferes with normal occlusion. Minor discrepancies with an unfilled sealant are eliminated by normal masticatory processes.

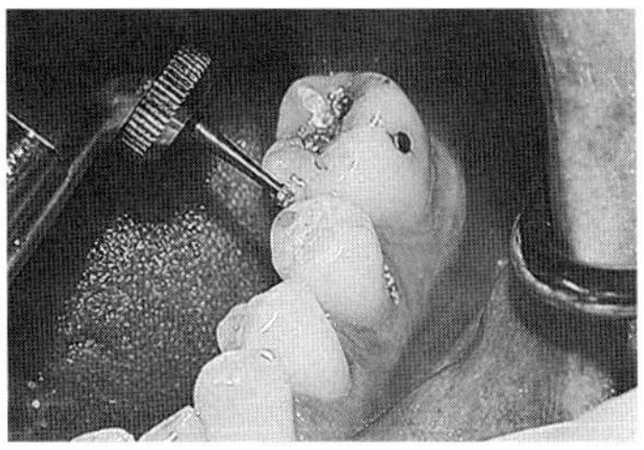

Figure 32-12.

17. Remove any residual unsealed liquid sealant with dry gauze. Floss treated teeth.
18. Apply topical fluoride.
19. Record type of sealant and teeth sealed in client's dental record.
20. Evaluate sealants 3 months after application and at every continued care appointment.

This ensures that the sealant has not blocked contact between the teeth.
Encourages remineralization of acid-etched surfaces.
Documentation allows for the proper monitoring of retention and serves as a legal record.
If the site was contaminated from faulty technique, partial or complete loss of the sealant material occurs within 6 to 12 months. Early sealant loss exposes the tooth to dental caries. Complete retention of sealants has been documented up to 10 years.

Copyright © 2010 by Saunders, an imprint of Elsevier Inc. All rights reserved.

Procedure 32-2 APPLYING SELF-CURED (AUTOPOLYMERIZING) SEALANTS

EQUIPMENT

Mouth mirror
Explorer
Saliva ejector
Self-cure sealant kit
Gauze
Cotton rolls and rubber dam
Air-water syringe tip

Dri-Angles
High-speed evacuation tube
Low-speed handpiece or air-polishing device
Bristled brush
Pumice
Floss
Personal protective equipment
Protective barriers

STEPS	RATIONALES
1. Follow steps 1 to 10 as described for light-cured sealants in Procedure 32-1.	
2. Mix one drop of universal liquid and one drop of catalyst liquid in mixing well. Follow manufacturer's directions, especially when sealing more than two teeth (Figure 32-13).	If a mix is prepared for more than two teeth, the mix sets prematurely and becomes thick and viscous. A viscous sealant does not allow for maximal flow into the pits and fissures. Bond strength and retention are compromised.

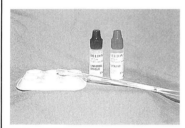

Figure 32-13.

STEPS	RATIONALES
3. Mix for 10 to 15 seconds or as specified by manufacturer's directions.	Manufacturer's directions may vary.
4. Apply sealant with brush over pits and fissures. Working time: 45 seconds.	A low-viscosity sealant that flows over the etched surfaces prevents air entrapment.
5. Allow sealant to set for 60 to 90 seconds or according to manufacturer's instructions.	Do not disturb sealant. Allow specified time for the sealant to cure.
6. Follow steps 14 to 20 as described for light-cured sealants in Procedure 32-1.	

Please refer to the Evolve website (http://evolve.elsevier.com/Darby/hygiene) for competency forms to help evaluate your mastery of each procedure in this chapter.

Copyright © 2010 by Saunders, an imprint of Elsevier Inc. All rights reserved.

Impressions, Study Casts, and Oral Stents

Procedure 35-1 | SELECTING THE CORRECT TRAY SIZE AND PREPARING IT FOR USE

EQUIPMENT (FIGURE 35-1)

Personal protective equipment
Antimicrobial mouth rinse
Lubricating gel
Maxillary and mandibular impression trays
Mouth mirror
Utility wax

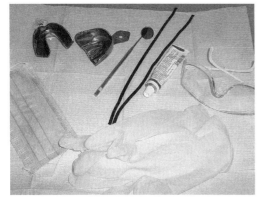

Figure 35-1. Equipment for selecting and preparing an impression tray. (Courtesy Gwen Essex.)

STEPS	RATIONALES
PREPARATION	
1. Gather all necessary supplies.	Prevents unnecessary interruptions to obtain supplies during the procedure.
2. Position self at side and in front of client, and seat the client in an upright position.	An upright position minimizes gagging. This positioning of clinician provides for good control of client and ease of insertion of tray.
3. Explain the procedure to the client. Have client remove any removable oral appliances.	The client who is familiar with the procedure is more manageable. Some may have had a negative experience; some may have a strong gag reflex.
4. Don personal protective equipment. Disinfect hands and don gloves.	Necessary for infection control.
5. Place protective eyewear on the client.	Protective eyewear prevents injury to the client.
6. Provide preprocedural antimicrobial mouth rinse.	Decreases surface microorganisms and saliva. Aids in achieving an accurate impression, provides a satisfying feeling for the client, and serves as a distraction.
7. Lubricate the client's lips with a small amount of lubricating gel.	Lubrication prevents the lips from cracking while impressions are made.
MANDIBULAR TRAY SELECTION	
8. Inspect client's mouth to estimate tray size. Note teeth out of alignment, tori, and length of dental arch that may require additional tray adaptation for client comfort.	A properly fitting impression tray will minimize tissue trauma and will hold an impression with all of the details of the mouth.

Copyright © 2010 by Saunders, an imprint of Elsevier Inc. All rights reserved.

Procedure 35-1   SELECTING THE CORRECT TRAY SIZE AND PREPARING IT FOR USE—*cont'd*

STEPS—*cont'd*	RATIONALES—*cont'd*
9. Instruct client to tilt chin down. Retract the client's lip and cheek with index and middle fingers of nondominant hand and at the same time turn the tray sideways and distend the lip and cheek on the opposite side of the mouth with the side of the tray to gain entry into the client's mouth. Insert the tray with a rotary motion (Figure 35-2).	Tilting the chin down minimizes gagging. Turning the impression tray sideways before insertion allows for the tray to be placed properly in the mouth with minimal tissue trauma.

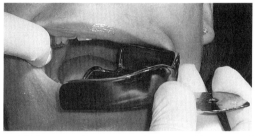

Figure 35-2.   Inserting impression tray. (Courtesy Gwen Essex.)

10. Make sure the tray is centered over the lower teeth by placing the handle at the midline, usually between the central incisors and in line with the center of the chin.	Ensures adequate fit for a symmetric impression of the dental arch.
11. Instruct client to raise tongue. Lower the tray and at the same time retract the cheek to make certain the buccal mucosa is not caught under the rim of the tray.	Raising the tongue ensures that it can pass by the rim of the tray without interference. Catching the buccal mucosa under the tray rim is painful.
12. Check to be sure that the tray covers the teeth and soft tissue. Lift the front of the tray to make certain that the area posterior to the retromolar pad is covered and that there is enough room to allow for ¼ inch of impression material in the facial and lingual surfaces of the teeth. If necessary, adapt the tray borders with utility (beading) wax to extend into the depth of the vestibule or extend the posterior length of the tray (Figure 35-3).	The tray should fit to the depth of the vestibule and should not impinge on the soft tissues.

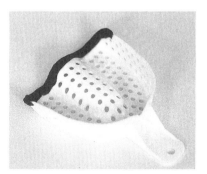

Figure 35-3.   Extending impression tray with utility wax. (From Bird DL, Robinson DS: *Torres and Ehrlich modern dental assisting,* ed 9, St Louis, 2009, Saunders.)

13. Reselect larger or smaller tray as needed.	Trays must fit properly to obtain a satisfactory impression.
MAXILLARY TRAY SELECTION	
14. Repeat steps 8 and 9.	See rationales with preceding steps.
15. Center the tray by placing the handle between the central incisors in line with the center of the nose.	Ensures adequate fit for a symmetric impression of the dental arch.

Copyright © 2010 by Saunders, an imprint of Elsevier Inc. All rights reserved.

(Continued)

Procedure 35-1   SELECTING THE CORRECT TRAY SIZE AND PREPARING IT FOR USE—*cont'd*

STEPS—*cont'd*	RATIONALES—*cont'd*
16. Bring the front of the tray about ¼ inch anterior to the incisors.	Ensures room for impression material when fitting the tray to the anterior teeth.
17. Seat the tray first by lowering the handle toward the mandibular teeth.	Allows for viewing the access to posterior teeth and associated structures.
18. Make certain all the posterior teeth and soft tissue, including the maxillary tuberosity, are covered. Check that laterally there is enough room to allow for ¼ inch space between the inside of the tray and the facial and lingual surfaces of the teeth.	Ensures proper fit to obtain adequate detail of all needed structures and that there is enough room for impression material on the facial and lingual surfaces of the teeth.
19. Retract the lip and raise the anterior portion of the tray into place. The tray should fit to the depth of the vestibule and not impinge on soft tissue.	Ensures proper and comfortable fit to obtain necessary detail of the anterior teeth and associated structures.
20. Reselect larger or smaller tray as needed.	Trays that are "tried" but not used must be sterilized before storage or discarded.
TRAY PREPARATION	
21. Spray smooth trays with adhesive. Wait 15 minutes before use.	Smooth trays have no porous openings to create a mechanical lock. They require adhesive to hold the impression in the tray after gelation so that the impression material does not stay in the client's mouth. If the adhesive has not had time to dry, the impression will pull away from the tray and distort the impression.
22. Record service in "Services Rendered" section of the client's dental chart, and date the entry.	Ensures integrity of the client's record for both the client's health and the legal protection of the practitioner.

Copyright © 2010 by Saunders, an imprint of Elsevier Inc. All rights reserved.

Procedure 35-2   MIXING ALGINATE

EQUIPMENT (FIGURE 35-4)
Personal protective equipment
Alginate powder
Water
Measuring scoop
Vial for measuring water
Wide-blade spatula
Rubber mixing bowl
Timer
Thermometer

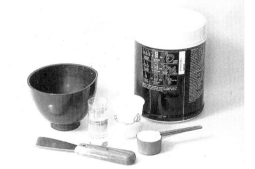

Figure 35-4. Equipment for mixing alginate impression material. (From Bird DL, Robinson DS: *Torres and Ehrlich modern dental assisting,* ed 9, St Louis, 2009, Saunders.)

STEPS	RATIONALES
1. Read the manufacturer's directions for the dispensing and manipulation of the alginate.	Following instructions will decrease the likelihood of errors in mixing and setting time.
2. Place one measure of room-temperature water into the mixing bowl for each scoop of alginate. Check temperature of water with thermometer.	Room-temperature water is important for proper setting time.
3. Shake or fluff the alginate by tipping the container two or three times.	It is essential to have correct amount of alginate to obtain an accurate impression. Alginate tends to settle and pack down in the can. If the container holding the alginate is not fluffed before measuring, too much powder may be dispensed, causing a grainy impression.
4. Overfill the correct scoop with powder; tap the scoop with the side of the spatula. Scrape the excess from the scoop with the spatula.	Overfilling and tapping the scoop before scraping the excess from the scoop help to avoid air pockets to ensure a proper measure.
5. Sift the powder into the water, and stir with the spatula until all the powder has been moistened.	Moistening all powder facilitates adequate mixing.

(Continued)

Copyright © 2010 by Saunders, an imprint of Elsevier Inc. All rights reserved.

Procedure 35-2 | MIXING ALGINATE—*cont'd*

STEPS—*cont'd*	RATIONALES—*cont'd*
6. Cup the rubber bowl in your hand with the mouth of the bowl next to the wrist. Firmly spread the alginate between the spatula and the side of the rubber bowl. Spatulate the mixture vigorously using a back-and-forth hand motion, spreading the material against the sides of the bowl. Use both sides of the spatula, and turn the bowl with your fingers during spatulation (Figure 35-5).	This position stabilizes the bowl. Vigorous mixing and spreading of material against the sides of the bowl while turning the bowl facilitate the breakage of powder crystals.

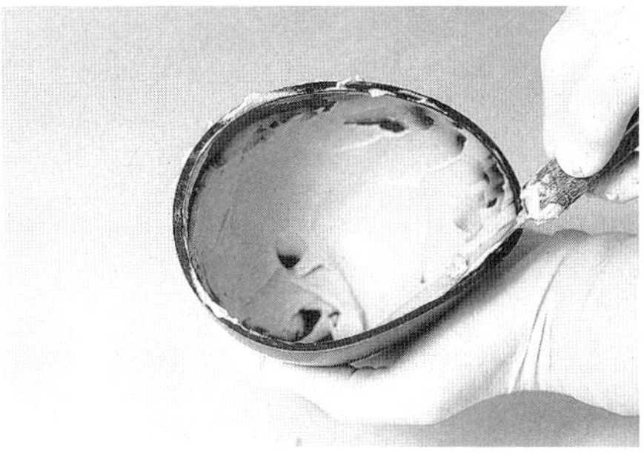

Figure 35-5. Proper consistency of mixed alginate impression material. (From Bird DL, Robinson DS: *Torres and Ehrlich modern dental assisting,* ed 9, St Louis, 2009, Saunders.)

STEPS—*cont'd*	RATIONALES—*cont'd*
7. Spatulate vigorously for 30 seconds and gather the material together. Use the spatula to crush the mixture and spread it out again. Repeat until a smooth, creamy consistency is achieved within the designated mixing time for either the normal-set or fast-set alginate.	Vigorous spatulation minimizes trapped air bubbles and promotes a smooth mix. A smooth mixture of alginate is important for an accurate impression.
8. Gather the material into one mass, and wipe on the inside edge of the mixing bowl.	Positions the material for easy access to fill the tray.

Copyright © 2010 by Saunders, an imprint of Elsevier Inc. All rights reserved.

Procedure 35-3   MAKING A MANDIBULAR PRELIMINARY IMPRESSION

EQUIPMENT (Figure 35-6)
Personal protective equipment
Antimicrobial rinse
Occupational Safety and Health Administration (OSHA)–approved disinfectant
Alginate powder
Water
Measuring scoop
Vial for measuring water
Wide-blade spatula
Utility wax
Rubber mixing bowl
Selected mandibular impression tray
Saliva ejector

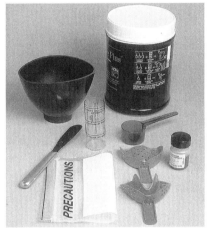

Figure 35-6. Scoop for alginate powder, water dispensers, mixing bowl, spatula, and stock impression tray. (From Bird DL, Robinson DS: *Torres and Ehrlich modern dental assisting*, ed 9, St Louis, 2009, Saunders.)

STEPS	RATIONALES
PREPARATION	
1. Gather all necessary supplies. Seat the client upright and explain the procedure. Have client remove any removable oral appliances.	Prevents unnecessary interruptions to obtain needed supplies. An upright position minimizes gagging. The client who is familiar with the procedure is more manageable. A removable oral appliance when left in place prevents an impression of all the anatomic details of the mouth.
2. Check the client's health history to determine any risk factor that may complicate the procedure.	Keeps client safe.
3. Don personal protective equipment, safety glasses, mask, and bonnet. Disinfect hands and don gloves.	Infection control procedures prevent the transmission of disease.
4. Place protective eyewear on the client.	Protective eyewear prevents injury to the client.
5. Provide preprocedural antimicrobial mouth rinse.	An antimicrobial mouth rinse decreases surface microorganisms and saliva. This aids in achieving an accurate impression, provides a satisfying feeling for the client, and serves as a distraction.
6. Lubricate the client's lips with a small amount of moisturizer.	Lubrication prevents the lips from cracking during impression making.
7. Dry the teeth with compressed air.	Drying the teeth removes saliva from the teeth, which can cause irregularities in the study cast.
8. Measure two measures of room-temperature water with two scoops of alginate, and mix the alginate.	Initiates the chemical reaction.

(Continued)

Copyright © 2010 by Saunders, an imprint of Elsevier Inc. All rights reserved.

Procedure 35-3 | MAKING A MANDIBULAR PRELIMINARY IMPRESSION—*cont'd*

STEPS—*cont'd*	RATIONALES—*cont'd*
LOADING THE TRAY	
9. Quickly gather half the alginate in the bowl onto the spatula. Wipe the alginate into one side of the tray from the lingual side, working from the posterior toward the anterior. Fill to an area just below the rim. Quickly press the material down to the base of the tray.	Mandibular impression trays are loaded one half at a time to ensure complete filling of the impression tray. Pressing the material down to the base of the tray removes any air bubbles trapped in the tray.
10. Gather the remaining half of the alginate in the bowl onto the spatula and load the other side of the tray in the same way.	Loading one half of the tray at a time ensures proper fill of tray.
11. Moisten fingers with cold water and smooth over alginate. Make a slight indentation where teeth will insert (Figure 35-7).	Wiping the impression with wet fingers before insertion in the mouth smoothes the alginate and minimizes voids in the impression. Making slight indentations for teeth guides insertion of the tray.

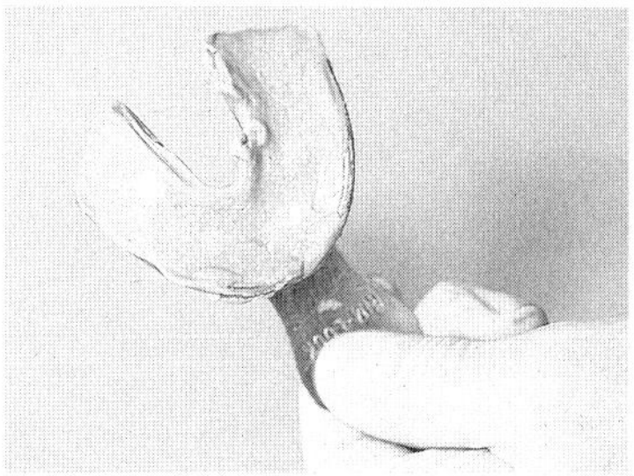

Figure 35-7. The mandibular impression tray is filled with alginate and is smoothed. (From Bird DL, Robinson DS: *Torres and Ehrlich modern dental assisting,* ed 9, St Louis, 2009, Saunders.)

STEPS—*cont'd*	RATIONALES—*cont'd*
12. Take a small amount of impression mixture from the spatula and quickly apply to the occlusal surfaces of the teeth, undercut areas, and vestibular areas.	Precoating potential areas provides for accurate anatomy of the impression.
SEATING THE TRAY	
13. Place yourself at the 8-o'clock position (4-o'clock position if left-handed), and ask the client to tilt the chin down.	Tilting the chin down minimizes gagging.
14. Turn the impression tray sideways.	Turning the impression tray sideways before insertion allows for the tray to fit through the opened lips comfortably.
15. Retract the client's lip and cheek with fingers of nondominant hand. Turn the tray sideways when placing it in the mouth, distending the lip and cheek on the opposite side of the mouth with the side of the tray.	Allows for insertion of tray with minimum discomfort to soft tissue.
16. Center the tray over the teeth, and center the handle in line with the center of the client's chin.	Ensures symmetric impression and adequate detail of anterior teeth, vestibule, and labial frenum.
17. Align the tray ¼ inch anterior to the incisors. Press down the posterior portion of the tray first and then seat the anterior portion of the tray directly down. Instruct client to raise the tongue (Figure 35-8).	Seating the posterior border of the tray first forms a seal. Seating the tray in a posterior to anterior direction avoids triggering the gag reflex and moves the impression material forward, ensuring complete coverage of the oral structures with alginate. The vibratory motion helps to fill in all crevices and between the teeth. Asking the client to extend the tongue helps the clinician to be sure the mandibular tray is seated on the floor of the mouth and allows the alginate to make an impression of the lingual aspects of the alveolar process.

Copyright © 2010 by Saunders, an imprint of Elsevier Inc. All rights reserved.

Procedure **35-3**	MAKING A MANDIBULAR PRELIMINARY IMPRESSION—*cont'd*

STEPS—*cont'd*	**RATIONALES**—*cont'd*

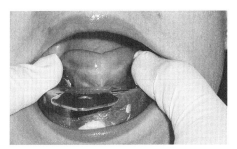

Figure 35-8. The mandibular impression tray is seated in the arch with the tongue out of the way. (Courtesy Gwen Essex.)

18. Instruct client to move the lips and to breathe normally.	Moving the lips ensures that the impression material flows into the depth of the vestibule. Breathing normally enhances client comfort and management.
19. Hold the tray steady in place until the material has gelled. Apply firm bilateral pressure with the middle fingers, and use the thumbs to support the jaw (Figure 35-9).	Holding the tray steady prevents a double impression. Facilitates clear impression of structures.

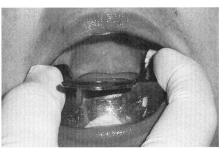

Figure 35-9. Holding the mandibular tray. (Courtesy Gwen Essex.)

REMOVING THE IMPRESSION

20. Place fingers of nondominant hand on top of the tray. The index finger of the nondominant hand rests on the incisal surface of the maxillary anterior teeth.	Protects maxillary teeth from damage during removal of the tray.
21. Move index finger of other hand along the buccal mucosa posteriorly between the impression and the peripheral tissues. The index finger is placed under the posterior facial portion of the tray to lift the tray and break the seal between the impression and the teeth. Grasp the handle of the tray with the thumb and index finger of the dominant hand, and use a firm lifting motion.	Breaking the seal between the impression and the peripheral tissues and teeth before removal of the impression avoids injury to the impression. The finger-thumb grasp of the handle allows for control of the tray, and placement of the index finger of the opposite hand as described protects the anterior teeth in the opposite arch from being injured by the tray.
22. Remove the tray by turning it sideways to take it out of the client's mouth.	The straight snapping motion promotes obtaining an intact impression, and turning it sideways facilitates tray removal from mouth.

(Continued)

Copyright © 2010 by Saunders, an imprint of Elsevier Inc. All rights reserved.

Procedure 35-3 | MAKING A MANDIBULAR PRELIMINARY IMPRESSION—*cont'd*

STEPS—*cont'd*	**RATIONALES—*cont'd***
23. Evaluate the impression for accuracy (Figure 35-10).	Determines need for remaking of the impression.

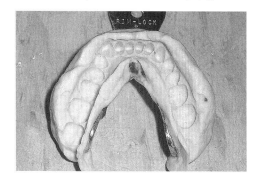

Figure 35-10. How a mandibular impression must look. (Courtesy Gwen Essex.)

POSTIMPRESSION CARE

24. Give the client water to rinse the mouth.	Removes any excess alginate material from mouth; promotes client comfort.
25. Gently rinse debris from the impression under a stream of cold water (Figure 35-11).	Rinsing the impression removes blood, saliva, and food debris that would interfere with the setting of the gypsum product.

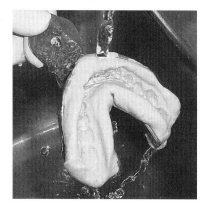

Figure 35-11. Rinsing the impression. (From Bird DL, Robinson DS: *Torres and Ehrlich modern dental assisting,* ed 9, St Louis, 2009, Saunders.)

26. Spray the impression with an approved disinfectant (e.g., 1:213 iodophor or 1:10 sodium hypochlorite) within 10 to 15 minutes. Follow the manufacturer's recommended procedure (Figure 35-12).	Use of approved disinfectants prevents disease transmission with no distortion of the impression. The procedure determined by the manufacturer must be followed to prevent distortion of the impression.

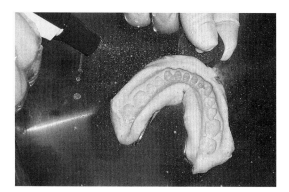

Figure 35-12. Spraying the impression. (Courtesy Gwen Essex.)

Copyright © 2010 by Saunders, an imprint of Elsevier Inc. All rights reserved.

Procedure 35-3   MAKING A MANDIBULAR PRELIMINARY IMPRESSION—*cont'd*

STEPS—*cont'd*	RATIONALES—*cont'd*
27. Wrap the impression in a moist paper towel and place it in a biohazard bag before pouring it up (Figure 35-13) or in a humidor; label with client's name. Prepare the laboratory prescription if sending the impressions to the dental laboratory.	Prevents syneresis or imbibitions.

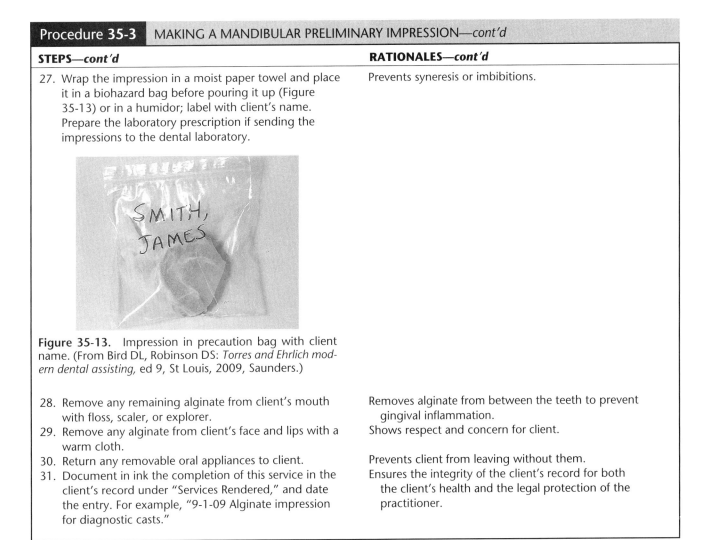

Figure 35-13. Impression in precaution bag with client name. (From Bird DL, Robinson DS: *Torres and Ehrlich modern dental assisting,* ed 9, St Louis, 2009, Saunders.)

28. Remove any remaining alginate from client's mouth with floss, scaler, or explorer.	Removes alginate from between the teeth to prevent gingival inflammation.
29. Remove any alginate from client's face and lips with a warm cloth.	Shows respect and concern for client.
30. Return any removable oral appliances to client.	Prevents client from leaving without them.
31. Document in ink the completion of this service in the client's record under "Services Rendered," and date the entry. For example, "9-1-09 Alginate impression for diagnostic casts."	Ensures the integrity of the client's record for both the client's health and the legal protection of the practitioner.

Copyright © 2010 by Saunders, an imprint of Elsevier Inc. All rights reserved.

Procedure 35-4 | MAKING A MAXILLARY PRELIMINARY IMPRESSION

EQUIPMENT
Personal protective equipment
Antimicrobial rinse
Occupational Safety and Health Administration (OSHA)–approved disinfecting solution
Alginate powder
Water
Measuring scoop
Vial for measuring water
Wide-blade spatula*
Bite registration wax (baseplate utility wax or wax wafer)
Rubber mixing bowl
Maxillary and mandibular impression trays
Saliva ejector

STEPS	RATIONALES
PREPARATION	
1. Gather all necessary supplies. Seat and prepare the client.	See Procedure 35-3, steps 1 through 7.
2. Measure three units of room-temperature water and three scoops of alginate, and mix the alginate.	Initiates the chemical reaction.
LOADING THE TRAY	
3. Load the maxillary tray in one large increment. Load from the posterior end of tray. Use a wiping motion to bring the material forward with the spatula, being careful to place the bulk of the material in the anterior palatal area of the tray. Fill to an area just below the edge of the wax rim.	Maxillary impression trays are loaded from the posterior to prevent the formation of air bubbles in the material. Placing the bulk of the material in the anterior area of the tray prevents the alginate from overflowing into the throat when the tray is seated.
4. Be careful not to overfill the posterior portion of the tray that rests against the palate.	Overfilling the posterior portion of the tray will trigger the gag reflex.
5. Moisten fingers with water, and smooth surface of the alginate (Figure 35-14).	Smoothing the surface with moistened fingers minimizes voids in the impression.

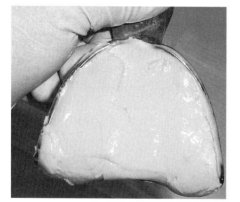

Figure 35-14. The maxillary impression tray is filled with alginate. The filled tray is smoothed on the alginate surface. (Courtesy Gwen Essex.)

SEATING THE TRAY	
6. Position yourself at the 11-o'clock position (1-o'clock position if left-handed), and instruct the client to tilt head forward and chin down.	Tilting the head forward and the chin down minimizes gagging.
7. Retract the client's lips and cheek with fingers of nondominant hand. With the dominant hand, turn the impression tray sideways and at the same time distend the lip and cheek on the opposite side of the mouth with the side of the tray.	Turning the impression tray sideways before insertion allows for the tray to be placed in the mouth with minimum impingement of soft tissue.

Copyright © 2010 by Saunders, an imprint of Elsevier Inc. All rights reserved.

Procedure 35-4   MAKING A MAXILLARY PRELIMINARY IMPRESSION—*cont'd*

STEPS—*cont'd*	RATIONALES—*cont'd*
8. Center the tray over the client's teeth, and center the handle at the midline in line with the center of the client's nose.	Centering the handle promotes a symmetric impression.
9. Seat the back of the tray against the posterior border of the hard palate to form a seal. Place the tray ¼ inch or 6 mm anterior to incisors, and seat posterior to anterior direction with a slight vibratory motion.	Seating the tray in a posterior to anterior direction avoids triggering the gag reflex, prevents the excess material from going toward the back of the mouth, and moves the impression material forward, ensuring complete coverage of the oral structures with alginate. The vibratory motion forces the material into crevices and proximal areas.
10. Gently move the client's lips out of the way as the tray is seated, and instruct the client to move the lips (Figure 35-15).	Retracting the lips allows the impression material to flow into the vestibule. Moving the lips ensures that the impression material flows into the depth of the vestibule.

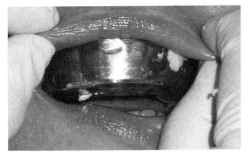

Figure 35-15. A maxillary alginate impression is placed in the arch. The maxillary lip is lifted and positioned outside of the tray. (Courtesy Gwen Essex.)

11. Place middle fingers over the premolar areas, and hold the lip out with the index finger and the thumb.	This stabilization protects opposing teeth and promotes clear impression of structures.
12. Instruct the client to breathe slowly through the nose and form an O with his or her lips.	Having the client form an O with the lips molds the impression material around the tray.
13. Hold the tray in place until the material has gelled.	Holding the tray steady prevents a double impression.

REMOVING THE IMPRESSION

14. Place an index finger under the posterior facial portion of the tray to break the seal between the impression and the teeth.	Breaking the seal before removal of the impression avoids injury to the impression and the teeth.
15. Place the index finger of the nondominant hand on the incisal surface of the mandibular anterior teeth.	This finger-thumb grasp allows for control of the tray. Placement of the index finger of the opposite hand as described protects the anterior teeth in the opposite arch from being injured by the tray during the tray removal process.
16. Move index finger of other hand along the buccal mucosa posteriorly between the impression and the peripheral tissues. The index finger is placed under the rim of the tray to lift and break the seal between the impression and the teeth. Grasp the handle of the tray with the thumb and index finger of the dominant hand to lower it from the maxillary teeth.	
17. Remove the tray by turning it sideways to take it out of the client's mouth.	The straight snapping motion promotes obtaining an intact impression, and turning the tray sideways facilitates tray removal from mouth.

(Continued)

Copyright © 2010 by Saunders, an imprint of Elsevier Inc. All rights reserved.

Procedure 35-4	MAKING A MAXILLARY PRELIMINARY IMPRESSION—*cont'd*

STEPS—*cont'd*	**RATIONALES**—*cont'd*
POSTIMPRESSION CARE	
18. Evaluate the impression for accuracy (Figure 35-16).	Determines need for retaking the impression. See Procedure 35-3, steps 24 through 31.

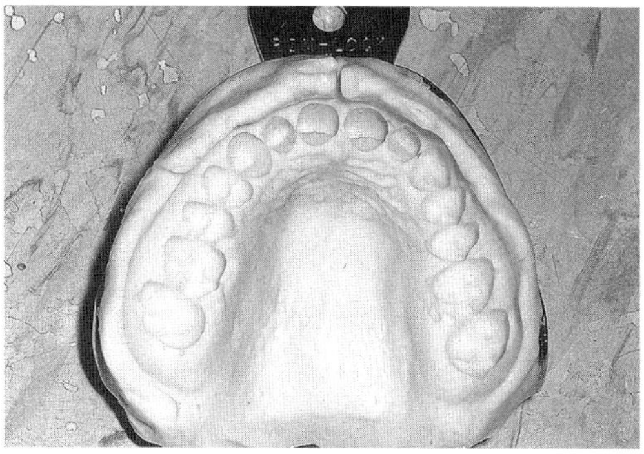

Figure 35-16. How a maxillary impression must look. (From Bird DL, Robinson DS: *Torres and Ehrlich modern dental assisting,* ed 9, St Louis, 2009, Saunders.)

*If the same bowl and spatula are used that were used for the mandibular impression, they must be thoroughly cleaned and dried to prevent contamination of the maxillary mix (see Figure 35-8).

Copyright © 2010 by Saunders, an imprint of Elsevier Inc. All rights reserved.

Procedure 35-5 MAKING A WAX-BITE REGISTRATION

EQUIPMENT (FIGURE 35-17)

Protective barriers (safety glasses, mask, gloves, hair bonnet)
Antimicrobial rinse
Bite registration wax (baseplate wax or wax wafer)
Wide-blade laboratory knife
Heat source (warm water, Bunsen burner, or torch)
Occupational Safety and Health Administration (OSHA)–approved disinfectant

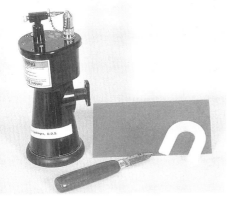

Figure 35-17. Supplies for taking a wax-bite registration. (From Bird DL, Robinson DS: *Torres and Ehrlich modern dental assisting,* ed 9, St Louis, 2009, Saunders.)

STEPS	RATIONALES
PREPARATION	
1. Gather all necessary supplies. Seat the client upright. Explain the procedure.	See Procedure 35-1, steps 1 through 7.
2. Reassure the client that the wax will be warm, not hot.	Reduces potential for client anxiety.
3. Measure the length of the wax needed by placing the wax over the biting surfaces of the teeth. If the wax extends past the last tooth, use the laboratory knife to shorten its length after removing the wax from the client's mouth.	This measurement ensures an accurate bite registration and client comfort.
4. Soften the bite registration wax in hot water or with another heat source (e.g., Bunsen burner or torch).	The softened wax allows the wax to make the bite registration.
SEATING	
5. Place the softened warm wax over the maxillary occlusal surfaces and instruct the client to bite together on posterior teeth gently and naturally into the wax (Figure 35-18).	Ensures that the correct position will be recorded in the wax.

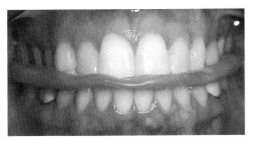

Figure 35-18. Wax-bite registration in client's mouth. (From Bird DL, Robinson DS: *Torres and Ehrlich modern dental assisting,* ed 9, St Louis, 2009, Saunders.)

6. Allow the wax bite to cool in the mouth. If necessary, air from the air-water syringe can cool the wax.	Cooled wax can be removed without distortion of the wax.

Copyright © 2010 by Saunders, an imprint of Elsevier Inc. All rights reserved.

(Continued)

Procedure 35-5	MAKING A WAX-BITE REGISTRATION—*cont'd*

STEPS—*cont'd*	**RATIONALES**—*cont'd*
REMOVAL	
7. Remove the wax carefully when it has cooled.	Removing the bite wax carefully prevents distortion.
POST–WAX-BITE CARE	
8. Inspect the wax to be sure it represents the client's bite (Figure 35-19). Chill in cold water until firm.	Chilling in cold water sets the registration.

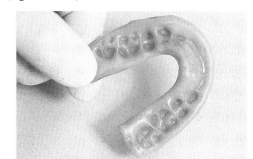

Figure 35-19. Wax-bite registration on a Wax Wafer. (From Bird DL, Robinson DS: *Torres and Ehrlich modern dental assisting,* ed 9, St Louis, 2009, Saunders.)

9. Write the client's name on a piece of paper and keep it with the wax-bite registration.	This process will identify whose bite the wax-bite registration represents.
10. Disinfect wax-bite registration with an OSHA-approved disinfectant.	
11. Store the wax-bite registration with the impressions or casts until it is needed for the trimming of the casts.	This storage will ensure that the wax-bite registration is available to articulate the client's models after the client has left the office.
12. Record service in "Services Rendered" section of the client's record, and date the entry.	Ensures integrity of the client's record for both the client's health and the legal protection of the practitioner.

Copyright © 2010 by Saunders, an imprint of Elsevier Inc. All rights reserved.

Procedure 35-6   POURING THE CAST AND THE BASE

EQUIPMENT (FIGURE 35-20)

Personal protective equipment
Rubber bowl
No. 7 wax spatula
Scale
Room-temperature water
Dental plaster
Two Plexiglas squares
Laboratory spatula
Disinfected alginate impressions
Water measuring device
Plaster knife
Vibrator covered with plastic
Occupational Safety and Health Administration (OSHA)–approved disinfectant

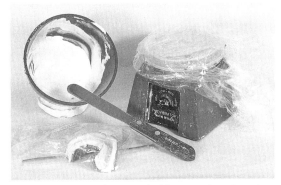

Figure 35-20. Supplies needed for pouring dental casts. (From Bird DL, Robinson DS: *Torres and Ehrlich modern dental assisting,* ed 9, St Louis, 2009, Saunders.)

STEPS	RATIONALES
PREPARATION	
1. Don personal protective equipment.	Safety procedures prevent injury and disease transmission to the clinician.
2. Disinfect the alginate impression following the manufacturer's instructions. Rinse with cool, running water, shake the excess water off in the sink, and gently dry with compressed air.	A rinsed impression reduces the surface tension of the alginate and allows the gypsum product to flow. Overdrying could distort the impression.
3. Use the laboratory knife to remove any excess impression material that will interfere with the pouring of the model, i.e., impression material past the end of the tray or excess material from the tongue area.	Excess impression material interferes with the pouring of the model. Removing the excess gypsum from the tongue area prevents having to scrape the area with a laboratory knife after hardening.
POURING THE MANDIBULAR IMPRESSION	
4. Measure 50 mL of room-temperature water, and place it into a clean mixing bowl.	This is the recommended amount of mixing water for dental plaster. Clean equipment prevents a contaminated mix of gypsum.
5. Place a paper towel on a scale, and make necessary adjustments. Obtain a measure of 100 g of dental plaster.	This is the recommended amount of dental plaster for mixing with 50 mL of water.
6. Add the powder into the water in steady increments to allow the powder to settle.	Prevents the trapping of air bubbles.
7. Use the spatula to incorporate the powder into the water. Use a wiping motion against the sides of the bowl. Spatulate 20 seconds to achieve a smooth, creamy mix (Figure 35-21).	Ensures a smooth mix of gypsum that is free of air bubbles, and avoids spilling the powder.

(Continued)

Copyright © 2010 by Saunders, an imprint of Elsevier Inc. All rights reserved.

Procedure 35-6 POURING THE CAST AND THE BASE—*cont'd*

STEPS—*cont'd*	**RATIONALES**—*cont'd*

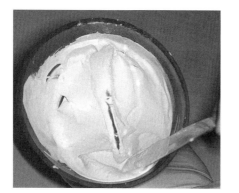

Figure 35-21. Smooth, creamy mix. (From Bird DL, Robinson DS: *Torres and Ehrlich modern dental assisting,* ed 9, St Louis, 2009, Saunders.)

8. Set the vibrator at low speed. Place the bowl on a vibrator and vibrate the material for 10 to 15 seconds. Lightly press and rotate the bowl on the vibrator.

Eliminates air bubbles in the mixture and in the final study model or diagnostic cast.

9. Gather the gypsum as a mass in the bowl. Remove bowl from vibrator (Figure 35-22).

Facilitates access for pouring the cast.

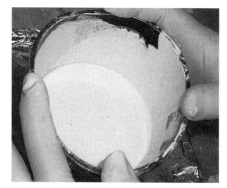

Figure 35-22. Mixing bowl on vibrator. (Courtesy Gwen Essex.)

10. Hold the impression tray by the handle, and press handle against the vibrator.

Positions the impression tray to begin to pour the impression.

11. Use the end of a wax spatula or laboratory knife to pick up about ½ teaspoon of mixed material. Allow mix to flow into the impression at the distal of the most posterior tooth while the impression is vibrated so that the material flows toward the anterior teeth. Turn the tray on its side to provide the continuous flow of material forward into each tooth. Tip the impression forward to make the gypsum mixture flow into the bottom of the alginate impression. Continue to add the gypsum product in small increments at the same place until the occlusal and incisal surfaces are filled. Vibrate continually (Figure 35-23).

The flowing of the material pushes out the air ahead of it and eliminates air bubbles. Adding small increments prevents trapping air in the occlusal or incisal areas of the impression, which would make the final outcome inaccurate. Filling all the occlusal and incisal areas first reduces the risk for trapped air.

12. When all tooth indentations are filled, use the laboratory spatula to add larger amounts of gypsum to fill the impression. Continue to vibrate until the entire impression is filled (Figure 35-24). Then set the poured impression aside.

The laboratory spatula helps to adequately fill the vestibule area of the impression. Vibrating eliminates air bubbles.

Copyright © 2010 by Saunders, an imprint of Elsevier Inc. All rights reserved.

Procedure 35-6   POURING THE CAST AND THE BASE—*cont'd*

STEPS—*cont'd*   **RATIONALES—*cont'd***

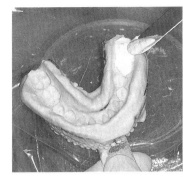

Figure 35-23. Initial placement of material in distal of most posterior tooth. (From Bird DL, Robinson DS: *Torres and Ehrlich modern dental assisting,* ed 9, St Louis, 2009, Saunders.)

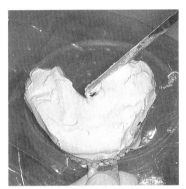

Figure 35-24. Impression filled with large amounts of gypsum. (From Bird DL, Robinson DS: *Torres and Ehrlich modern dental assisting,* ed 9, St Louis, 2009, Saunders.)

POURING THE BASE FOR THE MANDIBULAR CAST

13. Gather the remaining amount of mixed material together in the bowl.

The material flows and flattens; therefore mounding the gypsum product helps to ensure that a base 1 inch thick is constructed.

14. Place the mix in a mound on a Plexiglas square or tile. Shape the base to approximately 2 × 2 inches wide and 1 inch thick (Figure 35-25).

It is important to place the base on a smooth, nonabsorbent surface.

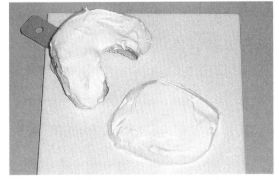

Figure 35-25. Filled impression tray and base on Plexiglas. (From Bird DL, Robinson DS: *Torres and Ehrlich modern dental assisting,* ed 9, St Louis, 2009, Saunders.)

15. Invert the firm, poured impression onto the firm base. Do not push the impression into the base.

The mix will flow out of the impression if inverted before the stone is firm.

Copyright © 2010 by Saunders, an imprint of Elsevier Inc. All rights reserved.

(Continued)

Procedure 35-6 POURING THE CAST AND THE BASE—*cont'd*

STEPS—*cont'd*	RATIONALES—*cont'd*
16. Position impression tray on the center of the mound to provide a uniform thickness all around it. Position the occlusal plane of posterior teeth parallel with the table top as judged by the handle of the tray.	This position will provide for a symmetric base.
17. Hold the tray steady, and with the laboratory spatula or a moistened finger, smooth the sides around the base onto the margins of the impression tray (Figure 35-26).	This technique will provide for a symmetric base with uniform thickness.

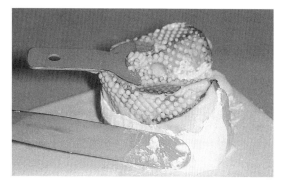

Figure 35-26. Smoothing the plaster base mix up into the margins of the tray. (From Bird DL, Robinson DS: *Torres and Ehrlich modern dental assisting,* ed 9, St Louis, 2009, Saunders.)

18. Remove excess stone or plaster above the edge of the tray rim.	A locked tray is very difficult to remove from the study model or diagnostic cast. Excess stone above the tray rim locks the tray in the model.
19. Allow the gypsum to reach the initial set before moving the Plexiglas square.	Moving the Plexiglas before initial set will cause the base of the model or cast to flatten out, making the base too thin.

POURING THE MAXILLARY IMPRESSION AND BASE

20. Repeat steps 2 through 19 above for the maxillary impression to create an anatomic and art portion of a dental cast. Use clean equipment for the fresh mix of plaster.	Remnants of material from the earlier mix or other debris will adversely affect setting time.

SEPARATING THE IMPRESSIONS FROM THE CASTS

21. Wait 45 to 60 minutes after the base has been poured before attempting to separate the impression from the cast.	Final set occurs after the exothermic reaction has completed. The model or cast will feel cool to the touch. Separating after the final set occurs prevents damage to the teeth.
22. Use a plaster knife to remove excess material from the edges of the impression tray and to gently separate the margins of the tray from the cast (Figure 35-27).	Removal of excess material frees the tray from the model.

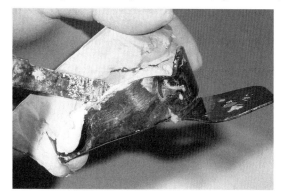

Figure 35-27. Plaster knife used to free tray from stone. (Courtesy Gwen Essex.)

Copyright © 2010 by Saunders, an imprint of Elsevier Inc. All rights reserved.

Procedure 35-6 | POURING THE CAST AND THE BASE—*cont'd*

STEPS—*cont'd*	**RATIONALES**—*cont'd*
23. If the teeth are in good alignment, remove tray and impression material together. First release the anterior portion by gently pulling downward and forward one time. Then make a firm, straight pull upward. Do not apply lateral pressure or rock the tray (Figure 35-28).	Forces created by lateral pressure and rocking of the tray may break teeth.

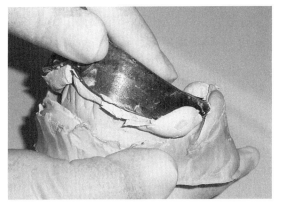

Figure 35-28. Removing impression from cast. (Courtesy Gwen Essex.)

24. If the tray does not separate, check to see where the tray may be locked by the gypsum. Use the plaster knife to free the tray from the gypsum.	Excess stone above the tray rim locks the tray in the model.
25. If teeth are misaligned, remove the tray first, then cut the impression material carefully along the occlusal line and gently peel off.	Prevents the accidental breakage of teeth on the cast.

POSTSEPARATION PROCEDURES

26. Use a pencil or permanent marker to label the base (bottom) of the model or cast with the client's name. Keep the wax bite with the gypsum models and casts.	Proper labeling prevents unidentifiable models and casts.
27. Store the casts until they can be trimmed.	Prevents distortion.
28. Remove gypsum material from the vibrator, spatula, and mixing bowl, and clean with cool water.	It is easier to clean the equipment immediately, before the gypsum product sets.

Copyright © 2010 by Saunders, an imprint of Elsevier Inc. All rights reserved.

Procedure 35-7	CONSTRUCTING A CUSTOM-MADE STENT (A SINGLE-LAYER MOUTH GUARD, FLUORIDE TRAY, OR TOOTH-WHITENING TRAY)

EQUIPMENT (FIGURE 35-29)

Personal protective equipment
Petrolatum lubricant, silicone lubricant
Polyurethane
Mouth guard 4 × 4 square
Long-shank acrylic burr in a laboratory engine
Matches
Diagnostic casts
Crown and collar scissors
Hanau torch
Vacuum forming machine
Laboratory knife

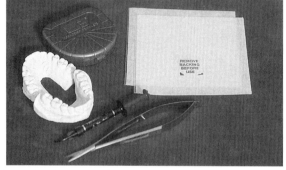

Figure 35-29. Supplies for constructing a custom-made stent. (From Bird DL, Robinson DS: *Torres and Ehrlich modern dental assisting,* ed 9, St Louis, 2009, Saunders.)

STEPS

RATIONALES

1. Don personal protective equipment.

Safety glasses protect eyes from debris. The mask protects from breathing burning organic material and acrylic dust. The bonnet protects hair from fire and from getting caught in the machine.

2. Trim the diagnostic cast so that the base extends 3 to 4 mm past the gingival border and the vertical height is minimal. Spray the cast with silicone lubricant (Figure 35-30).

Casts made of stone must be used for stent manufacturing. Plaster casts are not strong enough to withstand the suction of the vacuum former. The smaller the base of the diagnostic cast, the more likely it is that the vacuum former can suck the material down around the cast. Lubricant helps in the removal of the stent.

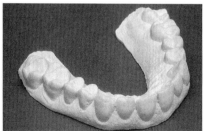

Figure 35-30. Trimmed diagnostic cast. (From Bird DL, Robinson DS: *Torres and Ehrlich modern dental assisting,* ed 9, St Louis, 2009, Saunders.)

3. Place the vacuum forming machine under a hood fan for control of organic emissions.

Constructing a stent involves the burning of organic material. Occupational Safety and Healthy Administration (OSHA) safety regulations for the burning of organic compounds require that fumes be removed from the air by use of a hood fan.

4. Prepare the machine. The perforated vacuum plate and the sides of the hinged frame must be lightly sprayed with silicone lubricant.

Lubricating the vacuum former prevents the stent material from sticking when warm. Overspraying will clog the suction holes.

Copyright © 2010 by Saunders, an imprint of Elsevier Inc. All rights reserved.

| Procedure 35-7 | CONSTRUCTING A CUSTOM-MADE STENT (A SINGLE-LAYER MOUTH GUARD, FLUORIDE TRAY, OR TOOTH-WHITENING TRAY)—*cont'd* |

STEPS—*cont'd* | **RATIONALES—*cont'd***

5. Open the hinged frame, and center the polyurethane material onto the lower frame (Figure 35-31).

Holds the material securely in place.

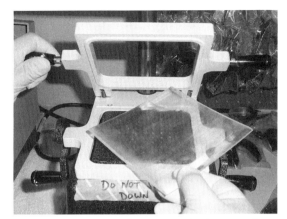

Figure 35-31. Opening hinge and placing mouth guard material. (Courtesy Gwen Essex.)

6. Close the frame and secure the frame with the latch knob.

Ensures proper placement of material.

7. Grasp both handles of the locked, hinged frame and lift it until it clicks into position approximately 3 inches above the vacuum plate.

Ensures frame is locked into place.

8. Swing the heating unit to the center position and turn on the heating element switch at the base of the unit.

Ensures source of heat and proper distance of heating unit from material.

9. Center cast on the vacuum plate. Some units have extra holes at the front and back of the machine; place the cast between these holes.

Ensures proper placement of material over cast.

10. Do not leave the machine unattended. Watch the material as it heats for 1 to 2 minutes until it sags ½ inch below the hinged frame (Figure 35-32).

The material heats quickly and may be sucked into the motor if overheated.

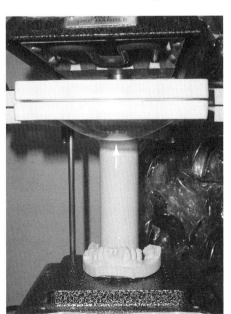

Figure 35-32. Sagging mouth guard material. (Courtesy Gwen Essex.)

Copyright © 2010 by Saunders, an imprint of Elsevier Inc. All rights reserved.

(Continued)

Procedure 35-7	CONSTRUCTING A CUSTOM-MADE STENT (A SINGLE-LAYER MOUTH GUARD, FLUORIDE TRAY, OR TOOTH-WHITENING TRAY)—*cont'd*

STEPS—*cont'd*	**RATIONALES**—*cont'd*

11. Grasp both handles of the hinged frame and pull it down over the vacuum plate. The material will be draped over the cast (Figure 35-33).

Grasping with both handles allows for proper force.

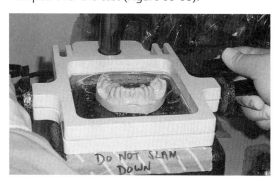

Figure 35-33.   Hinged frame pulled over vacuum plate. (Courtesy Gwen Essex.)

12. Turn on the vacuum motor for 10 seconds.

Applying the vacuum adapts the material to the cast.

13. Swing the heating unit out of the way and turn the switch off.

There is no more need for the heating unit.

14. Turn off the vacuum switch. Release the hinged frame knob and open the frame and hold by the edges to remove it from the vacuum plate.

Holding the polyurethane by the edges prevents getting fingerprints on the stent.

15. Hold the splint and cast under running, cold water for at least 30 seconds.

Cooling the stent hardens the thermoplastic material. The stent will become opaque in color.

16. Cut excess material just below the depth of the periphery to remove it from the cast (Figure 35-34).

Begins the tray trimming process. If the stent cannot be cut with the scissors, a hot instrument can melt through the material, or a laboratory knife can be used to separate it from the cast.

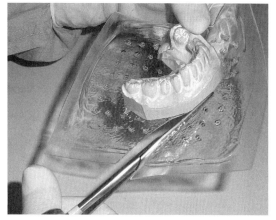

Figure 35-34.   Cutting away gross excess material. (From Bird DL, Robinson DS: *Torres and Ehrlich modern dental assisting,* ed 9, St Louis, 2009, Saunders.)

17. Use small, sharp crown and collar scissors to trim approximately 0.5 mm away from the gingival margin (Figure 35-35).

This trimming prevents the stent from irritating the client's soft tissues.

18. Place the mouth guard back on the cast.

This replacement allows the checking of gingival extensions.

19. If necessary, place a thin coat of petroleum jelly on the facial surfaces. Use a low flame to gently readapt the margins so that they cover the entire tooth, but do not overlap the gingivae.

This readaptation of the margins of the stent to the model ensures complete coverage of client's teeth and comfort.

Copyright © 2010 by Saunders, an imprint of Elsevier Inc. All rights reserved.

| Procedure 35-7 | CONSTRUCTING A CUSTOM-MADE STENT (A SINGLE-LAYER MOUTH GUARD, FLUORIDE TRAY, OR TOOTH-WHITENING TRAY)—*cont'd* |

STEPS—*cont'd*   **RATIONALES**—*cont'd*

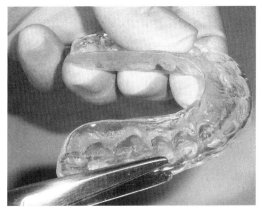

Figure 35-35. Trimming material away from the gingival margin. (Courtesy Gwen Essex.)

20. Wearing a mask and safety goggles, trim the mouth guard with an acrylic burr in a laboratory engine (Figure 35-36).

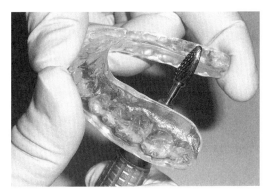

Figure 35-36. Trimming mouth guard with an acrylic burr. (Courtesy Gwen Essex.)

21. Use the Hanau torch to smooth the edges from the peripheral border of the mouth guard.   Enhances client comfort.

Please refer to the Evolve website (http://evolve.elsevier.com/Darby/hygiene) for competency forms to help evaluate your mastery of each procedure in this chapter.

Copyright © 2010 by Saunders, an imprint of Elsevier Inc. All rights reserved.

Restorative Therapy

| Procedure 36-1 | APPLYING A RUBBER DAM |

EQUIPMENT
Personal protective equipment
Protective eyewear for client
Rubber dam material
Dental floss or tape
Rubber dam punch
Petrolatum
Rubber dam retainers
Water-soluble lubricant
Rubber dam forceps
Spoon excavator
Rubber dam frame
Air-water syringe
Mouth mirror

STEPS	RATIONALES
1. Explain procedure to client. Instruct client to breathe through the nose after application of the rubber dam and to maintain an open mouth after placement of the rubber dam retainer.	Client is less apprehensive and more able to appreciate value of the rubber dam to the ultimate success of the restorative treatment. Maintaining an open mouth prevents biting on the bow of the retainer.
2. Put on protective eyewear and mask; wash hands and put on gloves.	Prevents transmission of microorganisms.
3. Place protective eyewear on client.	Prevents client injury from airborne objects.
4. Lubricate client's lips with petrolatum, especially corners of mouth.	Prevents lips from becoming chapped during isolation.
5. Use a bite block to maintain an open mouth position when individuals are unable to do this unassisted.	Facilitates client comfort.
6. Assess client's dentition and soft tissues. Confirm tooth or teeth to be restored.	Influences operator's application of the rubber dam.
7. Remove oral biofilm, debris, and supragingival calculus.	Removal of oral debris simplifies application process.
8. If determined to be necessary, infiltrate a small amount of anesthetic solution adjacent to area of retainer placement.	Routine injections for pulpal anesthesia may not anesthetize areas where the retainer retracts gingiva. Lingual gingiva of maxillary molars and facial gingiva of mandibular molars may require supplemental anesthesia. Anterior soft tissue is typically not a concern because anterior rubber dams can be successfully retained without retainers.
9. Select correct size, color, and weight of rubber dam material for the procedure.	These features vary based on client dimensions and operator preference.
10. Mark holes on the rubber dam.	Individual placement of holes permits operator to take into consideration factors such as missing teeth, extra teeth, tight contacts, and misaligned teeth.
11. Punch holes as marked with sharp, determined punching action.	Makes clean holes free of tears and tags.

Copyright © 2010 by Saunders, an imprint of Elsevier Inc. All rights reserved.

Procedure **36-1**	APPLYING A RUBBER DAM—*cont'd*

STEPS—*cont'd*	**RATIONALES**—*cont'd*
12. Select appropriate rubber dam retainer for anchor tooth (Figure 36-1). 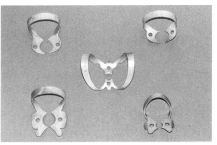 **Figure 36-1.** Rubber dam retainer variations: wingless molar retainers *(upper left and right),* winged premolar retainer *(lower right),* winged molar retainer *(lower left),* and anterior retainer *(center).*	A stable rubber dam requires the selection of a retainer that securely adapts to the tooth.
13. Tie approximately 18 inches of dental floss to retainer (Figure 36-2). Tie floss through lingual forceps hole, wrap it around the bow, and then tie it through facial forceps hole. 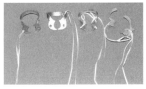 **Figure 36-2.** Retainer ligation progressing from lingual *(left)* to facial *(right),* and a broken ligated retainer at far right.	Ensures that both sides of the retainer are secured in event of retainer breakage (see Figure 36-2); permits operator to recover the retainer in event of dislodgment or breakage and prevents aspiration of retainer.
14. If using the "one-step" placement technique, fixate the anchor tooth hole over the retainer bow before placement in the oral cavity.	By carrying the retainer and rubber dam to the mouth in one piece, extra effort to stretch the rubber dam over the retainer is eliminated; risk of retainer going down the client's throat is minimized.
15. Seat the rubber dam and retainer on the anchor tooth with the rubber dam forceps.	Provides stabilization for rubber dam; secures rubber dam in place to expedite placement of remainder of dam.
16. Place rubber dam frame.	Removes edges of the rubber dam from isolation site.
17. Isolate remainder of teeth, working from front to back, through the holes; tease small amount of rubber dam at a time through tight contacts.	Provides an established regimen that provides for isolation of the easiest teeth first.
18. Pass floss through contacts using double floss technique to assist in sliding rubber dam material through proximal contacts (Figure 36-3). 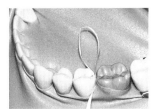 **Figure 36-3.** Dental floss is used to carry the septa between the teeth using the double flossing technique.	Facilitates faster rubber dam placement; enables movement of rubber dam through tight contacts.

(Continued)

Copyright © 2010 by Saunders, an imprint of Elsevier Inc. All rights reserved.

Procedure 36-1 | APPLYING A RUBBER DAM—*cont'd*

STEPS—*cont'd*	RATIONALES—*cont'd*
19. Invert rubber dam material when all teeth are completely isolated and rubber dam is between all contacts. (Several instruments can be used to invert, or tuck, the dam; however, the spoon excavator is the instrument of choice.) Use an air stream to support the inversion process. When the teeth are properly isolated, secure the floss safety ligature to the frame or remove (Figures 36-4 and 36-5).	Ensures a dry, isolated field. Prevents entangling in the handpiece and interfere with the operation. Removal of ligature is acceptable because risk of client swallowing the retainer after rubber dam is in place is minimal.

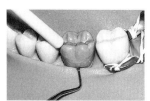

Figure 36-4.   The spoon excavator is supported by an air stream to invert the dam and create a seal.

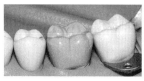

Figure 36-5.   A well-sealed, properly inverted rubber dam.

STEPS	RATIONALES
20. Center rubber dam frame on client's face, with the upper lip covered and nose revealed. If the nose is inadvertently covered, fold or cut the rubber dam at the top of frame to expose the nose. If the client is experiencing nasal congestion or difficulty in breathing through the nasal passage, cut an incision in the rubber dam away from the surgical site to allow air passage.	Facilitates access to the surgical site while still allowing the client to breathe comfortably.
21. Place saliva ejector under the rubber dam if client reports or exhibits signs of difficulty in swallowing.	Supports client's efforts to remove saliva from the oral cavity.

Copyright © 2010 by Saunders, an imprint of Elsevier Inc. All rights reserved.

Procedure 36-2 REMOVING A RUBBER DAM

EQUIPMENT
Personal protective equipment
Protective eyewear for client
Scissors
Rubber dam forceps
Dental floss or tape

STEPS	RATIONALES
1. Cut safety ligature, if still present. Replace beaks of the rubber dam forceps in the retainer forceps holes, and spread jaws of rubber dam retainer. Raise the facial jaw of the retainer over the contour of the tooth, then raise the lingual jaw (Figure 36-6) to remove the retainer.	Provides improved access to cut the septa.

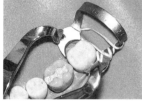

Figure 36-6.   The retainer is removed from the tooth with forceps.

STEPS	RATIONALES
2. Cut each septum between teeth with sharp, blunt scissors. On mandibular arch, stretch septa facially to improve access for cutting: place a finger under dam to protect oral tissues (Figure 36-7). On maxillary arch, stretch rubber dam lingually to improve access for cutting.	Expedites removal of the dam without concern for passage through contacts.

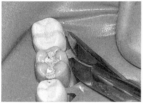

Figure 36-7.   Rubber dam is stretched, and septa are cut with scissors.

STEPS	RATIONALES
3. Remove dam and frame together.	Removal of parts at one time is done for efficiency.
4. Wipe client's lips to remove excess saliva and debris; rinse and evacuate the mouth.	Enhances client comfort.
5. Briefly massage client's facial muscles.	Relieves tension in the muscles from prolonged opening; clients appreciate the show of concern for comfort.
6. Examine rubber dam to ensure removal of all rubber dam fragments and septa (Figure 36-8).	If left between teeth, small fragments can produce discomfort, inflammation, and potential eventual tooth loss (see Figure 36-8).

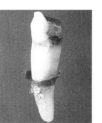

Figure 36-8.   Tooth lost to undetected band of rubber dam left after dental treatment.

STEPS	RATIONALES
7. Floss dental contacts to remove any dam fragments as necessary.	Done if necessary to remove fragments.

Copyright © 2010 by Saunders, an imprint of Elsevier Inc. All rights reserved.

Procedure 36-3 | PLACING A TOFFLEMIRE MATRIX SYSTEM

EQUIPMENT
Personal protective equipment
Protective eyewear for client
Tofflemire retainer
Matrix bands
Wooden wedges
Metal-cutting scissors
Cotton forceps
Modeling compound
Burnishing instrument
Tofflemire matrix system

STEPS	RATIONALES
1. Evaluate the prepared tooth.	Create a mental picture to aid in selection of a matrix band.
2. Select a matrix band that best encloses all lateral aspects of the cavity and extends 1 to 2 mm above the adjacent marginal ridge and 1 mm beyond the gingival margin.	Simplifies the procedure: Class II cavities that have short proximal boxes can be enclosed with a standard band, tall proximal boxes may require a band with gingival extensions, and a single tall box may need a band with one gingival extension.
	All gingival margins must be sealed against the band; band must extend occlusally high enough to enclose missing ridges and cusps.
3. Select a matrix retainer.	The contra-angle Tofflemire retainer fits most situations; design allows it to be positioned from the lingual side if necessary.
	The straight Tofflemire retainer is usually limited to facial applications.
4. Loop band in fingers so that ends match. The convergent opening (smaller) of the loop should be positioned next to the gingiva (rubber dam) (Figure 36-9).	Convergent opening is smaller and matches the converging area of the crown (cementoenamel junction [CEJ]).

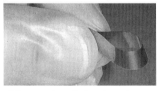

Figure 36-9. The ends of the band are placed evenly together to form a loop. The loop is tapered to permit adaptation at the gingival aspect.

5. Position locking vise approximately ¼ inch from end of retainer and free locking screw (spindle) from band slot in the locking vise (Figure 36-10).	Prepares the retainer to receive the matrix band.

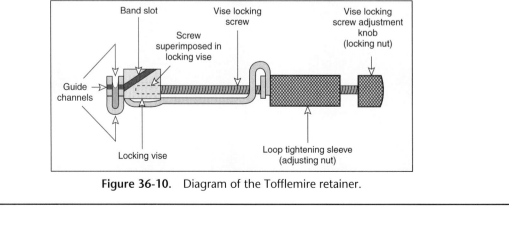

Figure 36-10.   Diagram of the Tofflemire retainer.

Copyright © 2010 by Saunders, an imprint of Elsevier Inc. All rights reserved.

Procedure 36-3   PLACING A TOFFLEMIRE MATRIX SYSTEM—*cont'd*

STEPS—*cont'd*	RATIONALES—*cont'd*
6. Position loop in retainer (leading with the occlusal edge of the band); insert matched ends into the slots in the locking vise and the loop into the appropriate guide channel. When positioned, the guide channels of the retainer open toward the gingiva. The loop of band should exit guide channel to allow the loop to be positioned from the preferred side of the tooth (usually the facial side). Assuming that the seated retainer will be most commonly positioned on the facial aspect of the prepared tooth, use left channel guide for dentition in the maxillary left and mandibular right; use right channel guide for dentition in the maxillary right and mandibular left. When inserting band into the retainer, first insert the wider occlusal aspect of the band so that the retainer is seated with the slots of the retainer toward the gingiva (Figure 36-11).	Allows the Tofflemire to be lifted occlusally when the matrix is being disassembled. If the Tofflemire is inverted (guide channels open occlusally), the retainer is trapped because it cannot be removed in a gingival direction. If this happens, the locking screw must be loosened and the Tofflemire totally removed before the band can be removed.

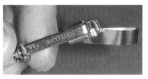

Figure 36-11. Initial placement of band in retainer slot with occlusal aspect of loop being inserted first.

7. Secure matrix band by advancing the locking screw (smaller nut) (Figure 36-12).	The band must be secured in the retainer or it may loosen during condensation, ruining the restoration.

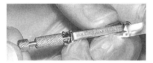

Figure 36-12. The locking nut is tightened to secure the band in the retainer.

8. Shape matrix loop into a rounded form: (1) insert an instrument handle through the loop, (2) pinch the band between the instrument handle and your thumb, and (3) rotate your wrist as you pinch the band (Figure 36-13).	The opened loop slips over the tooth easily.

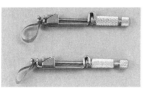

Figure 36-13. Inserted band before shaping *(bottom)* and band shaped to rounded form to facilitate placement *(top)*.

9. Position loop around tooth with slots of the Tofflemire and narrow aspect of band toward the gingiva (Figure 36-14); brace lingual aspect of loop with thumb of opposite hand; gently tighten band by rotating the adjusting nut (larger nut).	Adapts the band against the lingual aspect of the tooth. Extreme tightening of the band tends to pull it away from adjacent teeth, which could result in open proximal contacts.

(Continued)

Copyright © 2010 by Saunders, an imprint of Elsevier Inc. All rights reserved.

Procedure 36-3	PLACING A TOFFLEMIRE MATRIX SYSTEM—*cont'd*

STEPS—*cont'd* | **RATIONALES—*cont'd***

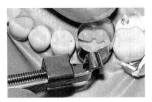

Figure 36-14. Initial placement of band over prepared tooth. Finger pressure supports lingual aspect of band.

Examine placement of band to ensure that band extends occlusally 1 to 2 mm beyond the adjacent marginal ridge; it should also extend apically approximately 1 mm beyond the gingival margin without impinging on soft tissue.

10. Moisten wedge(s) and place into the lingual embrasure between band and adjacent tooth, slightly beyond the gingival margin (Figure 36-15). Apply steady pressure on base of the wedge to move it in a facial direction to desired position (Figure 36-16). Numerous pretrimmed wedges are available for selection.

Moisture lubricates the wedge so that it is easier to position, will not stick to the rubber dam, and remains securely in place. Wedge(s) adapt the band at the gingival margin(s); wedge should not encroach on the proximal contact area, because an open contact may result, or proximal surface will be undercontoured (these defects could result in food impaction and gingival irritation).

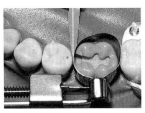

Figure 36-15. Wedge is inserted into lingual embrasure between band and adjacent tooth using cotton forceps.

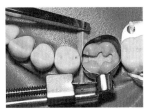

Figure 36-16. The handle of the cotton forceps is used to firmly position the wedge.

Copyright © 2010 by Saunders, an imprint of Elsevier Inc. All rights reserved.

Procedure 36-3	PLACING A TOFFLEMIRE MATRIX SYSTEM—*cont'd*
STEPS—*cont'd*	**RATIONALES**—*cont'd*

11. Burnish internal aspect of band against the adjacent tooth (or teeth) with a thin, rigid instrument (Figure 36-17).

Facilitates achieving proximal contact(s) and proper proximal contour in the final restoration.

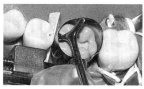

Figure 36-17.   The band is firmly burnished against the adjacent tooth.

12. Conduct a final evaluation of cavity preparation with matrix system in place (Figure 36-18).

This evaluation verifies that the preparation for a high-quality restoration has been completed.

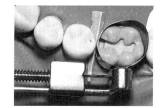

Figure 36-18.   Final preparation and matrix system.

Copyright © 2010 by Saunders, an imprint of Elsevier Inc. All rights reserved.

Procedure 36-4 PLACING AN AMALGAM RESTORATION

EQUIPMENT
Personal protective equipment
Protective eyewear for client
Isolation materials
Triturator
Amalgam well
Amalgam carrier
Amalgam capsules
Condensing instruments
Tofflemire matrix system
Carving and burnishing instruments
Articulating paper

STEPS	RATIONALES
1. Pretest access to cavity by holding condenser nibs in confined areas of preparation to verify accurate condenser selection.	Condensers that are too large cannot adapt the amalgam to the internal aspects of the cavity.
2. Adjust triturator settings for speed and time of mix, according to manufacturer's recommendations.	Triturators vary in speeds; amalgam alloys also vary in composition and mixing requirements.
3. Secure amalgam capsule in triturator locking device; close protective lid.	If not securely placed, capsule may be propelled from the locking device, injuring someone or breaking open.
4. Mix amalgam, then remove capsule; open it over a catch tray and dispense mix into the amalgam well.	Tray catches loose fragments of amalgam; on occasion, amalgamation may not occur and free mercury could spill out when the capsule is opened.
5. Examine mixed amalgam; note time, or set a timer for 3 minutes.	Amalgam should be a soft, round, shiny ball of material. A dry, crumbly mix or a >3-minute-old mix should be placed in scrap container and a new mix prepared. Old amalgam cannot be properly condensed and will not produce a homogeneous mass.
6. Load small end of amalgam carrier; dispense a portion into the most confined area of the preparation (Figure 36-19).	Produces voids in critical parts of the restoration, which invite leakage, sensitivity, and recurrent caries.

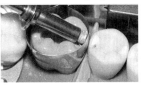

Figure 36-19.   A small increment of amalgam is expressed into the proximal box of the cavity preparation.

7. Using small condensers and a stable hand position, firmly adapt the amalgam into all internal cavity features and over margins (Figure 36-20).	Firm pressure with smaller condensers is less likely to produce voids in confined areas. Firm condensation adapts material intimately to cavity walls, eliminates voids, and expresses excess mercury from the mass.

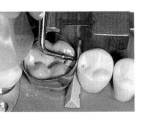

Figure 36-20.   Initial condensation is begun with a small condenser in the proximal box.

8. Continue to add increments; gradually increase condenser size; remove any "mercury-rich" surface by lateral scooping motions of the condenser nib.	Expresses mercury; its removal creates a dense, more durable restoration.
9. Triturate fresh amalgam as needed; continue to add increments and condense, to build a moderate excess over cavity margins (Figures 36-21 and 36-22).	Larger cavities may require several mixes; if mix begins to harden, discard it. Overpacking ensures coverage of all margins and, when the material is heavily burnished, draws excess mercury to the surface so it can be carved away.

Copyright © 2010 by Saunders, an imprint of Elsevier Inc. All rights reserved.

| Procedure 36-4 | PLACING AN AMALGAM RESTORATION—*cont'd* |

STEPS—*cont'd*	RATIONALES—*cont'd*

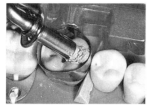

Figure 36-21. Additional increments of amalgam are carried to the cavity preparation.

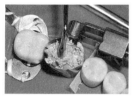

Figure 36-22. The cavity is overfilled with amalgam, and a large condenser is used to complete condensation.

10. Rub and grossly shape the occlusal surface with a few firm strokes using a large ball or egg-shaped burnisher (Figure 36-23).

Excess mercury is brought to the surface for easy removal.

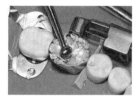

Figure 36-23. Burnishing of the overpacked amalgam.

11. Carve and suction away excess amalgam.

Removal of mercury-rich amalgam leaves a dense, durable alloy.

12. Establish marginal ridge height and outer contours next to matrix band by carving with an explorer or similar fine, sharp instrument. Excess amalgam is rapidly carved away, and occlusal margins recovered (Figures 36-24 to 36-26).

Marginal ridge contours, the most difficult to form, should be shaped while amalgam is carvable with matrix in place.

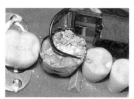

Figure 36-24. Marginal ridge height and outer contours are established with an explorer.

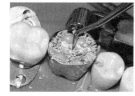

Figure 36-25. Excess amalgam is removed with a carver.

(Continued)

Copyright © 2010 by Saunders, an imprint of Elsevier Inc. All rights reserved.

Procedure **36-4**	PLACING AN AMALGAM RESTORATION—*cont'd*

STEPS—*cont'd*	**RATIONALES**—*cont'd*

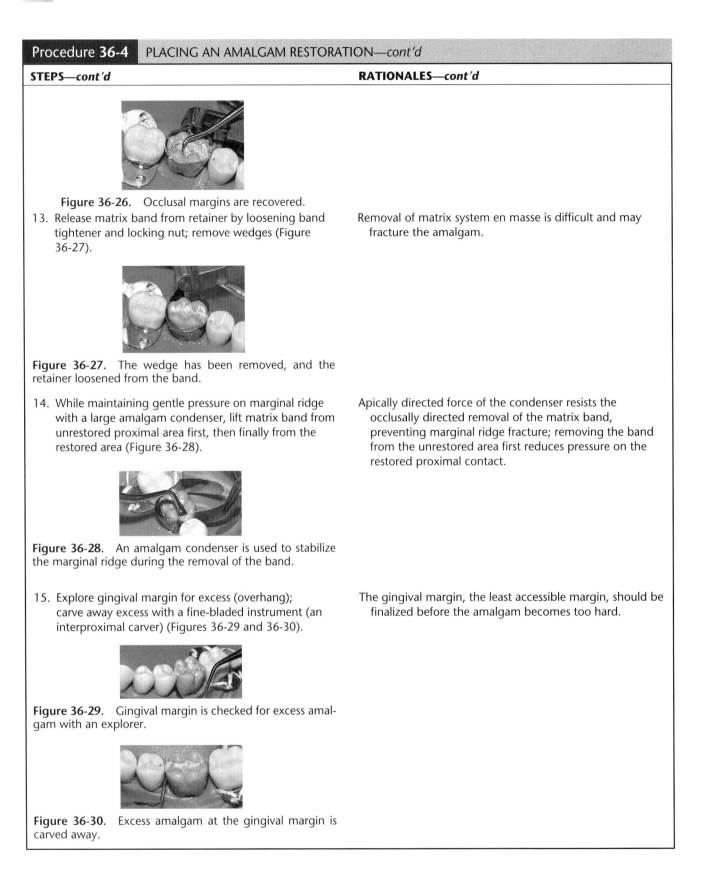

Figure 36-26. Occlusal margins are recovered.

13. Release matrix band from retainer by loosening band tightener and locking nut; remove wedges (Figure 36-27).

Removal of matrix system en masse is difficult and may fracture the amalgam.

Figure 36-27. The wedge has been removed, and the retainer loosened from the band.

14. While maintaining gentle pressure on marginal ridge with a large amalgam condenser, lift matrix band from unrestored proximal area first, then finally from the restored area (Figure 36-28).

Apically directed force of the condenser resists the occlusally directed removal of the matrix band, preventing marginal ridge fracture; removing the band from the unrestored area first reduces pressure on the restored proximal contact.

Figure 36-28. An amalgam condenser is used to stabilize the marginal ridge during the removal of the band.

15. Explore gingival margin for excess (overhang); carve away excess with a fine-bladed instrument (an interproximal carver) (Figures 36-29 and 36-30).

The gingival margin, the least accessible margin, should be finalized before the amalgam becomes too hard.

Figure 36-29. Gingival margin is checked for excess amalgam with an explorer.

Figure 36-30. Excess amalgam at the gingival margin is carved away.

Copyright © 2010 by Saunders, an imprint of Elsevier Inc. All rights reserved.

Procedure 36-4 | PLACING AN AMALGAM RESTORATION—*cont'd*

STEPS—*cont'd* | **RATIONALES**—*cont'd*

16. Carve proximal and outer contours to final form. Re-cover all margins. At margins, all cutting strokes should be directed parallel to margins to maintain a seal and avoid overcarving.

Steep anatomy in amalgam leads to marginal breakdown.

Tooth surface is used as a guide by resting the carving edge on it as shaving strokes are made. Carve occlusal anatomy to general form, keeping pits and grooves shallow (Figure 36-31).

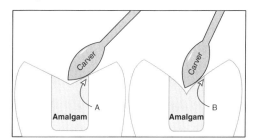

Figure 36-31. Amalgam anatomy should be carved to shallow form whenever possible. Doing so produces stronger margins *(A)*. Thin angles seen in *B* will eventually fracture from occlusal stress.

17. Remove rubber dam; caution client against biting at this time.

Inadvertent biting may fracture amalgam because occlusal surface has not yet been refined.

18. Wipe client's lips; suction mouth to remove saliva; isolate operating site with cotton rolls.

Occlusal marking ribbon (articulation paper) does not mark well on wet surfaces.

19. Insert articulating paper over area and have client "gently tap back teeth together."

Forceful biting on fresh amalgam will cause fracture; tapping is done to examine centric occlusion.

20. Carve away marking spots on the amalgam until centric occlusion is reestablished as it was before the procedure; re-mark the occlusion as necessary, carving away high spots each time with a carver or round burr, if the amalgam has set up (Figure 36-32).

Centric occlusion is re-established by noting that wear facets on the remaining tooth structure as well as on adjacent and opposing teeth imprint even marks.

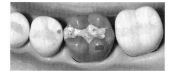

Figure 36-32. The occlusal markings show that the contact on amalgam, although present, is lighter than that on the natural tooth. As a result the operator does not need to further reduce the occlusal contact.

21. Insert ribbon and have client gently grind the back teeth; make sure the client moves teeth in all functional directions. Remove markings until presurgical contacts are restored.

Eccentric prematurities are removed.

22. Finalize carving and burnish carved amalgam to create smooth finish.

Creates a smooth finish that retains less oral biofilm and resists tarnish and corrosion.

Rinse and suction away all debris; caution client to avoid chewing on restored tooth for 24 hours.

Amalgam requires several hours to achieve its maximal hardness.

23. After putting client in an upright position, have client "tap-tap-tap" again, then look at the new restoration for shiny spots.

A shift from the prone position of the dental chair to an upright position can produce a different bite pattern because the mandible changes position.

Repeat procedure; have client grind the teeth for lateral movement.

Adjust high spots as necessary.

24. Caution client that discernible high spots should be adjusted to avoid fracture.

Client may later be aware of a high spot when local anesthesia has worn off.

Copyright © 2010 by Saunders, an imprint of Elsevier Inc. All rights reserved.

Procedure 36-5   FINISHING AND POLISHING AMALGAM RESTORATIONS

EQUIPMENT
Personal protective barriers
Isolation materials
Finishing burrs
Carving instruments
Handpiece
Rubber polishing cups and points (or flour of pumice and polishing powders)

STEPS	RATIONALES
1. Question client regarding occlusion and tooth sensitivity since restoration was placed.	Sensitivity may indicate premature centric and/or eccentric contacts; delay polishing for very sensitive teeth.
2. Explain value of polished versus unpolished restoration to the client.	Polished restoration resists oral biofilm retention, corrosion, and tarnish.
3. Examine amalgam for burnish marks; adjust occlusion as necessary with a round finishing burr.	Burnish marks indicate occlusal contacts; large areas and areas on inclines should be reduced, consistent with the client's natural occlusion.
4. Refine occlusal margins with a sharp discoid carver, drawn in shaving strokes parallel to margins (Figure 36-33).	Excess amalgam is shaved flush with the margins, preventing fracture; parallel strokes reduce the possibility of enamel microfractures and overcarving of the amalgam.

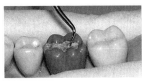

Figure 36-33. Using a stroke parallel to the margin, a sharp carver refines occlusal margins of the amalgam.

5. Using low-to-moderate speeds and intermittent brief strokes, polish amalgam with abrasive-impregnated rubber cups and points (Figures 36-34 and 36-35). Begin with most abrasive, end with least abrasive. Maintain wet field during polishing procedures; avoid overpolishing established occlusal contacts.	Minimizes heat caused by friction, which can create pulpal sensitivity and damage the amalgam restoration. Once proper occlusal contacts are established, they should be maintained.

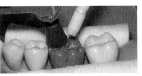

Figure 36-34. A rubber polishing cup is used to polish the marginal ridge and cusp slopes. An air stream is used as a coolant.

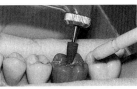

Figure 36-35. A rubber polishing point is used to polish pits and grooves.

6. Rinse mouth of debris.	Debris and excess saliva are annoying to the client.
7. Show client the polished restoration(s); reiterate value of the procedure (Figure 36-36). Record service.	Instills confidence; motivates client to take better oral care; demonstrates professionalism and pride in work. Accurate record keeping improves quality of care and protects practitioner from legal risks.

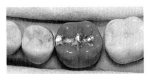

Figure 36-36. A polished amalgam.

Copyright © 2010 by Saunders, an imprint of Elsevier Inc. All rights reserved.

Procedure 36-6 PLACING AND FINISHING A RESIN COMPOSITE RESTORATION

EQUIPMENT
Personal protective equipment
Protective eyewear for client
Isolation materials
Glass ionomer cavity liner or sealer as needed
Conditioning agent (acid gel)
Priming agent
Bonding resin
Resin composite
Resin surface coating
Matrix system
Dispensing syringe
Curing light and protective shields
Plastic instruments
Finishing burrs and disks
Articulating paper

STEPS	RATIONALES
1. Query client regarding expectations; explain nature of resin composites.	Resin composites may stain and fracture, resulting in need for replacement in time; shades may not be perfect.
2. Select composite shade, place small amount of material on the tooth near the lesion and cure it; involve client in shade selection.	Cured resin may have a slight shade difference from the shade guide (one to two shades). Client preapproval is always a good idea, especially where esthetics is concerned.
3. Place rubber dam.	A dry operating field is essential.
4. After cavity preparation, apply cavity liner, sealer, and/or base as needed.	Protects pulp from undue irritation caused by the procedure.
5. Position a clear, plastic matrix strip between the preparation and the adjacent tooth.	Prevents acid from etching the adjacent tooth surface.
6. Dry tooth and apply etchant to the entire cavity surface according to manufacturer's instructions. Rinse with an air-water spray for at least 15 seconds; dry with forced-air drying. Reposition matrix as necessary; position a wedge interproximally.	Enamel etching is the primary retentive feature of most resin composite cavity preparations. Times vary from 10 to 60 seconds. The wedge stabilizes the matrix and adapts it to the gingival margin, preventing overhangs.
7. Inspect the peripheral etched pattern.	Chalky appearance over the entire bevel and enamel surface identifies adequate etching; if not present, repeat etching procedure.
8. Apply thin coats of primer to etched surfaces according to manufacturer's instructions, and lightly dry.	Some systems combine etchant and primer, others combine the primer and bonding agent or all three agents, and others keep all separate. Following manufacturer's instructions is mandatory to achieve maximum bonding.
9. Apply a thin coat of bonding resin to primed surface; spread resin over etched enamel with a small brush or sponge and a gentle stream of air (Figure 36-37).	Fluid resin flows into minute enamel irregularities. The stream of air evenly spreads resin over the preparation, prevents pooling of resin, and ensures a more uniform coating.

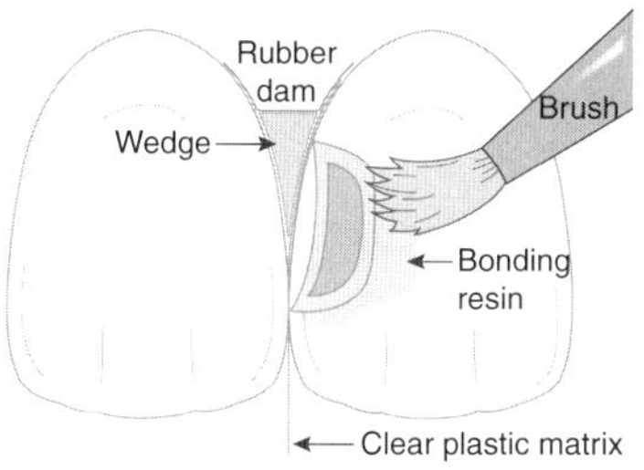

Figure 36-37. The etched enamel receiving a coating of bonding resin. A matrix separates the cavity from the adjacent tooth and is contoured and stabilized by a wedge placed interproximally.

(Continued)

Copyright © 2010 by Saunders, an imprint of Elsevier Inc. All rights reserved.

Procedure 36-6 | PLACING AND FINISHING A RESIN COMPOSITE RESTORATION—*cont'd*

STEPS—*cont'd*	**RATIONALES**—*cont'd*
10. Place special protective eyeshield on operator, assistant, and client to avoid eye damage during the curing that is about to start.	Protects eyes from damaging effects of curing light.
11. Polymerize bonding resin with curing light for 15 to 20 seconds; light wand should be as close as possible without direct contact. Careful inspection of cured bonding resin will reveal a slightly tacky surface. This very thin layer of resin is unable to completely polymerize because of the influence of air. It will rapidly polymerize once covered by resin composite or a matrix strip and reexposed to the curing light.	Establishes bond of resin composite to enamel. For systems using separate steps, light-curing is not done until application of bonding resin. For systems combining primer with bonding resin, curing is done after placement. Surface layer, called the *air-inhibited layer,* responsible for facilitating bonding to resin composite restorative material.
12. Remove cap from resin composite dispensing device; express small amount of selected resin composite onto a small paper pad; replace cap. Many systems are pre-encapsulated.	Pad is convenient for loading the placing instrument, can be covered with an opaque lid to protect resin from sunlight; replacing cap prevents material in dispenser device from polymerizing.
13. With a plastic instrument, or pre-encapsulated mixture placed in dispensing gun, place increment of resin (no more than 2 mm thick) in preparation; adapt to walls and margins; cure this first increment for 20 to 30 seconds (Figure 36-38).	Eliminates voids; enhances retention and marginal seal; larger increments and dark shades of composite require longer curing times to ensure penetration of light waves.

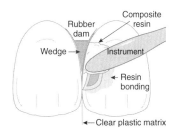

Figure 36-38. Placement of increments of resin composite into the preparation. The resin must be adapted into the recesses of the cavity and built against the matrix and cavity walls.

14. Continue to add and cure increments, building form to a slight excess in contour. In small cavities final form may be achieved by firmly wrapping clear matrix against tooth and curing through it (Figure 36-39); remove wedge and matrix.	Allows finishing without leading to undercontouring.

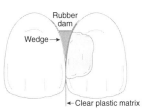

Figure 36-39. Cavity filled to slight excess, cured, and prepared for finishing.

Copyright © 2010 by Saunders, an imprint of Elsevier Inc. All rights reserved.

Procedure **36-6** | PLACING AND FINISHING A RESIN COMPOSITE RESTORATION—*cont'd*

STEPS—*cont'd*	**RATIONALES**—*cont'd*
15. Contour restoration with finishing burrs and disks, exercising care to avoid tooth damage (Figures 36-40 and 36-41).	Avoids removal of tooth structure.

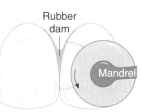

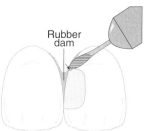

Figure 36-40.   Contouring the resin composite with a disk to achieve the final form. The wedge and matrix have been removed.

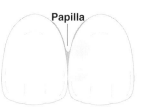

Figure 36-41.   Damage to the tooth structure occurs if due caution is not exercised with the use of a burr in the finishing procedure.

16. Remove rubber dam and check for occlusal prematurities on restoration. Lingual high spots can be carefully reduced with a large, round finishing burr or a football-shaped fine diamond.

In particular, lingual aspects of maxillary Class III restorations may require occlusal adjustment.

17. Polish accessible parts of restoration with polishing disks; examine gingival sulcus and remove debris.

Enhances oral hygiene and reduces biofilm accumulation.

18. Condition restoration surface with conditioning agent.

Cleans and prepares surface for final resin surface coating.

19. Apply resin surface coating with a cotton pellet or foam applicator; cure for 10 seconds.

Resin surface coating fills any rough surfaces or voids in resin composite.

20. Show client restoration; explain shade discrepancies (Figure 36-42). Record service.

Dried isolated teeth appear lighter; blending with the new resin restoration.

Accurate record keeping improves quality of care and protects practitioner from legal risks.

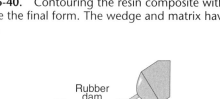

Figure 36-42.   Finished Class III resin composite restoration.

Copyright © 2010 by Saunders, an imprint of Elsevier Inc. All rights reserved.

Procedure 36-7	PLACING A RESIN-MODIFIED GLASS IONOMER (RMGI) CEMENT RESTORATION OF CLASS V ABRASION LESIONS

EQUIPMENT
Personal protective equipment
Protective eyewear for client
Isolation materials
RMGI
Polyacrylic acid/conditioner
Flour of pumice
Polishing cup
Plastic instruments
Carving instrument
Bonding resin
Special protective varnish
Curing light and protective shields
Matrix system

STEPS	RATIONALES
1. Examine lesions; assess need for local anesthetic agent.	Treatment of nonsensitive, easily accessed, noncarious lesions that are easily accessible may not require an anesthetic agent.
2. Select shade of restorative material to be used; involve client in selection.	Client preapproval is always a good idea, especially where esthetics are concerned.
3. Place rubber dam.	Rubber dam is the best device to control contamination of cavity.
4. Briefly, debride cavity and adjacent tooth structure with nonfluoridated flour of pumice and water slurry in a rubber polishing cup; rinse thoroughly and dry.	Oral biofilm and debris compromise adherence of restorative material. Residual fluoride may inhibit or decrease bonding.
5. According to manufacturer's instructions, apply conditioner to abrasion lesion (approximately 15 seconds); rinse thoroughly for 15 seconds with a strong air-water spray, and dry lightly, ensuring a moist surface.	Brief exposure to polyacrylic acid removes microscopic debris (smear layer) without opening dentinal tubules; desiccation of dentin causes collapse of the tender collagen fibrils, decreasing bonding strength of cement. Cement is also very sensitive to moisture changes.
6. Mix glass ionomer according to manufacturer's directions or triturate pre-encapsulated RMGI (Figure 36-43).	Directions should be followed closely because powder/liquid ratios and mixing times are critical.

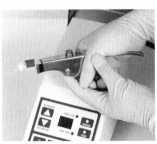

Figure 36-43. Glass ionomer products are supplied in various forms, including base and catalyst for hand mixing and triturated pre-encapsulated. (From Bird DL, Robinson DS: *Torres and Ehrlich modern dental assisting,* ed 9, St Louis, 2009, Saunders).

7. Rapidly fill cavity to slight excess, using a plastic instrument to place material (Figure 36-44); position cervical matrix over cavity to hold cement against tooth (Figure 36-45); light-cure per directions using protective shields.	Expeditious placement is important. Matrix prevents material from slumping or running out of cavity and from drying out and crazing as it hardens. Protects eye from damaging effects of curing light.

Copyright © 2010 by Saunders, an imprint of Elsevier Inc. All rights reserved.

Procedure 36-7	PLACING A RESIN-MODIFIED GLASS IONOMER (RMGI) CEMENT RESTORATION OF CLASS V ABRASION LESIONS—*cont'd*

STEPS—*cont'd*

RATIONALES—*cont'd*

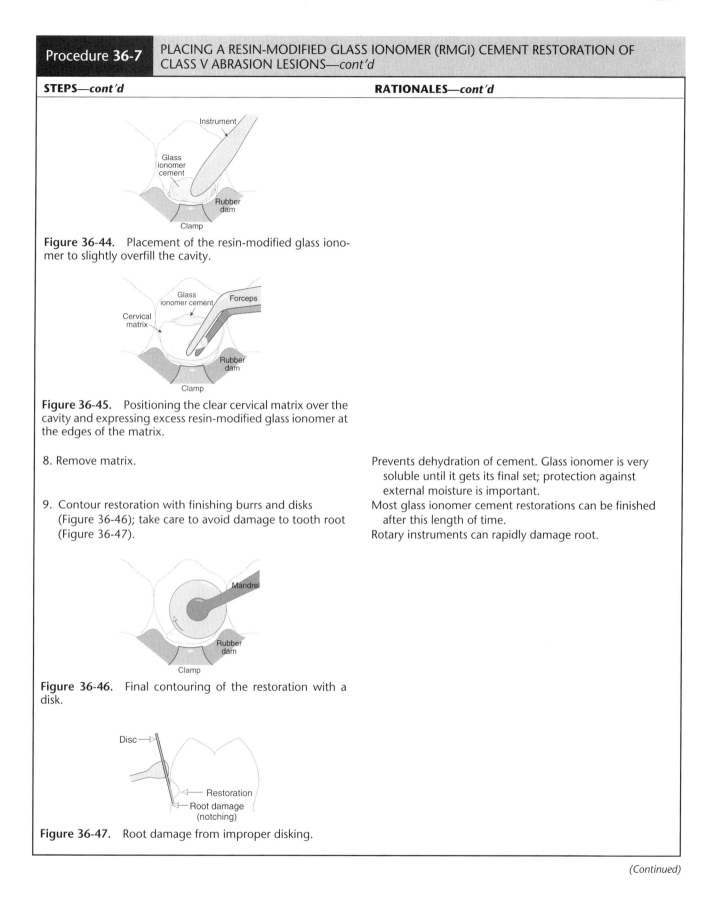

Figure 36-44. Placement of the resin-modified glass iono-mer to slightly overfill the cavity.

Figure 36-45. Positioning the clear cervical matrix over the cavity and expressing excess resin-modified glass ionomer at the edges of the matrix.

8. Remove matrix.

Prevents dehydration of cement. Glass ionomer is very soluble until it gets its final set; protection against external moisture is important.

9. Contour restoration with finishing burrs and disks (Figure 36-46); take care to avoid damage to tooth root (Figure 36-47).

Most glass ionomer cement restorations can be finished after this length of time.
Rotary instruments can rapidly damage root.

Figure 36-46. Final contouring of the restoration with a disk.

Figure 36-47. Root damage from improper disking.

(Continued)

Copyright © 2010 by Saunders, an imprint of Elsevier Inc. All rights reserved.

Procedure 36-7	PLACING A RESIN-MODIFIED GLASS IONOMER (RMGI) CEMENT RESTORATION OF CLASS V ABRASION LESIONS—*cont'd*

STEPS—*cont'd*	RATIONALES—*cont'd*
10. Apply thin coat of bonding resin to cement restoration surface and cure resin for 15 to 20 seconds.	Protect cement from excess moisture or drying for several hours.
11. Remove rubber dam; examine gingival sulcus and remove debris.	Cured bonding resin debris is very difficult to see because it is transparent.
12. Show final result to client (Figure 36-48). Record service.	Instills confidence; motivates client to better oral care; demonstrates professionalism and pride in work.
	Accurate record keeping improves quality of care and protects practitioner from legal risks.

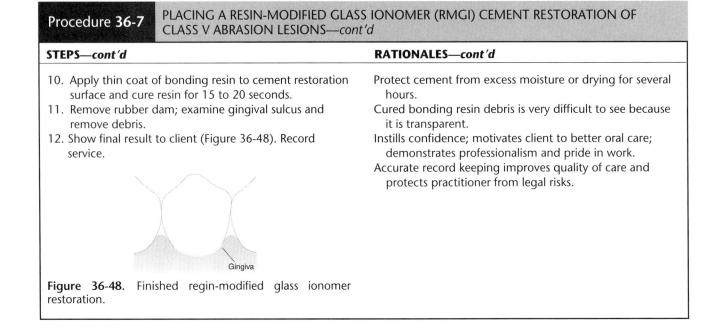
Gingiva

Figure 36-48. Finished regin-modified glass ionomer restoration.

Copyright © 2010 by Saunders, an imprint of Elsevier Inc. All rights reserved.

Procedure 36-8   RESTORING A CARIOUS LESION USING ATRAUMATIC RESTORATIVE THERAPY

EQUIPMENT
Cotton rolls, dry angles (dry aids)
Dental hatchet
Dental excavator
Cotton pellets
Glass ionomer conditioner
Glass ionomer restoration material (self-cure or light-cure)
Cotton tipped applicators
Petroleum jelly
Curing light
Articulating paper
Dental carver

STEPS	RATIONALES
1. Clean the tooth surface to be free of plaque.	Keeping the area plaque-free prevents the introduction of oral bacteria into the lesion.
2. Isolate the site as appropriate.	Cotton roll isolation may be sufficient.
3. Initiate the cavity preparation by using a dental hatchet to widen the entrance to the lesion (if necessary).	Some lesions may have only a small opening on the surface but a larger cavitated area just below the surface of the enamel.
4. Perform the cavity preparation using an excavator to remove the outer layer of carious dentin.	
5. Clean the cavity preparation with a wet cotton pellet, and dry with a cotton pellet.	A clean preparation will facilitate a successful restoration. Air-water syringes are often not available when using atraumatic restorative therapy (ART).
6. Apply conditioning liquid to prepare the dentin.	
7. Mix glass ionomer according manufacturer's instructions.	Several glass ionomer delivery systems are available.
8. Fill the preparation, keeping the applicator tip at the bottom of the preparation.	Keeping applicator tip at the bottom of the preparation will help avoid introduction of air into the glass ionomer.
9. Do not overfill.	Overfilling will require the cured restoration to be altered. ART is often performed without motorized handpieces.
10. Adapt the glass ionomer to the preparation using light pressure with a damp cotton-tipped applicator or a gloved finger coated in petroleum jelly.	Detailed anatomy is not needed.
11. Expose with a curing light for 30 seconds. If using self-cure glass ionomer, wait until material hardens.	Glass ionomer is available in light-cure and self-cure varieties.
12. Check the bite with articulating paper.	High spots will result in premature occlusion.
13. Remove excess material with a carver.	A carver is used because motorized instruments are not used for ART.
14. Advise client not to eat for 1 hour.	One hour ensures the self-cure glass ionomer will completely set.

From Frencken JE, van Amerongen E: Phantumvanit P, et al: *Manual for the atraumatic restorative treatment approach to control dental caries,* ed 3, Groningen, The Netherlands, 1997, World Health Organization Collaborating Centre for Oral Health Services Research.

Copyright © 2010 by Saunders, an imprint of Elsevier Inc. All rights reserved.

Procedure 36-9 | PLACING A STAINLESS STEEL CROWN

EQUIPMENT
Personal protective equipment
Protective eyewear for client
Isolation materials
Stainless steel preformed crowns
Crown trimming scissors
Crimping pliers
Resin-modified glass ionomer cement
Floss
Articulating paper

STEPS	RATIONALES
1. Evaluate prepared tooth for size.	Aids in the selection of the preformed crown.
2. Correct size is selected by measuring the mesiodistal width between contact points of a matching tooth in mouth.	
3. Choose smallest crown that will fit	If crown is too large, it will be time-consuming to adjust its size, and its retention will not be as good.
4. To seat, place crown lingually and adapt it over the occlusal and buccal aspects of prepared tooth.	Seat buccal aspect after the lingual aspect because visibility is better.
5. Use firm pressure to seat crown. May hear an audible click as it springs over gingival undercut area of preparation.	If the crown seats too easily, it is probably too big.
6. To evaluate fit, observe marginal gingiva. It will blanch somewhat with a well-fitting crown. If excess blanching is observed, crown will have to be trimmed.	
7. In a properly seated crown, margin should extend approximately 1 mm subgingivally. To trim crown, scribe a line where marginal gingival hits crown with an explorer.	Seating crown margin below gingival margin is desirable so susceptible tooth structure is not exposed.
8. Trim crown 1 mm below scribed line. Use crown scissors or an abrasive wheel to trim crown (Figure 36-49).	

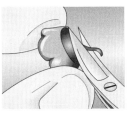

Figure 36-49.   Trim the margin of the crown with crown scissors.

9. Use crimping pliers to adapt edge of crown for a tighter fit (Figure 36-50).	Crimping pliers ensure a tight-fitting crown.

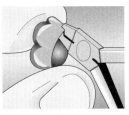

Figure 36-50.   Crimping pliers are used to adapt the margin of the crown.

Copyright © 2010 by Saunders, an imprint of Elsevier Inc. All rights reserved.

| Procedure 36-9 | PLACING A STAINLESS STEEL CROWN—*cont'd* |

STEPS—*cont'd*	RATIONALES—*cont'd*
10. Seat crown once more to evaluate fit.	
11. Crown is now ready to be cemented.	
12. Use resin-modified glass ionomer cement. Fill entire crown with cement (Figure 36-51).	Fluoride-releasing property of RMGI decreases caries risk.

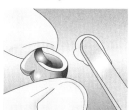

Figure 36-51. Overfill the crown with cement.

| 13. Excess cement will flow out from margins as crown is seated. | Stainless steel crowns are tight only at margin. If inadequate cement is used it will not flow out and may lead to early crown failure. |
| 14. Use an explorer, a scaler, and knotted floss to remove excess cement (Figure 36-52). | Removal of excess cement helps prevent gingival irritation. |

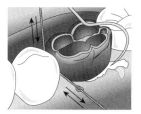

Figure 36-52. Use knotted floss and a scaler or explorer to remove excess cement after seating the crown.

15. Check occlusion using articulating paper.

Copyright © 2010 by Saunders, an imprint of Elsevier Inc. All rights reserved.

Procedure 36-10 | PLACING RETRACTION CORD

EQUIPMENT
Personal protective equipment
Protective eyewear for client
Examination kit (mouth mirror, explorer, periodontal probe, cotton pliers)
Dappen dish
Scissors
2 × 2 gauze
Cotton rolls or dry angles
Retraction cord hemostatic agent
Retraction cord of various sizes
Astringent and coagulation liquid

STEPS	RATIONALES
1. Estimate circumference of preparation; cut a piece of bottom cord (e.g., Deknatel No. 00, 0, 1, 2, or 3) to encompass preparation margins.	Ensures complete coverage of preparation with a single piece of bottom retraction cord. Cord size is dependent on status of gingival tissue.
2. Cut a piece of top cord that is approximately ½ inch longer than bottom cord and thicker in diameter. The top cord is longer and thicker than the bottom cord because it provides primary lateral tissue displacement necessary for satisfactorily allowing injection of impression material.	The top cord is longer and thicker than the bottom cord because it provides primary lateral tissue displacement necessary for satisfactory injection of impression material.
3. Soak bottom and top cords in hemostatic agent; place cord on a dry 2 × 2 gauze to remove excess solution.	Serves as a lubricant during placement of cord into sulcus, minimizing damage to friable gingival tissues. Hemostatic agent minimizes hemorrhagic seepage during impression procedure, which could distort final impression.
4. Isolate site with cotton rolls and/or dry angles.	Having a moist but not wet environment is critical to achieving necessary replication of tooth preparation margins.
5. Using bottom cord, lasso tooth with loop around lingual aspect of the tooth (Figure 36-53).	Cord approximates its ultimate location on the tooth and simplifies the placement process.

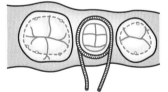

Figure 36-53.   Retraction cord looped around the lingual of the prepared tooth.

6. Start placement of bottom cord in one of the interproximal areas using a periodontal probe; while periodontal probe holds packed cord in place, side of the explorer rotates the cord into sulcus (Figure 36-54). Cord placement is achieved by gently rolling cord down tooth into the gingival sulcus and below gingival margin of the preparation (Figure 36-55). Avoid forceful apical pressure on cord.	Explorer offers excellent control; following along with periodontal probe to hold down the cord that has just been packed ensures a methodic retraction with minimal necessity to repack. Explorer easily locates the gingival margin of the preparation so the operator receives immediate feedback on whether cord is correctly placed apical to margin.

Copyright © 2010 by Saunders, an imprint of Elsevier Inc. All rights reserved.

Procedure 36-10 | PLACING RETRACTION CORD—*cont'd*

STEPS—*cont'd*

RATIONALES—*cont'd*

Other retraction instruments have rounded ends that encourage cord movement in wrong direction if not carefully monitored (see Figure 36-90).

Bottom cord remains in place during the impression procedure.

Excess apical pressure could traumatize tissue, causing bleeding and gingival recession.

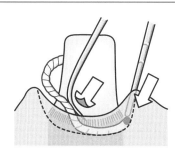

Figure 36-54. Periodontal probe holds packed cord in place while side of explorer rotates cord into place in the sulcus.

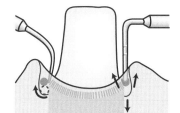

Figure 36-55. Explorer on left properly permits the cord to roll into place, but the round-ended instrument on the right permits the cord to improperly pop up on the sides.

7. Proceed in a methodic manner around the tooth, ending on the facial surface. Work from one end of cord to other; avoid skipping around.
   Excess cord should be cut at this point to avoid overlapping.

8. With bottom cord in place, take top cord and lasso tooth, with loop around the lingual aspect of tooth.

9. Start placement of top cord in one of the interproximal areas; proceed with placement technique described in steps 6 and 7. Depending on the gingival status, the top cord placement may not be below the gingival margin of the preparation. A small end of the top cord will extend out of the sulcus after it has been placed around circumference of tooth (Figure 36-56).

Ensures adequate placement of retraction cord.

Cord approximates its ultimate location on tooth and simplifies placement process.

Top cord removed before impression procedure.

Small end of top cord facilitates removal when impression material is ready for injection.

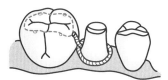

Figure 36-56. A small end of the top cord extends out of the sulcus.

Copyright © 2010 by Saunders, an imprint of Elsevier Inc. All rights reserved.

Procedure 36-11   PREPARING REINFORCED ZINC OXIDE AND EUGENOL TEMPORARY RESTORATIONS (CLASS II CAVITY PREPARATION)

EQUIPMENT

Personal protective equipment
Protective eyewear for client
Isolation materials
Tofflemire matrix system
Petrolatum
Reinforced zinc oxide and eugenol
Nonabsorbent mixing pad
Plastic instruments
Cotton pellets and rolls, dry aids
Finishing burrs
Carving instruments
Articulating paper

STEPS	RATIONALES
1. Isolate operating site as appropriate.	Isolation varies, depending on goals of therapy. Cotton roll isolation may be sufficient.
2. Prepare Tofflemire matrix system. Apply thin coat of petrolatum on the inside of the matrix band; position matrix, secure it, and place interproximal wedges as needed.	A matrix is useful to contain material in cavity preparation because walls are missing. Petrolatum prevents material from sticking to band. Excess material may be expressed into gingival sulcus if band is not supported interproximally.
3. Use manufacturer's instructions for measuring and mixing.	Products vary.
4. Prepare mix; when material reaches consistency of firm clay, carry an ample amount to cavity with a plastic instrument. Firmly adapt rubbery material to all walls of cavity with a placement instrument (Figures 36-57 and 36-58).	If material is too soft, it will not adapt well and it will stick to the instrument; if the material is too firm, it will not condense adequately, and voids and leakage may result.

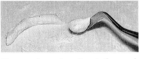

Figure 36-57.   Properly mixed reinforced zinc oxide with eugenol ready for placement.

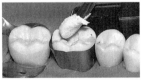

Figure 36-58.   Reinforced zinc oxide with eugenol being placed in cavity preparation.

STEPS	RATIONALES
5. Fill cavity to slight excess; shape occlusal anatomy by using a moist cotton pellet in cotton forceps to create a general anatomic form.	Excess material ensures margin coverage; moisture hastens set of zinc oxide–eugenol materials. Detailed anatomy is not needed.
6. When material has hardened, remove wedge(s), retainer, and matrix band; apply pressure apically on the temporary restoration to counteract removal of band.	Removing band before material has set may break marginal seal and dislodge temporary restoration.
7. Check proximal and gingival margins for excess material and remove with sharp, narrow-bladed carving instrument.	Excess material at gingival margins (overhang) could result in gingival irritation and hinder client's ability to maintain a plaque-free environment.

Copyright © 2010 by Saunders, an imprint of Elsevier Inc. All rights reserved.

Procedure 36-11	PREPARING REINFORCED ZINC OXIDE AND EUGENOL TEMPORARY RESTORATIONS (CLASS II CAVITY PREPARATION)—*cont'd*

STEPS—*cont'd*	RATIONALES—*cont'd*
8. Remove isolation materials; evaluate premature occlusion on temporary restoration with articulating paper and adjust as necessary with large, round burr and carving instruments (Figure 31-59). 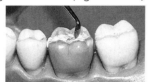 **Figure 36-59.** Final adjustment to the occlusal aspect of the temporary restoration with a carver.	Premature occlusion is very likely to fracture temporary restoration.
9. Examine gingival sulcus for debris and remove as necessary; excess material at gingival margin can be removed using a bladed instrument such as the ½ Hollenback or IPC carver.	Debris from restorative procedure can irritate the gingival tissues.

Please refer to the Evolve website (http://evolve.elsevier.com/Darby/hygiene) for competency forms to help evaluate your mastery of each procedure in this chapter.

Copyright © 2010 by Saunders, an imprint of Elsevier Inc. All rights reserved.

Behavior Management of Dental Fear and Anxiety

37

CHAPTER

Procedure 37-1	PREPARING THE CLIENT FOR RELAXATION THERAPY

The dental hygienist should not begin relaxation therapy without thoroughly explaining the process to the client and obtaining informed consent.

STEPS	RATIONALES
1. "If you would like to feel more relaxed during dental procedures, I can help you focus on feelings other than how tense you are."	Phrasing the concept permissively gives client control of the situation. Client must give informed consent to proceed with the relaxation therapy.
2. "It may help you feel better."	Positive phrasing contributes to the idea that clients will be helped if they participate.
3. "With your permission, I'll help you focus on how your muscles are feeling now and guide you into relaxation. Tension and relaxation cannot exist at the same time, so you will slowly become accustomed to feeling a warm heaviness in your arms and legs and a sense of well-being. You will be in control of yourself at all times."	Cooperation is needed for clients to be helped. If clients give their consent, you may proceed with the progressive relaxation. If they do not, you may offer other strategies. Explaining the process eliminates the fear of the unknown and validates clients' knowledge that they are in control of the experience.
4. "Several methods are perfectly suited for the dental situation. One focuses on mentally touching your muscles to target tension; one allows you to take a "mental vacation." Which one do you prefer?"	Explaining the different scenarios for relaxation allows the individual a choice.

Copyright © 2010 by Saunders, an imprint of Elsevier Inc. All rights reserved.

Procedure 37-2   TEACHING DEEP BREATHING TO A FEARFUL CLIENT

STEPS	RATIONALES
1. "I would like to share with you how to perform a deep breathing exercise to help you relax. Deep breathing floods the body with oxygen and other chemicals that work on your brain to help you relax. Would it be okay with you to take some time to show you how to do this exercise?"	Allows the client to understand the relationship between deep breathing and relaxation. Asking permission conveys respect and client control.
2. "Place your hands on your abdomen."	Allows the client to feel proper breathing from the diaphragm.
3. "Close your mouth, relax your shoulders, and inhale slowly and deeply through your nose to the count of six."	Walks the client through a deep breathing exercise to experience desired behavior.
4. "Push your abdomen out as you inhale as you allow the air to fill your diaphragm (the muscle between your abdomen and your chest)."	
5. "Pause for a second and exhale, slowly releasing the air through your mouth as you count to six and push out the tension that you feel."	
6. "Pause for a second, then repeat this exercise four or five times or until you feel more relaxed."	Allows the client to practice and experience relaxation.
7. "You are doing very well. Deep breathing is performed correctly when your abdomen (not your chest) moves with each breath."	Encourages the client and provides feedback.

Copyright © 2010 by Saunders, an imprint of Elsevier Inc. All rights reserved.

Procedure 37-3   GUIDED IMAGERY

STEPS	RATIONALES
1. "To begin, allow yourself to ease into a comfortable position in the chair."	Permits the client to move around and settle in before initiation of care.
2. "If you were able to go anywhere and do anything you choose to relax, where would you go and what would you do?"	Asks the client to become introspective and think about how he or she relaxes. Depending on response, the dental hygienist begins to construct a mental scene based on information offered by the client.
For purposes of this exercise, we will assume that the client verbalized enjoying lying in the sand at the beach.	
3. "You may find it easier to imagine the beach if you close your eyes to block out external sights, but that is entirely up to you. We will just talk quietly for a few minutes before doing any work."	Provides the client with the option of keeping the eyes open if mistrustful of closing them. Informs the client of what to expect.
4. "Picture in your mind's eye your favorite beach, what you're wearing, what you are sitting or lying on, and what the sand looks like."	Focuses the client's attention on visual cues of the beach. Since the client chose the scene, the client can begin constructing the setting. Most individuals are visually oriented, so these details are usually easy to imagine.
5. "Now look at the water. Notice what color it is and what the waves look like: their height, where they break, how far they roll up the beach toward you."	Deepens the client's attention on visual cues.
6. "Now feel the ocean breeze blow across your skin. Is it cool or warm, harsh or soft? Notice the sand now. Is it hot, warm, or cool? Is the sand powdery, coarse, or pebbly?"	Focuses the client's attention on the sense of temperature and touch.
7. "Try to pick up on the scents of the ocean: the salty tang in the air, the whiff of seaweed, the freshness of the breeze."	Focuses the client's attention on the sense of smell.
8. "Now look at the horizon and sky. Pick out a cloud if there are any present, and allow yourself to float as it is. Allow the breeze to carry you softly and safely until you feel like you're floating."	Deepens relaxation by suggesting a floating sensation.
9. "Now as you continue relaxing, allow yourself to become more and more a part of the scene, blending into the scene more and more with every breath. As you continue relaxing, I will begin my treatment. You may find your jaw slackens and your mouth opens while you stay just as deeply relaxed as you are now."	Deepens relaxation for mouth to open and for treatment to begin.

Copyright © 2010 by Saunders, an imprint of Elsevier Inc. All rights reserved.

Procedure 37-4   GUIDING THE CLIENT INTO PROGRESSIVE MUSCLE RELAXATION

STEPS	RATIONALES
1. Explain the process and gain informed consent (see Procedure 37-1). "All right, I am going to help you feel more relaxed by focusing on progressive muscle relaxation to reduce muscle tension. Your body cannot be physically relaxed and mentally anxious at the same time, so we will focus on relaxing each muscle group and then move to the next muscle group."	Conveys respect for the client.
2. "Let's begin by finding as comfortable a position as possible for you. Rest comfortably against the back of the chair, arms at your side, and let your hands rest comfortably on the armrests. Keep your legs separated with toes pointed slightly outward. Keep your head in line with your spine. Move until you feel at ease."	Promotes relaxation.
3. "If you would like to close your eyes, feel free. If you would rather keep them open, that's fine, too."	Promotes client autonomy.
4. "Take a deep breath. Feel your stomach and chest slowly rise…. Relax…. Now breathe out slowly… slowly…and relax. Count to 6, inhaling on 1, 2, and 3, exhaling on 4, 5, and 6…continue to breathe slowly…. Your body is beginning to relax…. Think *relax*…. Feel the parts of your body…. Notice any tension in your muscles…. Continue to breath slowly…and relax."	Teaches the client proper technique.
5. "As you settle back into the chair, in your mind's eye, focus on your feet as they rest against the chair. Curl your toes up and out. Now allow them to become warm and relaxed. Allow them to feel limp and heavy…. Good! Notice how your feet feel. Think *relax*."	Promotes relaxation.
6. "Now bend your ankles so that your toes point toward the ceiling. Notice any tension in your lower legs. Relax your lower legs. Repeat. Feel your body relaxing."	
7. "You are doing very well. Now squeeze your knees together and relax. Notice how the muscle feels when you relax."	Reinforces desired behavior.
8. "Now tighten your stomach muscles and then relax them. Feel calm. Breathe in warmth and relaxation."	Promotes relaxation of the stomach.
9. "Concentrate on any tension in your shoulders. Try to make your shoulders touch. Relax. Feel your body relaxing."	Promotes relaxation of the shoulders.
10. "You're doing very, very well. Now focus on any tension in your hands. Notice how it feels. Make a fist, a tight fist. As you begin to exhale, relax your fist…. Good! Now notice how your hand feels. Think *relax*. Your hands feel warm, heavy or light…. Just relax more…and more."	Promotes relaxation of hands and feet and allows the client to relate to the experience of progressive muscle relaxation.
11. "Now focus on your forearms…. Notice any tension…. Relax your arms…. Feel your body relaxing. Let the feelings of relaxation spread from your fingers and hands through the muscles of your arms."	Promotes relaxation of the arms.
12. "Gently touch your right ear to your right shoulder. Feel the pull in the back of your neck. Relax. Now gently touch your left ear to your left shoulder. Again feel the pull in the back of your neck. Now relax…. Feel your body relaxing."	Promotes relaxation of the neck.

(Continued)

Copyright © 2010 by Saunders, an imprint of Elsevier Inc. All rights reserved.

Procedure 37-4	GUIDING THE CLIENT INTO PROGRESSIVE MUSCLE RELAXATION—*cont'd*
STEPS—*cont'd*	**RATIONALES—*cont'd***
13. "Now concentrate on your face…your jaws. Notice any tightness…. Raise your eyebrows and relax. Breathe in warmth and relaxation…. Close your eyes tightly and then relax them, feeling the tension leave your face. Now relax your face. Notice how it feels when your muscles are relaxed."	Promotes relaxation of the face.
14. "You did very well. Now permit your jaw to slack so that I can look in your mouth. Please continue relaxing and softening your muscles as I begin to work. If you want me to stop for any reason just raise your hand, and I will stop immediately. Allow the feeling of muscle relaxation to intensify the longer we work. All is well."	Promotes relaxation of the lower jaw and mouth. Reinforces client control and autonomy.

Adapted from Potter PA, Perry AG: *Fundamentals of nursing,* ed 7, St Louis, 2009, Mosby.

Copyright © 2010 by Saunders, an imprint of Elsevier Inc. All rights reserved.

Procedure 37-5 | GUIDING THE CLIENT INTO PROGRESSIVE RELAXATION

STEPS	RATIONALES
1. "Rest comfortably against the back of your chair; let your hands rest in your lap or on the armrests."	Helps clients focus on how their body feels; begins introspection.
2. "If you would like to close your eyes, feel free. If you'd rather keep them open, that's fine, too."	Gives clients control over how the experience will begin.
3. "As you settle back into the chair, in your mind's eye, focus on your feet as they rest against the chair."	Heightened awareness of the feet moves attention from the dental procedures.
4. "Try to feel every muscle. Feel each toe. Feel the way your shoes cradle and hold your feet securely. Allow them to become warm and relaxed. Allow them to feel limp and heavy."	Suggesting feelings and sensations helps the client to create the relaxation.
5. "Now allow that feeling of limp, heavy warmth to move up into your calves and lower legs. Just let them feel like cooked spaghetti noodles (or other similar metaphors)."	Working from the extremities confines the sensation and gives clients a chance to develop deeper levels of relaxation so that when the head and inner organs are approached, the phenomenon is noticeable.
6. "And now let the feeling of loose, limp relaxation move into your hips and lower back. Allow yourself to be supported by the chair. Let it push against you to hold you in calm quietness."	Constant use of metaphors provides cues of how clients should feel. Reinforcement of the relaxed state should happen frequently.
7. "As the calmness flows up your back, vertebra by vertebra can soften and ease into the chair, to be cradled and supported as you go even deeper into relaxation."	"Softening" the back reinforces the suggestion that relaxation cannot coexist with tension.
8. "Allow that limp, warm relaxation to flow up into and across your shoulders. Go deeper and deeper into relaxation with every breath."	Suggestions allow clients to feel more profound relaxation and sense of well-being as additional muscle groups are targeted.
9. "Now let the feeling of warm, limp muscles ease up the back of your neck into the base of your skull. Let your head rest comfortably into the headrest."	Same as above.
10. "As your head and neck rest even more deeply into the chair, allow that sense of tranquility to ease into your scalp and forehead. Allow your jaw to slacken and your tongue to relax. You may notice that your eyelids are getting heavier and heavier as you breathe evenly and deeply."	Same as above. Using verbiage phrased permissively, such as "you may notice," not only guides the attention of the subjects but also suggests in an optional manner how they might feel.
11. "Now turn your attention inward to your heart, diaphragm, stomach, and intestines. Your brain is able to tell your organs to slow down, to become smooth, calm, and stress-free yet retain healthy functioning."	Using many synonyms allows a choice of words to cue the subjects. Wording for one subject may not work for another.
12. "Just take a few moments now to scan your body for any pockets of tension. Your brain knows what to do to find them. Focus on them now and allow warmth and relaxation to soften and release them. Breathe out the tension. Get rid of it and become even more peaceful, tranquil, warm, and cozy, feeling more relaxed than you ever thought possible."	The last suggestion acknowledges that the first pass over the body may not have relieved all of the tension. Clients may now return to be certain or continue deepening their state of relaxation. The scanning of the body for residual tension should take 30 to 60 seconds.
13. "Now, if you could stay that relaxed and keep scanning your body, permit your jaw to slacken so that I can look in your mouth."	The suggestion for clients to open the mouth is combined with jaw relaxation as a transition into treatment.
14. "You're doing very, very well. Please continue relaxing and softening as we begin to work. Allow that feeling of well-being to intensify the longer we work. You're doing so well."	Always reinforce any positive behavior to encourage its continuance.

Copyright © 2010 by Saunders, an imprint of Elsevier Inc. All rights reserved.

Procedure 37-6 AWAKENING THE CLIENT AFTER RELAXATION THERAPY

STEPS	RATIONALES
1. "Now that we have completed treatment, I'd like for you to begin the process of coming back from relaxing so well."	Alerts the client that treatment is complete and the relaxation session is terminating.
2. "As you begin to waken, do so at your own pace. You may find that a few deep breaths will arouse you, with lots of oxygen getting to your body."	Deep breaths will arouse clients.
3. "When you are ready, you may open your eyes, feeling completely refreshed. Retain as much of the relaxation as you choose as you continue your day."	Permissive phrasing allows clients to pace their awakening and alerts them that they may feel more relaxed than when they began their appointment.

Please refer to the Evolve website (http://evolve.elsevier.com/Darby/hygiene) for competency forms to help evaluate your mastery of each procedure in this chapter.

Copyright © 2010 by Saunders, an imprint of Elsevier Inc. All rights reserved.

Dentinal Hypersensitivity Management

38

Procedure 38-1	ADMINISTRATION OF DESENSITIZING AGENTS

EQUIPMENT
Isolating materials (cotton rolls, gauze, or dry angles)
Cotton applicators
Dappen dish
Personal protective equipment
Desensitizing agent

STEPS	RATIONALES
1. Assemble armamentarium for desensitization.	Preparation results in less chair time and greater comfort for client.
2. Explain rationale, procedure, and limitations of desensitizing agent to client.	Dispels any confusion regarding consent, purpose, extent, duration, and consequences of treatment. Client is actively involved in decision making.
3. Identify sensitive sites requiring desensitization treatment.	Site-specific application of desensitizing agent is prudent and acceptable. Follow manufacturer directions.
4. Remove oral biofilm and debris from tooth surfaces before desensitizing agent is applied.	Allows for greater retention and effectiveness.
5. Isolate area with cotton rolls, and dry dentin surface by blotting with gauze.	Prevents flow and ingestion of product; maximizes uptake where needed.
6. Dispense desensitizing agent and apply according to manufacturer's instructions.	Different products require different application procedures. Note instructions for maximum effectiveness.
7. Evaluate treated areas for success; reapply if necessary.	Reapplication may be necessary to achieve adequate amounts of the active agent at specific sites in order to overcome pain threshold.
8. Discard materials according to infection control procedures.	Prevents cross-contamination.
9. Record treatment in services-rendered section of client record, including tooth number, region of treatment, agent used, and client response.	Manages legal risks and facilitates evaluation at next appointment.
10. Educate client about supplementary procedures for controlling sensitivity.	Prevents further incidences of hypersensitivity and manages the problem long term.

Please refer to the Evolve website (http://evolve.elsevier.com/Darby/hygiene) for competency forms to help evaluate your mastery of each procedure in this chapter.

Copyright © 2010 by Saunders, an imprint of Elsevier Inc. All rights reserved.

Local Anesthesia

Procedure 39-1	LOADING THE METALLIC OR PLASTIC CARTRIDGE-TYPE SYRINGE

EQUIPMENT
Personal protective equipment
Syringe
Needle
Gauze
Anesthetic cartridge
Topical anesthetic
Cotton-tip applicator
Hemostat or cotton pliers

STEPS	**RATIONALES**

1. Assemble armamentarium (Figure 39-1).

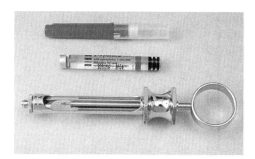

Figure 39-1. Armamentarium. From top: needle, cartridge, syringe. (From Malamed SF: *Handbook of local anesthesia,* ed 5, St Louis, 2004, Mosby.)

2. Remove the sterilized syringe from its container and inspect to ensure the harpoon is sharp and straight.   Ensures armamentarium is free of defects and in working order.
3. Retract the piston (Figure 39-2).   Allows room for the cartridge to fit into the syringe.

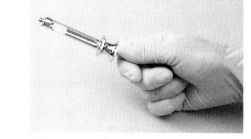

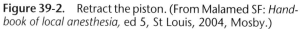

Figure 39-2. Retract the piston. (From Malamed SF: *Handbook of local anesthesia,* ed 5, St Louis, 2004, Mosby.)

Copyright © 2010 by Saunders, an imprint of Elsevier Inc. All rights reserved.

Procedure 39-1   LOADING THE METALLIC OR PLASTIC CARTRIDGE-TYPE SYRINGE—*cont'd*

STEPS—*cont'd*	RATIONALES—*cont'd*
4. Insert the cartridge (Figure 39-3).	Cartridge fits into the syringe without being damaged.

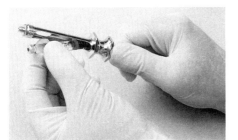

Figure 39-3.   Insert the cartridge. (From Malamed SF: *Handbook of local anesthesia,* ed 5, St Louis, 2004, Mosby.)

5. Engage the harpoon in plunger with gentle finger pressure (Figure 39-4)	Secures the cartridge in the barrel of the syringe.

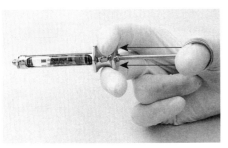

Figure 39-4.   Engage the harpoon in the plunger with gentle finger pressure. (From Malamed SF: *Handbook of local anesthesia,* ed 5, St Louis, 2004, Mosby.)

6. Do not exert forced on plunger; the glass may crack (Figure 39-5).	Too much force on the syringe may cause the cartridge glass to crack.

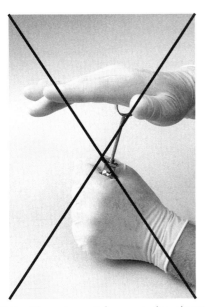

Figure 39-5.   Do not exert force on the plunger. (From Malamed SF: *Handbook of local anesthesia,* ed 5, St Louis, 2004, Mosby.)

(Continued)

Copyright © 2010 by Saunders, an imprint of Elsevier Inc. All rights reserved.

| Procedure 39-1 | LOADING THE METALLIC OR PLASTIC CARTRIDGE-TYPE SYRINGE—*cont'd* |

STEPS—*cont'd*

RATIONALES—*cont'd*

7. Remove the clear or white plastic protective shield that covers the syringe and cartridge end of the needle (Figure 39-6).

This removal of the plastic cap allows for the needle to be screwed onto the rubber diaphragm of the anesthetic cartridge.

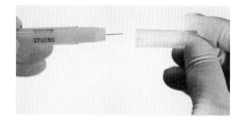

Figure 39-6. Remove the clear plastic protective cap from the opposite end of the colored plastic cap that hubs the needle.

8. Screw the colored plastic-hubbed needle onto the syringe while simultaneously pushing it into the metal needle adapter of the syringe *(arrow)* (Figure 39-7).

The plastic hub of the needle maintains the sterility of the needle and protects the clinician from a needle stick. Piercing the rubber diaphragm of the anesthetic cartridge ensures that anesthetic solution can be expelled from the cartridge.

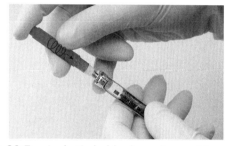

Figure 39-7. A plastic hubbed needle must be screwed onto the syringe while simultaneously being pushed into the metal needle adaptor of the syringe *(arrow)*. (From Malamed SF: *Handbook of local anesthesia,* ed 5, St Louis, 2004, Mosby.)

9. Directing the needle away from the body, keep the hand at the needle hub and loosen the colored plastic protective cap from the needle (Figure 39-8).

Facilitates removal of the colored plastic protective cap from the needle.

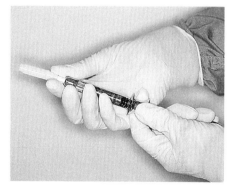

Figure 39-8. Directing the needle away from the body, keep the hand at the needle hub and loosen the colored plastic protective cap from the needle.

Copyright © 2010 by Saunders, an imprint of Elsevier Inc. All rights reserved.

Procedure 39-1   LOADING THE METALLIC OR PLASTIC CARTRIDGE-TYPE SYRINGE—*cont'd*

STEPS—*cont'd*	**RATIONALES—*cont'd***
10. Let the cap slide off the needle and onto a piece of sterile gauze (Figure 39-9).	Checks for needle sharpness to ensure an atraumatic insertion and withdrawal.

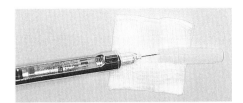

Figure 39-9.   Let the cap slide off the needle and onto a piece of sterile gauze.

11. Expel a few drops of solution to test for proper flow, and recap the needle using the scoop technique (Figure 39-10).	Ensures that the syringe, needle, and cartridge are properly prepared and functional.

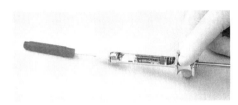

Figure 39-10.   "Scoop" technique for recapping needle after use. (From Malamed SF: *Handbook of local anesthesia,* ed 5, St Louis, 2004, Mosby.)

   a. Hold the syringe with one hand and glide the needle into the colored plastic cap lying on the instrument tray. Never attempt to hold cap with other hand because this may lead to an accidental needle stick exposure.
   b. Tilt the syringe upward to allow the cap to slide down to the hub and cover the needle. If the cap starts to slip off the needle, do not attempt to stop it with the other hand. Instead, let the cap fall on the instrument tray and begin the process again.

12. The syringe is now ready for use.	Keeps the needle in a sterile field and prevents needle stick exposure.

Copyright © 2010 by Saunders, an imprint of Elsevier Inc. All rights reserved.

Procedure 39-2   UNLOADING THE BREECH-LOADING METALLIC OR PLASTIC CARTRIDGE-TYPE SYRINGE

EQUIPMENT
See Procedure 39-1.

STEPS	**RATIONALES**
1. Retract the piston and pull the cartridge away from the needle with your thumb and forefinger as you retract the piston, until the harpoon disengages from the plunger (Figure 39-11).	Allows room for the cartridge to be disengaged from the syringe.

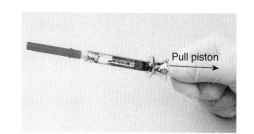

Pull piston

Figure 39-11. Retract the piston. (From Malamed SF: *Handbook of local anesthesia,* ed 5, St Louis, 2004, Mosby.)

2. Remove the cartridge from the syringe by inverting the syringe, permitting the cartridge to fall free (Figure 39-12).	Frees the cartridge from the barrel of the syringe.

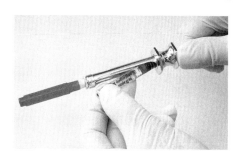

Figure 39-12. Remove the used cartridge. (From Malamed SF: *Handbook of local anesthesia,* ed 5, St Louis, 2004, Mosby.)

3. Carefully unscrew the recapped needle, being careful not to accidentally discard the metal needle adaptor (Figure 39-13).	Frees the needle from the syringe. Recapped needle protects the dental hygienist from needle stick exposure during needle removal and disposal.

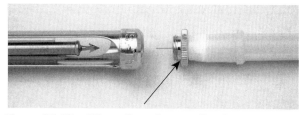

Figure 39-13. When discarding needle, check to be sure that the metal needle adaptor from the syringe is not inadvertently discarded too *(arrow).* (From Malamed SF: *Handbook of local anesthesia,* ed 5, St Louis, 2004, Mosby.)

Copyright © 2010 by Saunders, an imprint of Elsevier Inc. All rights reserved.

| Procedure **39-2** | UNLOADING THE BREECH-LOADING METALLIC OR PLASTIC CARTRIDGE-TYPE SYRINGE—*cont'd* |

STEPS—*cont'd*

4. Place the needle in a sharps container (Figure 39-14) and the cartridge in a separate sealed container (Figure 39-15).

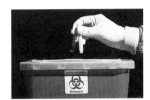

Figure 39-14. Used needles and cartridges are considered infectious. Sharps must be discarded in a rigid, puncture-proof, leak-resistant container.

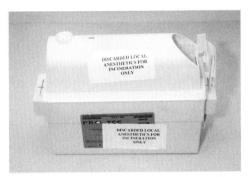

Figure 39-15. Separate sealed container. (From Malamed SF: *Handbook of local anesthesia,* ed 5, St Louis, 2004, Mosby.)

RATIONALES—*cont'd*

Used needles and cartridges are considered infectious. Sharps must be discarded in a rigid, puncture-proof, leak-resistant container.

Copyright © 2010 by Saunders, an imprint of Elsevier Inc. All rights reserved.

Procedure 39-3   BASIC TECHNIQUES FOR A SUCCESSFUL INJECTION

EQUIPMENT
See Procedure 39-1.

STEPS	RATIONALES
1. Assess health history. Take vital signs (include blood pressure, heart rate (pulse) and respiratory rate at a minimum).	Assists the dental hygienist in determining if the client is physiologically and psychologically able to tolerate the proposed treatment and local anesthetic administration and in modifying approach to care, if necessary, to decrease risks and prevent subsequent medical emergencies. Taking vital signs and following guidelines for dental hygiene care management minimize medical complications.
2. Confirm care plan.	Verifies with the client the dental hygiene care indicated.
3. Check armamentarium.	Ensures that all materials are properly assembled, prepared, and functional so the procedure is efficient.
4. Load the syringe and determine the syringe window and needle bevel orientation. The window of the cartridge should face the clinician, and the bevel of the needle should face the bone.	The large window of the syringe should face the operator so that she or he is able to see the amount of anesthetic being administered and detect a positive aspiration. The bevel of the needle should face the bone; therefore if the needle contacts bone, the bevel deflects over the periosteum, minimizing discomfort and trauma. If the bevel faces away from the bone, the point of the needle may tear the sensitive tissues, causing discomfort both during and after the injection.
5. Check that the needle is sharp with no fishhook-type barbs on the tip by placing the needle against a sterile 2 × 2 gauze square. If the gauze is snagged, indicating a barb is present, discard the needle.	A sharp needle free of barbs does not snag gauze and provides an atraumatic insertion and withdrawal.
6. Expel a few drops of the anesthetic solution to determine if a free flow of solution exists.	Ensures the syringe, needle, and cartridge are properly prepared and functional so the procedure is efficient.
7. Position the client in a supine position (head and heart parallel to the floor) with the feet elevated slightly (Figure 39-16).	Placing the client in a supine position provides better accessibility and visibility for the clinician and reduces the likelihood of syncope for the client. Position may vary with client's health status or clinician's preference.

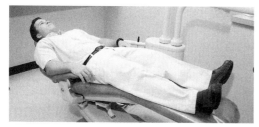

Figure 39-16. Physiologic position of patient for receipt of local anesthetic injection. (From Malamed SF: *Handbook of local anesthesia,* ed 5, St Louis, 2004, Mosby.)

8. Communicate with the client to place positive ideas in the client's mind about the injection. Tell the client about the reasons for topical anesthetic (e.g., "I am applying a topical anesthetic to the tissue so that the remainder of the procedure will be much more comfortable." Do not use words with a negative connotation, such as *injection, shot, pain,* or *hurt.* Instead, use less-threatening terms such as *administer the local anesthetic.*	Keeping the client informed about the procedure helps the client anticipate the operator's actions. A calm approach minimizes client anxiety.

Copyright © 2010 by Saunders, an imprint of Elsevier Inc. All rights reserved.

Procedure 39-3   BASIC TECHNIQUES FOR A SUCCESSFUL INJECTION—*cont'd*

STEPS—*cont'd*	RATIONALES—*cont'd*
9. Visualize or palpate to locate the penetration site.	Accurate injection of anesthetic requires insertion in correct site.
10. Dry the needle penetration site with gauze (Figure 39-17).	Removes saliva and debris from the penetration site, reducing the risk of infection.

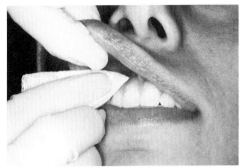

Figure 39-17. Sterilized gauze is used to gently wipe tissue at site of needle. (From Malamed SF: *Handbook of local anesthesia,* ed 5, St Louis, 2004, Mosby.)

11. Apply topical anesthetic to needle penetration site for 1 to 2 minutes (Figure 39-18).	Application of topical anesthetic results in a more comfortable penetration.

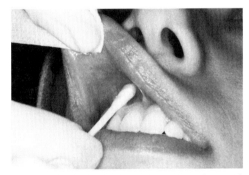

Figure 39-18. A small quantity of topical anesthetic is placed at the site of needle penetration and kept in place for at least 1 minute. (From Malamed SF: *Handbook of local anesthesia,* ed 5, St Louis, 2004, Mosby.)

(Continued)

Copyright © 2010 by Saunders, an imprint of Elsevier Inc. All rights reserved.

Procedure 39-3 BASIC TECHNIQUES FOR A SUCCESSFUL INJECTION—*cont'd*

STEPS—*cont'd*

RATIONALES—*cont'd*

12. In the case of palatal injections, when placing topical anesthetic on the injection site, apply considerable pressure with the cotton swab for a minimum of 1 minute before the injection. Move the swab immediately adjacent to the penetration site, and maintain pressure at this site during the injection (Figures 39-19 and 39-20).

Injections into the dense, tightly attached palatal tissue can be extremely painful to the client. Pressure anesthesia provides for a more comfortable procedure by producing ischemia and blocking pain impulses arising from the needle penetration.

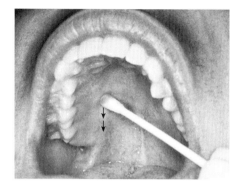

Figure 39-19. A cotton swab is pressed against the hard palate at the junction of the maxillary alveolar process and palatal bone. The swab is slowly moved distally *(arrows)* until a depression in the tissue is felt. This is the greater (anterior) palatine foramen. Apply pressure for a minimum of 30 seconds. (From Malamed SF: *Handbook of local anesthesia,* ed 5, St Louis, 2004, Mosby.)

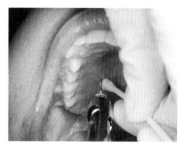

Figure 39-20. Notice the angle of needle entry into the mouth. The insertion is into ischemic tissues slightly anterior to the applicator stick. The barrel of the syringe is stabilized by the corner of the mouth and the teeth. (From Malamed SF: *Handbook of local anesthesia,* ed 5, St Louis, 2004, Mosby.)

13. After the topical anesthetic swab is removed from the tissue, dry the penetration site.
14. Pick up the prepared local anesthetic syringe and establish a firm hand rest. Never place the arm holding the syringe directly on the client's arm or shoulder.

Removes the saliva and excess topical anesthetic from the injection site.
Provides stability and control during the injection, thus ensuring greater client safety and comfort.

Copyright © 2010 by Saunders, an imprint of Elsevier Inc. All rights reserved.

Procedure 39-3	BASIC TECHNIQUES FOR A SUCCESSFUL INJECTION—*cont'd*

STEPS—*cont'd*

RATIONALES—*cont'd*

15. Make the tissue taut at the penetration site by retracting it (except on the palate) using sterile gauze, aiding both visibility and atraumatic needle insertion (Figure 39-21).

Gauze is used to aid in retraction and stability. Stretching the tissue tightly at the penetration site provides maximal visibility and allows the needle to enter the tissue with minimal resistance and discomfort. Avoid jiggling the soft tissues or pulling the lip over the needle tip, which may impair visibility of the penetration site.

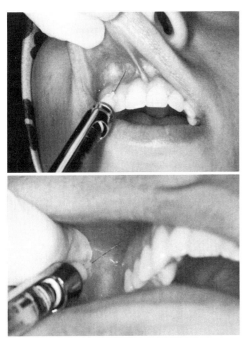

Figure 39-21.   Tissue at needle penetration site is pulled taut, promoting both visibility and atraumatic needle insertion. (From Malamed SF: *Handbook of local anesthesia,* ed 5, St Louis, 2004, Mosby.)

16. Keep syringe and needle out of the client's line of vision.

Minimizes client anxiety.

17. Gently insert the needle into the mucosa until the bevel is completely under the tissue (see Figure 39-21).

Initiates needle penetration with minimal discomfort.

18. Observe and communicate with the client. Watch for any signs of discomfort or distress.

Keeping the client informed about the procedure helps the client anticipate the operator's actions and minimizes anxiety. Careful observation of the client alerts the clinician to a potential behavioral problem or medical emergency.

19. Deposit a few drops of anesthetic solution, pause for 5 seconds, and then advance the needle a few millimeters. Repeat process as you slowly advance to the deposition site. Communicate with the client by saying, "To make you more comfortable, I will deposit a little anesthetic as I advance toward the target."

Anesthetizes the tissues in front of the needle before its advancement, thus minimizing discomfort. Pausing for several seconds allows the anesthesia to develop. At this point, aspiration is not necessary because of the small amount of solution being deposited over a changing injection site.

20. Aspirate on arrival at the deposition site by pulling the thumb ring back gently. Movement of only 1 or 2 mm is needed. Tip of needle must remain unmoved.

Minimizes the possibility of an intravascular injection by ascertaining if the needle tip is located within a blood vessel. Aspiration of blood into the cartridge indicates intravenous placement of the needle (see Figure 39-23).

(Continued)

Copyright © 2010 by Saunders, an imprint of Elsevier Inc. All rights reserved.

Procedure 39-3 | BASIC TECHNIQUES FOR A SUCCESSFUL INJECTION—*cont'd*

STEPS—*cont'd*

21. Rotate barrel of the syringe about 45 degrees, and aspirate a second time to ensure that the needle is not located inside a blood vessel but abutting against the wall of the vessel, providing a false-negative aspiration (Figures 39-22 and 39-23).

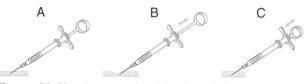

Figure 39-22. Intravascular injection of local anesthetic. **A,** Needle is inserted into lumen of blood vessel. **B,** Aspiration test is performed. Negative pressure pulls vessel wall against bevel of needle; therefore no blood enters syringe (negative aspiration). **C,** Drug is injected. Positive pressure on plunger of syringe forces local anesthetic solution out through needle. Wall of vessel is forced away from bevel, and anesthetic solution is deposited directly into lumen of blood vessel. (From Malamed SF: *Medical emergencies in the dental office,* ed 6, St Louis, 2007, Mosby.)

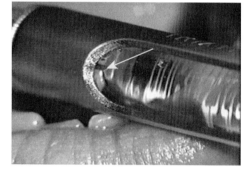

Figure 39-23. Positive aspiration. A slight reddish discoloration at the diaphragm end of the cartridge *(arrow)* on the aspiration usually indicates venous penetration. Reposition the needle, reaspirate, and if negative, deposit the solution. (From Malamed SF: *Handbook of local anesthesia,* ed 5, St Louis, 2004, Mosby.)

22. If no blood appears (negative aspiration), slowly deposit the local anesthetic solution at a rate of 1 mL/min for approximately 2 minutes for a full cartridge.

RATIONALES—*cont'd*

False-negative aspiration may occur if the needle bevel is occluded by the inner wall of the blood vessel. Multiple aspirations with the needle bevel in different planes prevent this potential problem.

Slow deposition reduces the risk of inadvertent intravascular injection and the severity of an overdose reaction in case inadvertent intravascular injection occurs, and prevents tearing and necrosis of the tissue and subsequent discomfort. If, despite slow introduction of the solution, blood levels of anesthetic become elevated, the severity and duration of the toxic reaction will be reduced. Slow injection of the anesthetic solution is critical to preventing an adverse drug reaction.

Copyright © 2010 by Saunders, an imprint of Elsevier Inc. All rights reserved.

Procedure **39-3** BASIC TECHNIQUES FOR A SUCCESSFUL INJECTION—*cont'd*

STEPS—*cont'd*	**RATIONALES**—*cont'd*
23. Observe and communicate with the client. Watch for any signs of discomfort or distress. Reassure the client with statements such as "I am depositing the solution slowly so this procedure will be comfortable for you."	Keeping the client informed about the procedure helps the client to anticipate the operator's actions and minimizes anxiety.
24. Slowly withdraw the needle when the indicated amount of anesthetic has been deposited.	Concludes the injection with minimal discomfort.
25. Replace the needle sheath using the scoop technique (Figure 39-24).	Prevents inadvertent needle stick injury with a contaminated needle to the hygienist and other oral healthcare personnel.

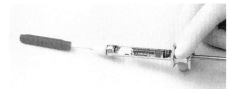

Figure 39-24. "Scoop" technique for recapping needle after use. (From Malamed SF: *Handbook of local anesthesia,* ed 5, St Louis, 2004, Mosby.)

26. Observe the client.	Most adverse reactions, such as syncope, occur either during the injection or within 5 to 10 minutes after completion of administration; therefore remaining with the client after the injection is imperative.
27. Rinse the client's mouth.	Washes out any anesthetic solution that may have dripped into the client's mouth.
28. Massage the tissue over the injection site when indicated.	Gives the client a sense of well-being.
29. Test for anesthesia by touching the rounded back of an explorer to both the area anesthetized and an area not anesthetized. The client should have little or no sensation in the anesthetized area.	Ensures that proper anesthesia is obtained before treatment is commenced.
30. Reassure the client that numbness, tingling, and a sense of swelling, or the tooth feeling different, are normal responses.	Gives the client a sense of well-being.
31. Record the injection(s) in the client's chart, including: a. Area anesthetized and specific injection(s) given b. Type of anesthetic used and type of vasoconstrictor and its concentration (ratio) c. Total amount of solution administered (in milliliters and/or total cartridges) d. Client reaction	Accurate documentation provides a reference for future appointments, provides essential information if the client exhibits any negative reactions, and is your best line of defense if a client challenges the care received.

See Tables 39-1 to 39-11 on pp. 228-244 for specific injection techniques.

Copyright © 2010 by Saunders, an imprint of Elsevier Inc. All rights reserved.

TABLE 39-1 Supraperiosteal Injection (Local Infiltration)

Nerves anesthetized	Large terminal branches of dental plexus
Areas anesthetized	Entire region innervated by the large terminal branches of the plexus: Pulp of the tooth Facial periosteum Connective tissue Mucous membranes overlying the tooth (Figure 39-25)
Needle gauge and length	25- or 27-gauge short
Operator position	8 or 9 o'clock
Penetration site	Height of the mucobuccal fold above the apex of the target tooth (Figure 39-26)
Landmarks	Mucobuccal fold Crown of tooth Root contour of tooth
Syringe orientation	Parallel to the long axis of the tooth (Figure 39-27)
Hand rests	Client's chin Forefinger, or wrist of operator's opposite hand (Figure 39-28)
Deposition site	Apical region of the target tooth
Penetration depth	Usually only a few millimeters, no more than 5 mm or one quarter of a short needle
Amount of anesthetic to be deposited	0.6 mL, or one third of a cartridge
Length of time to deposit	Approximately 30-60 seconds

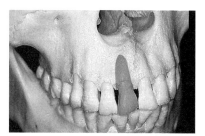

Figure 39-25. Areas anesthetized with a local infiltration of a maxillary central incisor. The deposition site is at the apical region of the target tooth.

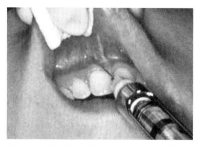

Figure 39-26. Penetration site for a supraperiosteal injection of the maxillary right central incisor.

Potential Problems

Anesthetic deposition below apex of target tooth, resulting in insufficient pulpal anesthesia.

Needle too far from bone, and therefore solution deposited into buccal tissue.

Dense bone may cover apices. Most often occurs on permanent maxillary first molars in children because the apex is located under the dense zygomatic bone. May occur on central incisors where the apex lies beneath the nose.

Pain on insertion with the needle against the periosteum.

Technique Tips

Increase depth of penetration so the needle is at the apical region of the target tooth.

Redirect needle closer to periosteum.

Administer a nerve block.

Withdraw the needle and reinsert farther away (laterally) from the periosteum.

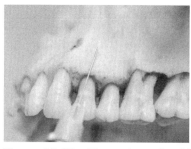

Figure 39-27. The syringe should be held parallel with the long axis of the tooth and inserted at the height of the mucobuccal fold over the tooth. (From Malamed SF: *Handbook of local anesthesia,* ed 5, St Louis, 2004, Mosby.)

Copyright © 2010 by Saunders, an imprint of Elsevier Inc. All rights reserved.

TABLE 39-1 Supraperiosteal Injection (Local Infiltration)—cont'd

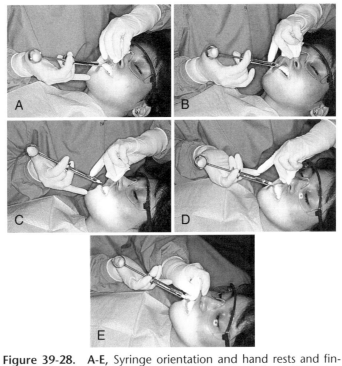

Figure 39-28. **A-E,** Syringe orientation and hand rests and finger rests that may be used for a maxillary supraperiosteal injection and anterior superior alveolar and middle superior alveolar nerve blocks. (From Malamed SF: *Handbook of local anesthesia,* ed 5, St Louis, 2004, Mosby.)

Copyright © 2010 by Saunders, an imprint of Elsevier Inc. All rights reserved.

TABLE 39-2 Anterior Superior Alveolar (ASA) Field Block

Nerves anesthetized	Anterior superior alveolar
Areas anesthetized	Pulpal tissue of the following maxillary teeth unilaterally: Central incisor Lateral incisor Canine Facial periodontal tissues and bones of these same teeth (Figure 39-29)
Needle gauge and length	25- or 27-gauge short
Operator position	8 or 9 o'clock
Penetration site	Height of the mucobuccal fold just mesial to the canine (Figure 39-30)
Landmarks	Mucobuccal fold Canine and canine eminence
Syringe orientation	Parallel to the long axis of the canine (Figure 39-31)
Hand rests	Client's chin Forefinger, or wrist of operator's opposite hand (see Figure 39-28)
Deposition site	Apical region of the canine
Penetration depth	Usually only a few millimeters, no more than 5 mm or one quarter of a short needle
Amount of anesthetic to be deposited	0.6-0.9 mL, or one third to one half of a cartridge
Length of time to deposit	Approximately 30-60 seconds

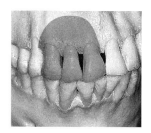

Figure 39-29. Areas anesthetized with the anterior superior nerve block.

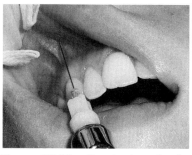

Figure 39-30. Penetration site for the anterior superior nerve block.

Potential Problems	*Technique Tips*
Anesthetic deposition below apex of target tooth, resulting in insufficient pulpal anesthesia.	Increase depth of penetration so the needle is at the apical region of the canine.
Needle too far from bone, and thus solution deposited into buccal tissue.	Redirect needle closer to periosteum.
Pain on insertion with the needle against the periosteum.	Withdraw the needle and reinsert farther away (laterally) from the periosteum.
Persistent sensitivity at mesial surface of central incisor resulting from cross-innervations.	Infiltrate contralateral central incisor.

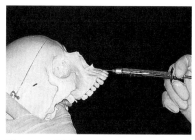

Figure 39-31. Syringe orientation for the anterior superior nerve block.

Copyright © 2010 by Saunders, an imprint of Elsevier Inc. All rights reserved.

TABLE 39-3 Middle Superior Alveolar (MSA) Nerve Block

Nerves anesthetized	Middle superior alveolar
Areas anesthetized	Pulpal tissue of the following maxillary teeth unilaterally:
	First premolar
	Second premolar
	Mesial root of first molar
	Buccal periodontal tissues and bones of these same teeth (Figure 39-32)
Needle gauge and length	25- or 27-gauge short
Operator position	8 or 9 o'clock
Penetration site	Height of the mucobuccal fold above second premolar (Figure 39-33)
Landmarks	Mucobuccal fold
	Second premolar
Syringe orientation	Parallel to the long axis of the second premolar (closer to vertical than in the anterior maxilla) (Figure 39-34)
Hand rests	Client's chin
	Client's cheek
	Forefinger, or wrist of operator's opposite hand (see Figure 39-28)
Deposition site	Above the apical region of the second premolar

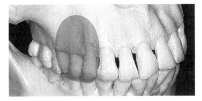

Figure 39-32. Area anesthetized by a middle superior alveolar nerve block.

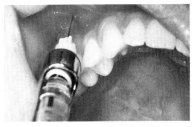

Figure 39-33. Needle penetration for a middle superior alveolar nerve block. (From Malamed SF: *Handbook of local anesthesia,* ed 5, St Louis, 2004, Mosby.)

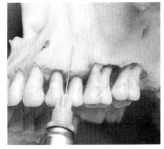

Figure 39-34. Position of needle between maxillary premolars for a middle superior alveolar nerve block. (From Malamed SF: *Handbook of local anesthesia,* ed 5, St Louis, 2004, Mosby.)

Penetration depth	Usually only a few millimeters, no more than 5 mm or one quarter of a short needle
Amount of anesthetic to be deposited	0.9-1.2 mL, or one half to two thirds of a cartridge
Length of time to deposit	Approximately 60-90 seconds

Potential Problems	*Technique Tips*
Anesthetic deposition below apex of target tooth, resulting in insufficient pulpal anesthesia.	Increase depth of penetration so the needle is at the apical region of the second premolar.
Needle too far from bone, and therefore solution deposited into buccal tissue.	Redirect needle closer to periosteum.
Pain on insertion with the needle against the periosteum.	Withdraw the needle and reinsert farther away (laterally) from the periosteum.
Dense bone of the zygomatic arch at the injection site prevents diffusion of anesthetic solution.	Administer an infraorbital block instead of the MSA block.
Buccal frenum present at preferred penetration site.	Penetrate slightly mesial to the frenum.

Copyright © 2010 by Saunders, an imprint of Elsevier Inc. All rights reserved.

TABLE 39-4 Infraorbital (IO) Nerve Block

Nerves anesthetized	Infraorbital Anterior superior alveolar Middle superior alveolar Inferior palpebral Lateral nasal Superior labial

Areas anesthetized	Pulpal tissue of the following maxillary teeth unilaterally:
	  Central incisor
	  Lateral incisor
	  Canine
	  First premolar
	  Second premolar
	  Mesial root of first molar
	  Buccal periodontal tissues and bone of these same teeth
	  Lower eyelid
	  Lateral aspect of the nose
	  Upper lip (Figure 39-35)

Needle gauge and length	25- or 27-gauge short (in rare instances a long needle may be preferred)
Operator position	8 or 9 o'clock (Figure 39-36)
Penetration site	Height of the mucobuccal fold above first premolar (Figure 39-37)

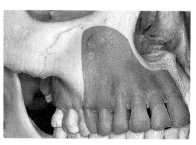

Figure 39-35. Area anesthetized by an infraorbital nerve block in approximately 60% of individuals.

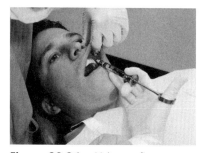

Figure 39-36. Using a finger over the foramen, lift the lip and hold the tissues in the mucobuccal fold taut. (From Malamed SF: *Handbook of local anesthesia,* ed 5, St Louis, 2004, Mosby.)

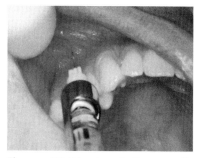

Figure 39-37. Insert the needle for infraorbital nerve block in mucobuccal fold over maxillary first premolar. (From Malamed SF: *Handbook of local anesthesia,* ed 5, St Louis, 2004, Mosby.)

Copyright © 2010 by Saunders, an imprint of Elsevier Inc. All rights reserved.

TABLE 39-4 Infraorbital (IO) Nerve Block—cont'd

Landmarks	Infraorbital notch Infraorbital ridge Infraorbital foramen Mucobuccal fold First premolar (Figure 39-38)
Syringe orientation	Parallel to the long axis of the first premolar; follow the angle (see Figures 39-36 and 39-37)
Hand rests	Client's chin Client's cheek Forefinger, or wrist of operator's opposite hand (see Figure 39-28)
Deposition site	Upper rim of the infraorbital foramen; the needle should gently contact bone before deposition (Figure 39-39)
Penetration depth	16 mm or three quarters of a short needle
Amount of anesthetic to be deposited	0.9-1.2 mL, or one half to two thirds of a cartridge
Length of time to deposit	Approximately 60-90 seconds

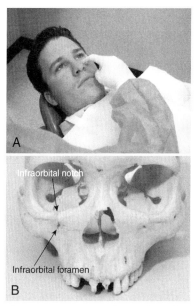

Figure 39-38. A, Palpate the infraorbital notch. **B,** Location of the infraorbital foramen in relation to the infraorbital notch. (From Malamed SF: *Handbook of local anesthesia,* ed 5, St Louis, 2004, Mosby.)

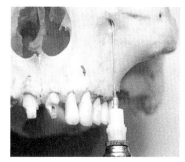

Figure 39-39. Position of the needle tip before deposition of local anesthetic at the infraorbital foramen. (From Malamed SF: *Handbook of local anesthesia,* ed 5, St Louis, 2004, Mosby.)

Technique Notes

1. Locate the infraorbital foramen: With your forefinger, palpate across the zygomatic arch; the foramen lies at the area of concavity directly below the medial border of the client's iris when the client gazes straight ahead.
2. Maintain finger pressure over the foramen throughout the injection and for 1 to 2 minutes after deposition. This will aid in directing the needle to the foramen and assist in directing the anesthetic solution to the foramen.

Potential Problems

Needle contacting bone below the infraorbital foramen; anesthesia of the lower eyelid, nose, or upper lip with little or no pulpal anesthesia.

Technique Tips

Keep needle in line with the infraorbital foramen during penetration; line the syringe up with your finger over the foramen.

Copyright © 2010 by Saunders, an imprint of Elsevier Inc. All rights reserved.

TABLE 39-5 Posterior Superior Alveolar (PSA) Nerve Block

Nerves anesthetized	Posterior superior alveolar
Areas anesthetized	(Figure 39-40)
Needle gauge and length	25- or 27-gauge short (in rare instances a long needle may be preferred)
Operator position	8 or 9 o'clock
Penetration site	Height of the mucobuccal fold posterior and superior to the last molar present (Figure 39-41)
Landmarks	Mucobuccal fold Maxillary tuberosity Maxillary occlusal plane Midsagittal plane Maxillary molars
Syringe orientation	45 degrees to the maxillary occlusal plane and 45 degrees to the midsagittal plane (Figure 39-42)
Hand rests	Forefinger, or thumb of opposite hand as it retracts client's buccal tissue

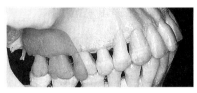

Figure 39-40. Area anesthetized by the posterior superior alveolar nerve block.

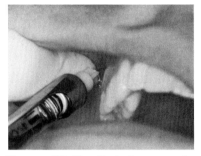

Figure 39-41. Posterior superior alveolar nerve block using a "short" dental needle (approximately 20 mm in length). (From Malamed SF: *Handbook of local anesthesia,* ed 5, St Louis, 2004, Mosby.)

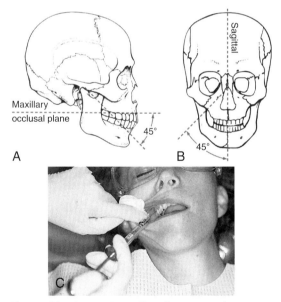

Figure 39-42. **A,** Forty-five degrees to the maxillary occlusal plane. **B,** Forty-five degrees to the midsagittal plane. **C,** Orientation of syringe during the posterior superior alveolar nerve block.

Copyright © 2010 by Saunders, an imprint of Elsevier Inc. All rights reserved.

TABLE 39-5 Posterior Superior Alveolar (PSA) Nerve Block—cont'd

Deposition site	Posterior and superior to the posterior border of the maxilla at the PSA nerve foramina (Figure 39-43)
Penetration depth	16 mm or three quarters of a short needle
Amount of anesthetic to be deposited	0.9-1.8 mL, or one half to one cartridge
Length of time to deposit	Approximately 60-120 seconds

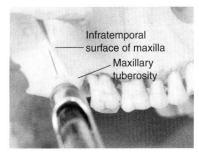

Infratemporal surface of maxilla
Maxillary tuberosity

Figure 39-43. Needle at the target area for a posterior superior alveolar nerve block. (From Malamed SF: *Handbook of local anesthesia,* ed 5, St Louis, 2004, Mosby.)

Technique Notes

Owing to the high vascularity of the deposition site for the PSA, a triple aspiration is recommended to ensure that the needle bevel is not against the interior wall of a vessel, thus providing a false-negative aspiration (see Figure 39-22). To aspirate in multiple planes, perform a single aspiration as usual, then rotate the body of the syringe toward you slightly, reaspirate, then rotate the body of the syringe back to the original position and perform a final aspiration. If all three aspiration tests are negative, it is safe to administer the anesthetic solution.

Potential Problems

Bone is contacted when the angle of needle is too great in reference to the midsagittal plane.

Mandibular anesthesia: The mandibular division of the trigeminal nerve is lateral to the PSA nerves.

Technique Tips

Withdraw the needle and bring the syringe closer to the midline.

Review landmarks and syringe orientation so as not to deposit lateral to the PSA nerves.

Copyright © 2010 by Saunders, an imprint of Elsevier Inc. All rights reserved.

TABLE 39-6 Greater Palatine (GP) Nerve Block (Anterior Palatine)

Nerves anesthetized	Greater palatine
Areas anesthetized	Hard palate and overlying soft tissue unilaterally from the maxillary third molar to the first premolar (Figure 39-44)
Needle gauge and length	25- or 27-gauge short
Operator position	8 or 9 o'clock
Penetration site	Just anterior to the greater palatine foramen (see Figure 39-19)
Landmarks	Greater palatine foramen Junction of alveolar process and palatine bone Maxillary second molar
Syringe orientation	Approaches from opposite the side being injected with the needle at a right angle to the penetration site (Figure 39-45)
Hand rests	Back of opposite hand Corner of client's mouth (Figure 39-46)
Deposition site	Just anterior to the greater palatine nerve foramen
Penetration depth	3-6 mm; often only the bevel is inserted
Amount of anesthetic to be deposited	0.45 mL, or one quarter of a cartridge; determine by development of blanching of palatal tissues
Length of time to deposit	Approximately 20-30 seconds

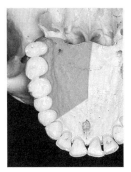

Figure 39-44. Area anesthetized with the greater palatine nerve block.

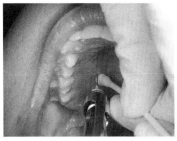

Figure 39-45. Notice the angle of needle entry into the mouth. The insertion is into ischemic tissues slightly anterior to the applicator stick. The barrel of the syringe is stabilized by the corner of the mouth and the teeth. (From Malamed SF: *Handbook of local anesthesia,* ed 5, St Louis, 2004, Mosby.)

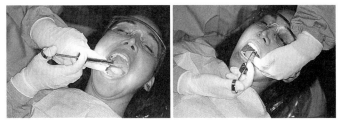

Figure 39-46. Hand rests for a greater palatine nerve block.

Technique Notes

1. To locate the greater palatine foramen, palpate the posterior palate with a cotton-tipped applicator or your forefinger at the junction of the hard palate and the alveolar process near the second molar until a depression is felt.
2. Topical anesthetics have very limited action on keratinized tissue such as the palate.
   To ensure client comfort, pressure anesthesia with a cotton-tipped applicator is recommended for a minimum of 1 minute before injection and throughout deposition (see Figure 39-16).

Potential Problems	*Technique Tips*
Deposition of the anesthetic solution too far anterior of the foramen, resulting in inadequate anesthesia.	Move the needle posteriorly.
Inadequate anesthesia of the first molar resulting from cross-innervation from the nasopalatine nerve.	Infiltrate palate in area of first molar.

Copyright © 2010 by Saunders, an imprint of Elsevier Inc. All rights reserved.

TABLE 39-7 Nasopalatine (NP) Nerve Block

Nerves anesthetized	Neopalatine
Areas anesthetized	Hard palate and overlying soft tissue bilaterally from the maxillary canine to canine (Figure 39-47)
Needle gauge and length	25- or 27-gauge short
Operator position	8 or 9 o'clock
Penetration site	Just lateral to posterior portion of the incisive papilla (Figures 39-48 and 39-49, D)
Landmarks	Central incisors Incisive papilla
Syringe orientation	Approaches from canine or premolar region at a 45-degree angle to the incisive papilla (see Figure 39-49, D)
Hand rests	Finger of opposite hand Syringe can be stabilized against the corner of the client's mouth (see Figure 39-46)
Deposition site	Incisive foramen, beneath incisive papilla
Penetration depth	3-6 mm; often only the bevel is inserted
Amount of anesthetic to be deposited	0.45 mL, or one quarter of a cartridge; determine by development of blanching of palatal tissues
Length of time to deposit	Approximately 20-30 seconds

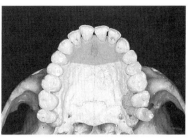

Figure 39-47. Area anesthetized with the nasopalatine nerve block.

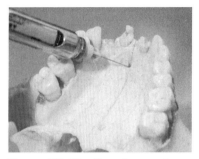

Figure 39-48. Target area for a nasopalatine nerve block. (From Malamed SF: *Handbook of local anesthesia,* ed 5, St Louis, 2004, Mosby.)

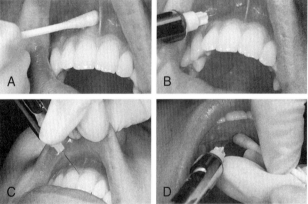

Figure 39-49. **A,** Topical anesthetic is applied to mucosa of the frenum. **B,** First injection, into the labial frenum. **C,** Use a finger of the opposite hand to stabilize the syringe during the second injection into the intended papilla between the central incisors. **D,** Pressure is maintained until the deposition of solution is completed. Needle penetration is just lateral to the incisive papilla. (From Malamed SF: *Handbook of local anesthesia,* ed 5, St Louis, 2004, Mosby.)

(Continued)

Copyright © 2010 by Saunders, an imprint of Elsevier Inc. All rights reserved.

TABLE 39-7 Nasopalatine (NP) Nerve Block—cont'd

Technique Notes

1. Topical anesthetics have very limited action on keratinized tissue such as the palate. To ensure client comfort, pressure anesthesia with a cotton-tipped applicator is recommended for a minimum of 1 minute before injection and throughout deposition (see Figure 39-21).

2. For greatest client comfort, the nasopalatine nerve block is best administered in a triple injection sequence as follows: infiltration of a central incisor, papillary infiltration of teeth 8 and 9, and then the nasopalatine. Each injection anesthetizes the area of the subsequent injection, resulting in an atraumatic procedure for the client (see Figure 39-49).

Potential Problems	Technique Tips
Unilateral anesthesia due to deposition of anesthetic solution to one side of incisive foramen.	Reinsert the needle until it is directly over the incisive foramen.
Inadequate anesthesia of canine or first premolar due to cross-innervation from the greater palatine nerve.	Infiltrate the palate at the area of the canine or first premolar.

Copyright © 2010 by Saunders, an imprint of Elsevier Inc. All rights reserved.

TABLE 39-8 Inferior Alveolar (IA) and Lingual (Li) Nerve Blocks

Nerves anesthetized	*IA:* Inferior alveolar Incisive Mental *Li:* Lingual
Areas anesthetized	*IA:* Mandibular teeth unilaterally to midline Body of mandible Inferior portion of the ramus Facial tissue anterior to the first molar Lower lip to midline *Li:* All lingual gingival tissue unilaterally to midline Anterior two thirds of the tongue Floor of the mouth unilaterally (Figure 39-50)
Needle gauge and length	25- or 27-gauge long
Operator position	8 or 9 o'clock
Penetration site	Middle of the pterygomandibular triangle (formed by the pterygomandibular raphe medially and the internal oblique ridge laterally) at the height of the coronoid notch, 6-10 mm above the mandibular occlusal plane (Figure 39-51)
Landmarks	Anterior border of the ramus External oblique ridge Coronoid notch Internal oblique ridge Pterygomandibular raphe Pterygomandibular triangle Mandibular occlusal plane (Figures 39-52 and 39-53)
Syringe orientation	Approaches from contralateral premolar area, parallel to the occlusal plane
Hand rests	Small finger on client's chin
Deposition site	*IA:* Superior to the mandibular foramen *Li:* Withdraw needle halfway after deposition for IA
Penetration depth	*IA:* Until bone is gently contacted (see Figure 39-25) Approximately 20-25 mm or two thirds to three quarters of needle (withdraw 1 mm before deposition) *Li:* Withdraw needle halfway after deposition for IA
Amount of anesthetic to be deposited	*IA:* 0.9-1.8 mL, or one half to one cartridge *Li:* 0.45 mL, or one quarter of a cartridge
Length of time to deposit	*IA:* 60-120 seconds *Li:* 10-15 seconds

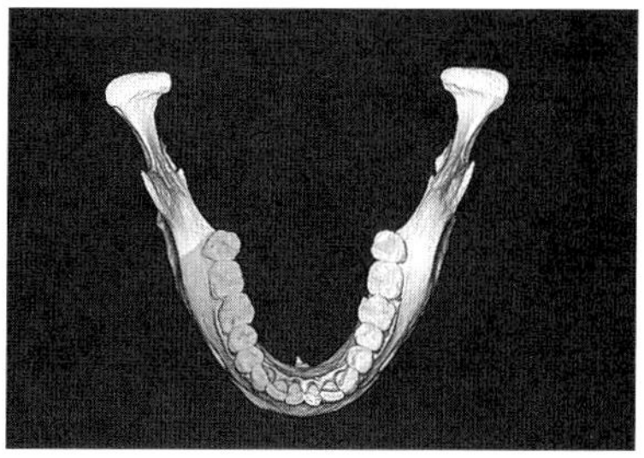

Figure 39-50. Area anesthetized with the inferior alveolar and lingual nerve blocks.

Figure 39-51. Notice the placement of the syringe barrel at the corner of the mouth, usually corresponding to the premolars. The needle tip gently touches the most distal end of the pterygomandibular raphe. (From Malamed SF: *Handbook of local anesthesia,* ed 5, St Louis, 2004, Mosby.)

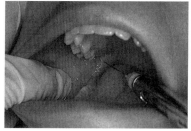

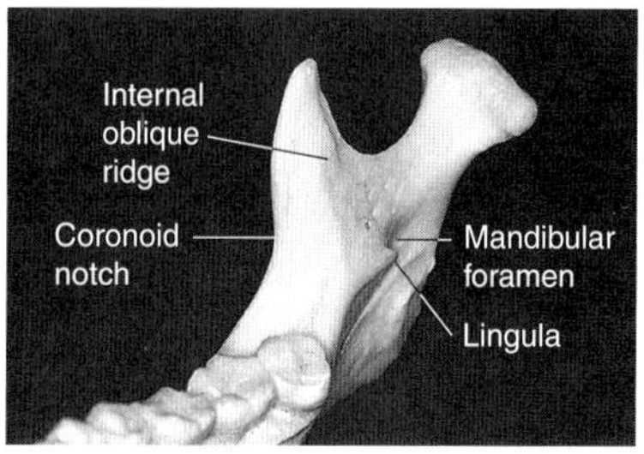

Figure 39-52. Landmarks on the mandible for the inferior alveolar and lingual nerve blocks.

(Continued)

Copyright © 2010 by Saunders, an imprint of Elsevier Inc. All rights reserved.

TABLE 39-8   Inferior Alveolar (IA) and Lingual (Li) Nerve Blocks—cont'd

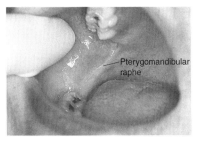

Figure 39-53. The posterior border of the mandibular ramus can be approximated intraorally by using the pterygomandibular raphe as it turns superiorly toward the maxilla.

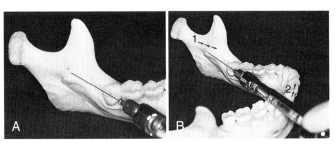

Figure 39-54. **A,** Premature bone contact on the lingula. **B,** Path of syringe orientation to correct for premature contact of bone.

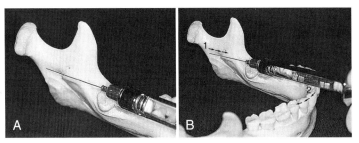

Figure 39-55. **A,** The needle is too far posterior; no bone is contacted. **B,** Path of syringe orientation to correct needle position.

Technique Notes
1. To locate the pterygomandibular triangle, place your thumb or index finger on the greatest depression on the anterior border of the ramus; this is the coronoid notch. Roll your finger medially to locate the internal oblique ridge. The point of penetration is between the internal oblique ridge and the pterygomandibular raphe (in the pterygomandibular triangle), 6-10 mm above the mandibular occlusal plane (see Figures 39-52 and 39-53). While inserting, advancing, and withdrawing the needle, it is important to place the thumb or index finger on the internal oblique ridge and at the same time grasp the posterior border of the mandible with the remainder of the hand. This technique provides stabilization and control in the event the client moves unexpectedly during the procedure.
2. Owing to the high vascularity of the deposition site for the IA, a triple aspiration is recommended to ensure that the needle bevel is not against the interior wall of a vessel, thus providing a false-negative aspiration (see Figure 39-22). To aspirate in multiple planes, perform a single aspiration as usual, rotate the body of the syringe toward you slightly and reaspirate, then rotate the body of the syringe back to the original position and perform a final aspiration. If all three aspiration tests are negative, it is safe to administer the anesthetic solution.
3. If bone is contacted prematurely, before half of the needle length has entered the tissues, it is likely that the needle is too far anterior and has contacted the lingululm, which covers the mandibular foramen (Figure 39-54, *A*). To correct, withdraw the needle halfway but do not remove from the tissues. Bring the body of the syringe over the mandibular anterior teeth and reinsert past the depth previously penetrated. Redirect the body of the syringe back over the contralateral premolars and continue to penetrate until bone is contacted (Figure 39-54, *B*).
4. If bone is not contacted and the penetration depth is nearing the hub of the needle, it is likely that the needle is too far posterior (Figure 39-55, *A*). To correct, withdraw the needle halfway but do not remove it from the tissues. Redirect the syringe further over the contralateral molars and continue insertion until bone is contacted (Figure 39-55, *B*).
5. At the deposition site, deposit two thirds of the solution. Withdraw the needle halfway and deposit the remaining one third of the solution to anesthetize the lingual nerve.

Potential Problems

Technique Tips

Deposition of anesthetic below the mandibular foramen.

Reinject at a higher penetration site.

Deposition of anesthetic too far anterior on the ramus, indicated by early bone contact, with less than one half the needle length inserted.

See technique note 3.

Copyright © 2010 by Saunders, an imprint of Elsevier Inc. All rights reserved.

TABLE 39-8 Inferior Alveolar (IA) and Lingual (Li) Nerve Blocks—cont'd

Incomplete pulpal anesthesia of the molars (often mesial root of the first molar) or premolars. Theorized that the mylohyoid nerve, which is not blocked by the IA, provides accessory innervations to these areas.	Using a 27-gauge long needle, direct syringe from opposite corner of mouth and penetrate the apical region of the tooth just distal to the unanesthetized tooth. Advance 3-5 mm and deposit 0.6 mL or one third of a cartridge over 20 seconds (Figure 39-56).
Incomplete anesthesia of the central or lateral incisors. May be due to cross-innervation from the opposite side inferior alveolar nerve.	Using a 27-gauge short needle, infiltrate the mucobuccal fold and advance to the apical region of the unanesthetized tooth. Deposit 0.6 mL or one third of a cartridge over 20 seconds (Figure 39-57).

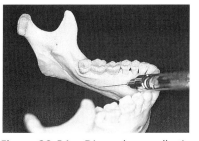

Figure 39-56. Direct the needle tip below the apical region of the tooth immediately posterior to the tooth in question.

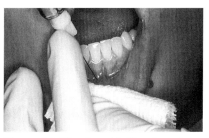

Figure 39-57. Local infiltration of the mandibular incisors.

Copyright © 2010 by Saunders, an imprint of Elsevier Inc. All rights reserved.

TABLE 39-9 Buccal Nerve Block (Long Buccal)

Nerves anesthetized	Buccal
Areas anesthetized	Soft tissues buccal to the mandibular molars unilaterally (Figure 39-58)
Needle gauge and length	25- or 27-gauge long
Operator position	8 or 9 o'clock
Penetration site	In the vestibule, distal and buccal to the most distal molar at the height of the occlusal plane (see Figure 39-32)
Landmarks	Mandibular molars Buccal vestibule Mucobuccal fold
Syringe orientation	Parallel to the mandibular occlusal plane on the buccal side of the teeth (Figure 39-59)
Hand rests	Client's cheek or chin Back of operator's opposite hand (Figure 39-60)
Deposition site	Buccal nerve as it passes over the anterior border of the ramus
Penetration depth	1-4 mm, often only the bevel is inserted
Amount of anesthetic to be deposited	0.3-0.45 mL, or one eighth to one quarter of a cartridge
Length of time to deposit	Approximately 10-20 seconds

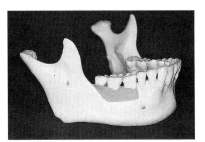

Figure 39-58. Area anesthetized with the buccal nerve block.

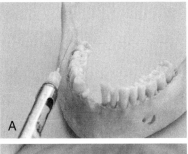

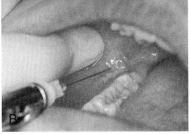

Figure 39-59. Syringe alignment. **A,** Parallel with the occlusal plane on the side of injection but buccal to it. **B,** Distal and buccal to the last molar. (From Malamed SF: *Handbook of local anesthesia,* ed 5, St Louis, 2004, Mosby.)

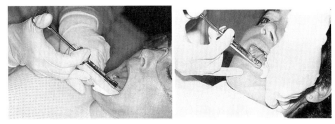

Figure 39-60. Hand rests for the buccal nerve block.

Technique Notes

The buccal nerve block can be administered immediately after the IA/Li. Therefore the penetration sites can be prepared simultaneously with topical anesthetic.

Copyright © 2010 by Saunders, an imprint of Elsevier Inc. All rights reserved.

TABLE 39-10 Mental Nerve Block

Nerves anesthetized	Mental (terminal branch of inferior alveolar nerve)
Areas anesthetized	Facial soft tissues unilaterally from the mental foramen anterior to midline Lower lip Skin of chin (Figure 39-61)
Needle gauge and length	25- or 27-gauge short
Operator position	8 or 9 o'clock or 11 or 1 o'clock
Penetration site	Mucobuccal fold directly over the mental foramen (Figure 39-62)
Landmarks	Mucobuccal fold Mandibular premolars Mental foramen
Syringe orientation	Directed toward the mental foramen
Hand rests	Client's chin Back of operator's opposite hand or wrist (Figure 39-63)
Deposition site	Directly over the mental foramen, between the apices of the premolars
Penetration depth	5-6 mm, or one quarter the needle length (do not enter the mental foramen)
Amount of anesthetic to be deposited	0.6 mL, or one third of a cartridge
Length of time to deposit	Approximately 30-60 seconds

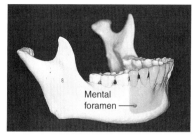

Figure 39-61. Area anesthetized with the mental nerve block.

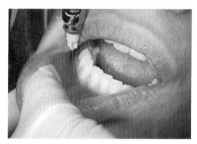

Figure 39-62. Mental nerve block needle penetration site. (From Malamed SF: *Handbook of local anesthesia*, ed 5, St Louis, 2004, Mosby.)

Technique Notes

1. To locate the mental foramen, place your forefinger in the mucobuccal fold against the body of the mandible near the first molar. Palpate anteriorly until a depression is felt or the bone feels irregular. This is the mental foramen, which is most often found between the apices of the first and second premolars (Figure 39-64).
2. Use radiographs to assist you in finding the mental foramen (Figure 39-65).

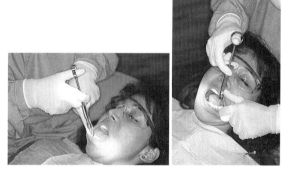

Figure 39-63. Hand rests for the mental and incisive nerve blocks. When possible, hold the arms close to the body to increase stabilization.

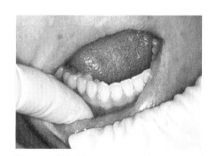

Figure 39-64. Locate the mental nerve foramen by palpating the vestibule at the premolars.

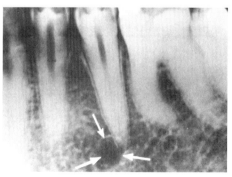

Figure 39-65. Radiographs can assist in locating the mental foramen.

Copyright © 2010 by Saunders, an imprint of Elsevier Inc. All rights reserved.

TABLE 39-11 Incisive Nerve Block

Nerves anesthetized	Incisive
	Mental (terminal branch of inferior alveolar)
Areas anesthetized	Mandibular second premolar to central incisor unilaterally
	Facial soft tissues unilaterally from the mental foramen anterior to midline
	Lower lip
	Skin of chin (Figure 39-66)
Needle gauge and length	25- or 27-gauge short
Operator position	8 or 9 o'clock or 11 or 1 o'clock
Penetration site	Mucobuccal fold directly over the mental foramen
Landmarks	Mucobuccal fold
	Mandibular premolars
	Mental foramen
Syringe orientation	Directed toward the mental foramen
Hand rests	Client's chin
	Back of operator's opposite hand or wrist (see Figure 39-65)
Deposition site	Directly over the mental foramen, between the apices of the premolars
Penetration depth	5-6 mm, or one quarter of the needle length (do not enter the mental foramen)
Amount of anesthetic to be deposited	0.6-0.9 mL, or one third to one half of a cartridge
Length of time to deposit	Approximately 30-60 seconds

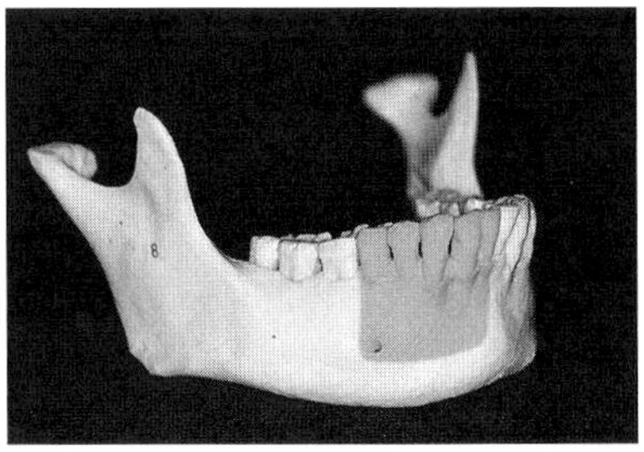

Figure 39-66. Area anesthetized with the incisive nerve block.

Technique Notes

1. The incisive nerve block is administered in the same manner as the mental, differing only in the application of pressure over the deposition site to direct the anesthetic solution into the mental foramen, resulting in pulpal anesthesia.
2. To locate the mental foramen, place your forefinger in the mucobuccal fold against the body of the mandible near the first molar. Palpate anteriorly until a depression is felt or the bone feels irregular. This is the mental foramen, which is most often found between the apices of the first and second premolars (see Figure 39-36).
3. Use radiographs to assist you in finding the mental foramen (see Figure 39-35).
4. Maintain pressure over the mental foramen with your finger for 1-2 minutes after the injection. This aids the flow of solution into the foramen, providing the pulpal anesthesia.

Potential Problems	*Technique Tips*
Incomplete anesthesia of the central or lateral incisors. May be due to cross-innervation from the opposite side inferior alveolar nerve.	Using a 27-gauge short needle, infiltrate the mucobuccal fold and advance to the apical region of the unanesthetized tooth. Deposit 0.6 mL or one third of a cartridge over 20 seconds (see Figure 39-31).
Incomplete pulpal anesthesia.	Redirect needle toward mental foramen and maintain pressure over the deposition site.

Please refer to the Evolve website (http://evolve.elsevier.com/Darby/hygiene) for competency forms to help evaluate your mastery of each procedure in this chapter.

Copyright © 2010 by Saunders, an imprint of Elsevier Inc. All rights reserved.

Nitrous Oxide–Oxygen Analgesia

Procedure 40-1	ADMINISTRATION OF NITROUS OXIDE–OXYGEN ANALGESIC USING THE CONSTANT LITER FLOW TECHNIQUE

EQUIPMENT

Personal protective barriers
Gas machine
Sterilized nasal mask
2 × 2 gauze
Saliva ejector
Suction calibrator

STEPS	**RATIONALES**
PREPARE EQUIPMENT	
1. Prepare the gas machine and related armamentaria before seating the client. Select appropriate sterilized nasal mask for size and attach it to mask tubing.	Preparation of equipment when the client is seated may raise the client's anxiety level.
2. Open gas cylinder valves and check gas supply. Open oxygen (O_2) tank slowly, then the nitrous oxide (N_2O) cylinder. (Centralized systems are turned on at the beginning of the day.) (Figure 40-1.)	This check enables the clinician to replenish the gas supply to ensure that adequate gas is available for the procedure.

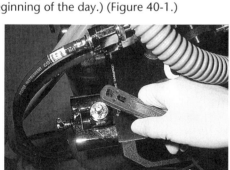

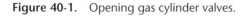

Figure 40-1. Opening gas cylinder valves.

(Continued)

Copyright © 2010 by Saunders, an imprint of Elsevier Inc. All rights reserved.

| Procedure **40-1** | ADMINISTRATION OF NITROUS OXIDE–OXYGEN ANALGESIC USING THE CONSTANT LITER FLOW TECHNIQUE—*cont'd* |

STEPS—*cont'd*

RATIONALES—*cont'd*

3. Obtain suction calibrator, attach it to the high-speed vacuum system, and adjust the suction until the steel ball in the calibrator is made to float in the green zone of the calibrator's window (Figure 40-2).

Adjusting the suction calibrator allows the clinician to obtain the optimal level of suction for the scavenger system.

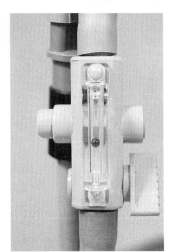

Figure 40-2. Suction calibration. (Courtesy Dr. Mark Dellinges and Cory Price.)

4. Remove the suction calibrator from the high-speed suction system, and tape in place the button used to adjust the suction.

Taping the button on the high-speed suction system after calibration ensures that the degree of suction will remove the exhaled N_2O-O_2 at an appropriate rate—not so quickly that gas is removed before air has been inhaled, and not so slowly that gas overaccumulates in the mask and leaks into the breathing zone of the clinician.

5. Connect the sterilized nose mask to two hoses coming off each side of it (Figure 40-3). Each pair of hoses is joined by an adaptor.

One pair of hoses delivers the N_2O-O_2 to the client, and the other pair carries away the exhaled N_2O-O_2 into the suction system, thus providing a scavenger system.

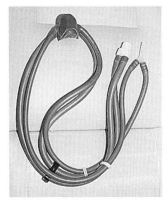

Figure 40-3. Nasal mask with two pairs of hoses.

Copyright © 2010 by Saunders, an imprint of Elsevier Inc. All rights reserved.

Procedure 40-1 ADMINISTRATION OF NITROUS OXIDE–OXYGEN ANALGESIC USING THE CONSTANT LITER FLOW TECHNIQUE—*cont'd*

STEPS—*cont'd*	**RATIONALES**—*cont'd*
6. Connect the larger adaptor on the nasal mask to the gas machine (Figure 40-4).	This connection carries the gas mixture (of proportions preset by the clinician) to the client from the reservoir bag.

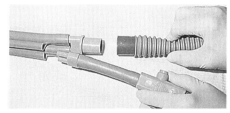

Figure 40-4. Attaching the larger adaptor of the sterilized nasal mask to the gas machine gas hose (held in right hand).

7. Connect the smaller adaptor on the nasal mask to the calibrated high-speed suction system (Figure 40-5).	This connection allows the exhaled N_2O-O_2 to be suctioned from the airway, ensuring that the N_2O-O_2 concentration breathed by the operator is reduced to 30 to 50 ppm from 900 ppm.

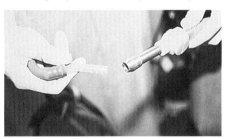

Figure 40-5. Attaching the smaller adaptor on the sterilized nasal mask to calibrated high-speed suction to provide for the scavenging system.

8. Turn on the gas machine.	This step ensures that the gas machine is ready for use.

PREPARE THE CLIENT

9. Seat the client; check and record the health history, blood pressure, and pulse (Figure 40-6).	To meet clients' human need for protection from health risks, it is essential that their health and vital signs are within normal limits before dental hygiene care is provided. Determine relative contraindications.

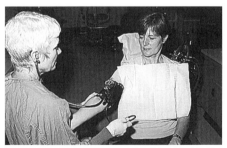

Figure 40-6. Checking client's vital signs.

10. Request that the client visit the restroom if necessary.	Prevents unnecessary interruption of care and ensures client comfort.
11. If client wears contact lenses, request that they be removed before the start of the sedation procedure.	Prevents drying out of contact lenses and eyes, which could potentially harm the cornea.

(Continued)

Copyright © 2010 by Saunders, an imprint of Elsevier Inc. All rights reserved.

Procedure 40-1	ADMINISTRATION OF NITROUS OXIDE–OXYGEN ANALGESIC USING THE CONSTANT LITER FLOW TECHNIQUE—*cont'd*

STEPS—*cont'd*

RATIONALES—*cont'd*

12. Familiarize client with procedures; discuss nasal breathing and nose mask, and describe sensations of warmth and tingling that will be experienced. Reaffirm the relaxing, comfortable feeling the client will experience. Assure clients that they will be aware of and in control of their actions (Figure 40-7).

Informing clients about what they can expect to experience with N_2O-O_2 sedation helps prevent behavior problems based on fear of the unknown or of becoming unconscious. In addition, studies report that providing information to individuals receiving a drug increases pain thresholds and tolerance of pain. These findings suggest that influencing the thought process in conjunction with giving analgesia can increase the depth of sedation.

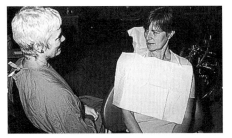

Figure 40-7. Familiarizing client with procedure.

13. Position client in comfortable, reclined position in dental chair.

Enhances client comfort and promotes relaxation.

14. Start O_2 flow at an estimated tidal volume of 6 L/min (Figure 40-8).

This estimate provides a reasonable amount of oxygen as a basis for determining the exact tidal volume.

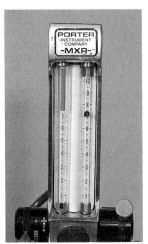

Figure 40-8. Start O_2 flow at estimated tidal volume. (Courtesy Dr. Mark Dellinges.)

15. Activate O_2 flush valve to fill the reservoir bag with O_2.

Filling the reservoir bag with oxygen ensures that there is enough oxygen available for the client's first couple of breaths.

Copyright © 2010 by Saunders, an imprint of Elsevier Inc. All rights reserved.

Procedure 40-1 ADMINISTRATION OF NITROUS OXIDE–OXYGEN ANALGESIC USING THE CONSTANT LITER FLOW TECHNIQUE—*cont'd*

STEPS—*cont'd*

RATIONALES—*cont'd*

16. Seat the nasal mask and have client hold the mask in a comfortable position while you adjust the slip ring to hold the mask in place (Figure 40-9).

Personal adjustment of the mask by the client ensures a comfortable fit; adjustment of mask tubing holds nose mask in place and ensures a minimum amount of gas leakage from the mask.

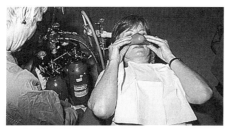

Figure 40-9. Client holding nasal mask in a comfortable position while dental hygienist adjusts the mask tubes to hold the mask in place.

17. Confirm comfortable mask fit with the client.
    If mask is impinging on a sensitive area on the face or if mask is too big, place a gauze square under the edge of the mask (Figure 40-10).

The gauze square makes the mask feel more comfortable if there is a sensitive area and closes any leakage if the mask is too big.

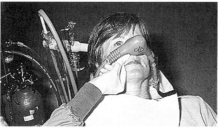

Figure 40-10. Placing gauze square under the edge of the mask.

DETERMINE EXACT TIDAL VOLUME

18. Remind the client to breath through the nose.
19. Ask the client if he or she has enough air to breathe comfortably. Adjust volume of O_2 as per client response. If client requests a greater volume, increase the O_2 by 1 L, wait a minute, and then ask the same question. This process is repeated until the client becomes comfortable and the exact tidal volume is established (Figure 40-11).

N_2O-O_2 is delivered through the nose.
This determination provides the client with an adequate and comfortable amount of gas per respiration. Documenting the tidal volume in the client chart serves as a record for future care.

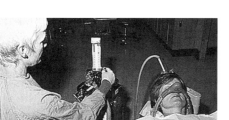

Figure 40-11. Determining the tidal volume.

(Continued)

Copyright © 2010 by Saunders, an imprint of Elsevier Inc. All rights reserved.

Procedure **40-1**	ADMINISTRATION OF NITROUS OXIDE–OXYGEN ANALGESIC USING THE CONSTANT LITER FLOW TECHNIQUE—*cont'd*

STEPS—*cont'd*	**RATIONALES**—*cont'd*
20. Observe the reservoir bag as an indicator of appropriate flow rate.	Slow introduction of N_2O allows the clinician to find the baseline for the client and ensures that the client is not oversedated. Decreasing O_2 by the same amount that N_2O is increased maintains the established tidal volume.
21. Write the established tidal volume in the client record.	There is a great deal of individual variation in the amount of N_2O one needs to achieve baseline. Usually the optimal concentration of N_2O does not exceed 35%.
Begin titration of N_2O	
22. Decrease O_2 by 0.5 L, and introduce 0.5 L/min of N_2O (Figure 40-12). Wait 60 to 90 seconds, and observe the client for signs of sedation. At the end of the 60- to 90-second waiting period, ask client, "What are you feeling?" It is important to ask open-ended question that requires the client to respond with more than a simple "yes" or "no."	Same as above.

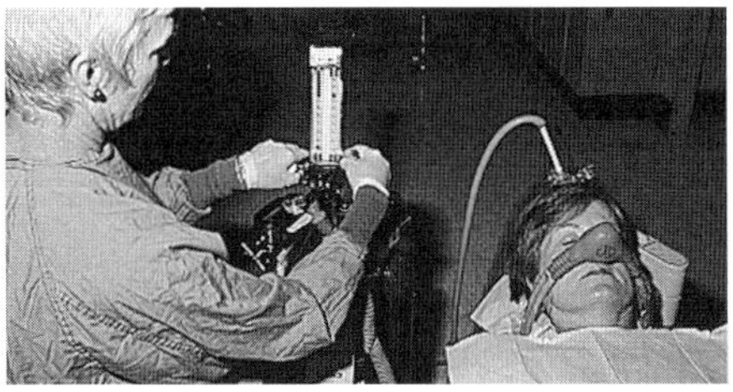

Figure 40-12.   Initiating titration of N_2O.

STEPS—*cont'd*	**RATIONALES**—*cont'd*
23. Continue titration of N_2O. If the initial concentration of N_2O proves inadequate, decrease the level of O_2 again by 0.5 to 1 L and increase N_2O by 0.5 to 1 L. Again wait 60 to 90 seconds, observing the client, then question the client to elicit signs and symptoms of baseline.	Same as above.
24. Continue titration (i.e., decreasing O_2 by 0.5 to 1 L and increasing N_2O by 0.5 to 1 L and waiting 60 to 90 seconds to observe for signs, then questioning to elicit symptoms) until observation and questioning elicit positive indications of baseline.	
25. Record the time baseline was reached and the associated percentages of N_2O and O_2 in the client's chart.	Documenting baseline levels provides a reference for future N_2O-O_2 sedation procedures. Noting time of baseline is necessary to determine oxygenation period before dismissing the client.
26. Monitor client and reassure as necessary; comment on how comfortable and relaxed the client seems.	Checking with clients periodically about their comfort level allows the operator to reduce or increase N_2O concentration as needed. The client should never be left alone while under N_2O-O_2 sedation in case the level of sedation needs to be lowered or in case of an emergency. Persons under N_2O-O_2 sedation are very suggestible.
27. Begin dental hygiene care and continue to observe the client and gas machine during the procedure.	At baseline level of sedation the client is relaxed and comfortable. If, however, nausea, sleepiness, dreaming, vertigo, repeated closing of the mouth, a rigid mandible, or restlessness are observed by the clinician or reported by the client, the concentration of N_2O needs to be reduced by 2 L/min to lighten the level of sedation.

Copyright © 2010 by Saunders, an imprint of Elsevier Inc. All rights reserved.

| Procedure **40-1** | ADMINISTRATION OF NITROUS OXIDE–OXYGEN ANALGESIC USING THE CONSTANT LITER FLOW TECHNIQUE—*cont'd* |

STEPS—*cont'd*	RATIONALES—*cont'd*

TERMINATE THE FLOW OF N$_2$O AND BEGIN OXYGENATION

| 28. Near the end of the appointment (e.g., during selective polishing), discontinue the N$_2$O and increase the O$_2$ concentration to 100%. | This action revives the client. |
| 29. Oxygenate 5 minutes for every 15 minutes of exposure to N$_2$O-O$_2$. | Oxygenating clients 5 minutes for every 15 minutes of N$_2$O exposure prevents diffusion hypoxia. |

DISCHARGE THE CLIENT, AND DOCUMENT PROCEDURE IN CHART

| 30. Remove the nose mask and slowly bring the client to an upright position (Figure 40-13). | Bringing the client to an upright position in an abrupt manner may cause syncope. |

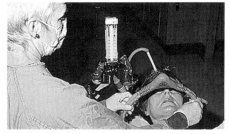

Figure 40-13.   Removing nasal mask.

| 31. If the client feels normal, discharge him or her (Figure 40-14). | After the appropriate oxygenation period, there is no additional recovery time needed if the client reports feeling normal. |

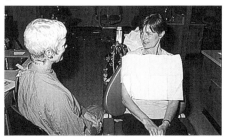

Figure 40-14.   Assessing client before discharge.

| 32. Document the experience in the client's record. Note vital signs, concentrations of N$_2$O and O$_2$ administered, length of time of sedation and oxygenation, the care provided, and the client's response to the sedation (Figure 40-15). | This documentation provides a legal record of care and serves as a reference for future care and administration of N$_2$O-O$_2$ conscious sedation. |

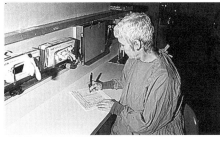

Figure 40-15.   Documenting care rendered.

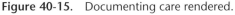

Please refer to the Evolve website (http://evolve.elsevier.com/Darby/hygiene) for competency forms to help evaluate your mastery of each procedure in this chapter.

Copyright © 2010 by Saunders, an imprint of Elsevier Inc. All rights reserved.

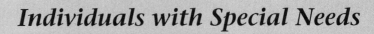
Persons with Disabilities

Procedure 41-1	TRANSFERRING CLIENT FROM WHEELCHAIR TO DENTAL CHAIR USING A ONE-PERSON LIFT

STEPS	RATIONALES
1. Position transfer belt around client's waist just below ribcage (Figure 41-1).	Ensures client safety.

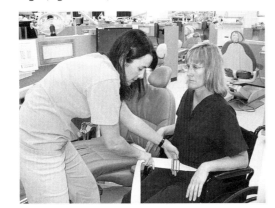

Figure 41-1. Transfer belt is placed around the client's waist and below the ribcage. (Courtesy Kathleen Muzzin, Caruth School of Dental Hygiene, Baylor College of Dentistry, Texas A&M University Health Science Center; and Bobi Robles, Baylor Institute for Rehabilitation, Dallas, Texas.)

Copyright © 2010 by Saunders, an imprint of Elsevier Inc. All rights reserved.

Procedure 41-1	TRANSFERRING CLIENT FROM WHEELCHAIR TO DENTAL CHAIR USING A ONE-PERSON LIFT—*cont'd*

STEPS—*cont'd* | **RATIONALES—*cont'd***

2. Insert your hands underneath client's thighs, and gently slide client forward in wheelchair seat so that client's buttocks are positioned on front portion of seat. Place sliding board under client so that one end of board is underneath client's thighs and other end is laid across the dental chair (Figure 41-2).

   Brings client's center of gravity closer to operator, facilitating transfer.

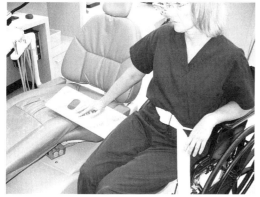

Figure 41-2. One end of the sliding board is placed underneath the client, and the other end is laid across the dental chair. (Courtesy Kathleen Muzzin, Caruth School of Dental Hygiene, Baylor College of Dentistry, Texas A&M University Health Science Center; and Bobi Robles, Baylor Institute for Rehabilitation, Dallas, Texas.)

3. Place client's feet together and hold them in place on either side by your feet. Close your knees or thighs on the client's knees, thus supporting and stabilizing client's leg, which allows client to bear some of own weight during the lift.

   Helps prevent client from falling forward onto operator during the lift.

4. Place client's arms on his or her lap or on the side of wheelchair; instruct client to rest the head over your shoulder so as to look in the opposite direction of the transfer (Figure 41-3).

   Allows operator to see behind client and to see the dental chair.

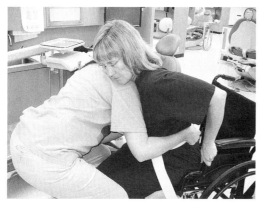

Figure 41-3. Client's hands are placed on side of wheelchair, and head is positioned on the operator's shoulder opposite the direction of the transfer. (Courtesy Kathleen Muzzin, Caruth School of Dental Hygiene, Baylor College of Dentistry, Texas A&M University Health Science Center; and Bobi Robles, Baylor Institute for Rehabilitation, Dallas, Texas.)

(Continued)

Copyright © 2010 by Saunders, an imprint of Elsevier Inc. All rights reserved.

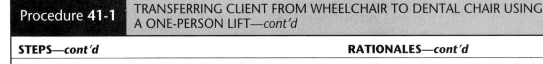

| **Procedure 41-1** | TRANSFERRING CLIENT FROM WHEELCHAIR TO DENTAL CHAIR USING A ONE-PERSON LIFT—*cont'd* |

STEPS—*cont'd*	**RATIONALES—*cont'd***
5. Grasp client around waist and hold transfer belt securely between both hands. If there is no transfer belt available, use an overlapping wrist grasp for greater stability.	Overlapping the arms to grasp the belt provides added stability.
6. Rock gently backward onto your heels and, using your leg muscles, lift client off seat. Client is now resting against you, the operator (Figure 41-4).	Provides momentum and minimizes operator back injury in the transfer.

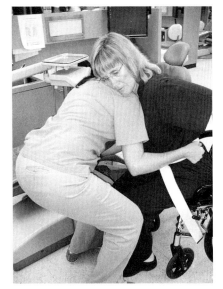

Figure 41-4. Client is lifted off the wheelchair and positioned for transfer to the dental chair. (Courtesy Kathleen Muzzin, Caruth School of Dental Hygiene, Baylor College of Dentistry, Texas A&M University Health Science Center; and Bobi Robles, Baylor Institute for Rehabilitation, Dallas, Texas.)

7. Pivot on your foot closer to the dental chair, and maneuver client over seat of dental chair. This should be done in a smooth motion.	Maximizes the clinician's strength; minimizes energy required for the transfer; protects operator's back.
8. Lower client onto dental chair by bending at your knees. Do not release transfer belt around client until client is securely placed into chair.	Reduces risk of operator injury; ensures client safety.
9. Release one hand to lift client's legs onto chair while still supporting client with the other hand. Reposition armrest of dental chair for client safety.	Establishes client stability and safety.

Copyright © 2010 by Saunders, an imprint of Elsevier Inc. All rights reserved.

Procedure 41-2	TRANSFERRING CLIENT FROM WHEELCHAIR TO DENTAL CHAIR USING A TWO-PERSON LIFT

STEPS	**RATIONALES**
1. First operator stands behind client and reaches around client's torso underneath armpits. Operator crosses her or his arms in front of client and grasps client's hands at the wrists with opposite hands (right over left, left over right). Operator then slides her or his arms down so that arms are positioned under the client's ribcage on the abdomen. Stronger and/or taller of two operators is placed behind client.	Supports the majority of the client's weight.
2. Second operator is positioned on the far side of the wheelchair at the client's knees or thighs. Bending at the knees, operator slides one arm underneath the client's thighs (approximately midway point) while other arm is placed slightly above the knees (Figure 41-5).	Provides support for the client's lower extremities during transfer.

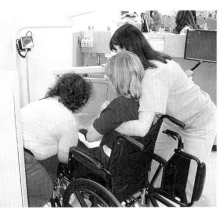

Figure 41-5. During the two-person transfer, the first operator stands behind the wheelchair and the second operator positions herself at the client's thighs. (Courtesy Kathleen Muzzin, Caruth School of Dental Hygiene, Baylor College of Dentistry, Texas A&M University Health Science Center; and Bobi Robles, Baylor Institute for Rehabilitation, Dallas, Texas.)

(Continued)

Copyright © 2010 by Saunders, an imprint of Elsevier Inc. All rights reserved.

| Procedure **41-2** | TRANSFERRING CLIENT FROM WHEELCHAIR TO DENTAL CHAIR USING A TWO-PERSON LIFT—*cont'd* |

STEPS—*cont'd*	**RATIONALES—*cont'd***
3. Client is lifted by both operators at a prearranged signal ("1, 2, 3, lift"). One person coordinates the lift, preferably the operator who is supporting the client's torso (the operator who is lifting the most weight) (Figure 41-6).	Minimizes risk of loss of client support by one or both operators; decreases client's and operators' risk for injury.

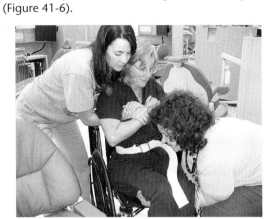

Figure 41-6. The operator who is supporting the client's torso coordinates the lift. (Courtesy Kathleen Muzzin, Caruth School of Dental Hygiene, Baylor College of Dentistry, Texas A&M University Health Science Center; and Bobi Robles, Baylor Institute for Rehabilitation, Dallas, Texas.)

STEPS—*cont'd*	**RATIONALES—*cont'd***
4. Client is lifted in one smooth motion and placed into dental chair (Figure 41-7).	Maximizes operators' strength; minimizes energy required for the transfer.

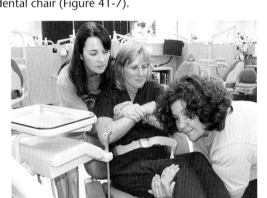

Figure 41-7. Client is lifted in one smooth motion and placed in the dental chair. (Courtesy Kathleen Muzzin, Caruth School of Dental Hygiene, Baylor College of Dentistry, Texas A&M University Health Science Center; and Bobi Robles, Baylor Institute for Rehabilitation, Dallas, Texas.)

STEPS—*cont'd*	**RATIONALES—*cont'd***
5. Operator holding the legs releases the grasp on the client and repositions client in chair. Other operator does not release client until the client is stabilized and arm of dental chair is replaced.	Establishes client stability and safety.

Please refer to the Evolve website (http://evolve.elsevier.com/Darby/hygiene) for competency forms to help evaluate your mastery of each procedure in this chapter.

Copyright © 2010 by Saunders, an imprint of Elsevier Inc. All rights reserved.

Persons with Human Immunodeficiency Virus Infection

Procedure 45-1	DENTAL HYGIENE CARE FOR THE HIV-INFECTED CLIENT

EQUIPMENT
Personal protective equipment
Mouth mirror
Explorer
Periodontal probe
Scalers
2 × 2 gauze
Saliva ejector
Disposable syringe with blunt needle
0.12% chlorhexidine gluconate
Ultrasonic scaling device (power scaler)
Syringe
Oral local and topical anesthetic agents
Cotton swabs

STEPS	RATIONALES
1. Assess client needs.	Ensures comprehensive, humanistic care.
2. Establish the dental hygiene care plan with client; determine need for consultation with other healthcare professionals.	Care must be integrated with the overall dental treatment plan.
	Additional medication may be needed during the course of care. Client's platelet count, prothrombin time, and partial prothrombin time may be needed to predict postoperative bleeding. Consultation with dentist and physician is necessary.
3. Provide oral disease control instructions.	Client responsibility for daily care is important for promoting and maintaining health.
4. Provide preprocedural oral rinse of 0.12% chlorhexidine gluconate.	Reduces oral microbial load.
5. Perform debridement procedures as needed (note that this may need to be done repeatedly for several consecutive appointments within a week.	Necessary for healing periodontal tissues.
6. Irrigate subgingivally with 0.12% chlorhexidine gluconate after scaling procedures.	Antibacterial properties promote soft-tissue healing by temporarily decreasing subgingival bacteria.
7. Postoperative recommendations include oral biofilm control and twice-daily use for 30 seconds of 0.12% chlorhexidine as an antibacterial mouth rinse. Slowly introduce mechanical daily oral care as pain subsides and healing occurs.	Provides for mechanical and chemical oral biofilm control.
8. Establish 2- to 3-month continued-care interval.	Close monitoring is required.

CLIENT WITH UNEXPECTEDLY SEVERE PERIODONTAL SIGNS AND SYMPTOMS AND/OR ORAL LESIONS

1. Consult with team members. Dentist may need to remove necrotic bone and prescribe medications.	Provides for optimal care.
2. Refer for lesion evaluation, dental diagnosis, periodontal consultation.	Determines extent of disease and appropriate care plan with other team members.

(Continued)

Copyright © 2010 by Saunders, an imprint of Elsevier Inc. All rights reserved.

Procedure 45-1 DENTAL HYGIENE CARE FOR THE HIV-INFECTED CLIENT—*cont'd*

STEPS—*cont'd*	RATIONALES—*cont'd*
3. Periodontal care requires irrigating tissues with an effective antimicrobial agent.	
4. Debride using hand-activated or ultrasonic instruments and topical or local anesthetic agent as needed.	Promotes healing of periodontal tissues and provides concurrent pain control if needed.
5. Use postoperative antibiotics or antifungal agents as needed.	Assists in healing.
6. Monitoring every 2 to 3 months by the team.	Close observation for preventive and treatment needs.
CASE DOCUMENTATION	
1. Record services rendered and client response to care at each treatment appointment in ink.	Ensures integrity of the client's record for client and dental practice and legal protection of practitioner.

Please refer to the Evolve website (http://evolve.elsevier.com/Darby/hygiene) for competency forms to help evaluate your mastery of each procedure in this chapter.

Copyright © 2010 by Saunders, an imprint of Elsevier Inc. All rights reserved.

Respiratory Diseases

49

Procedure 49-1   MANAGEMENT OF AN ACUTE ASTHMATIC EPISODE

STEPS	RATIONALES
1. Terminate the dental procedure and remove all materials from client's mouth immediately.	Client may inhale materials during asthma attack.
2. Place the client in a comfortable position as soon as signs are apparent—usually sitting with the arms thrown forward over the back of a chair.	This positioning allows for the most comfort during acute attack.
3. Remove all dental materials from mouth.	This helps client avoid aspiration.
4. Try to calm client and allay apprehension.	Anxiety can exacerbate symptoms, producing a "vicious cycle."
5. Evaluate ABCs (airway, breathing, circulation), and monitor vital signs.	Client remains conscious and breathing in most attacks; client usually has increased blood pressure and heart rate.
6. Definitive care:	
a. Administration of bronchodilator (client's prescribed medication preferred).	Bronchodilators are drugs used to manage the bronchospasm of an acute attack.
b. If attack persists, administer oxygen.	Clinical signs of low oxygen levels (confusion, anxiety, cyanosis, hypertension, hypotension, headache) warrant use of supplemental oxygen.
c. Call for emergency assistance if bronchodilators fail to resolve bronchospasm.	Emergency personnel may be needed to transport the client to the hospital if an attack is not controlled.
d. Administration of epinephrine if necessary (available in preloaded syringe).	Epinephrine may be needed if the bronchodilator does not arrest the attack.
7. Discharge of the client: alone, escorted, or with emergency personnel, depending on severity of attack.	The client may not be able to leave the office without an escort or may need hospitalization if the attack is severe.

Adapted from Malamed SF: *Medical emergencies in the dental office,* ed 6, St Louis, 2007, Mosby.

Please refer to the Evolve website (http://evolve.elsevier.com/Darby/hygiene) for competency forms to help evaluate your mastery of each procedure in this chapter.

Copyright © 2010 by Saunders, an imprint of Elsevier Inc. All rights reserved.

Persons with Fixed and Removable Dentures

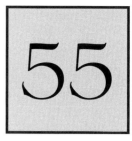

Procedure 55-1   PROFESSIONAL CARE FOR CLIENTS WITH FIXED AND REMOVABLE DENTURES

EQUIPMENT
Protective barriers
Prophy cup and bristled brush
Low-speed handpiece
Antimicrobial mouth rinse
Tin oxide
Mouth mirror
Hand mirror
Gauze
Disclosing solution
Tongue blades
Small plastic bag
Stain and calculus remover solution
Ultrasonic cleaning unit

STEPS	RATIONALES
ASSESSMENT	
1. Update client's health history to identify systemic disorders, current medications, and conditions that may affect care and ability to wear prostheses.	Systemic health affects oral health and success of prostheses.
2. Review client's personal history records; note details such as age, occupation, and culture.	The client's personal profile influences care and dictates priorities and self-care.
3. Review client's dental history.	Reflects previous oral disease, past dental and dental hygiene care, self-care priorities, and values.
4. Ask client to explain denture problems experienced; listen attentively to complaints.	Provides insight into nature of denture problems and client's beliefs and values.
5. Perform comprehensive assessment of head and neck.	Facilitates early recognition of abnormalities that may signal human need deficits related to oral health and disease.
6. Assess the temporomandibular joint (TMJ) and associated musculature as client opens and closes mouth and slides jaw from side to side.	TMJ disorders can develop from extended wear of ill-fitting dentures.
7. Assess extraoral soft tissues.	Adequate facial support by dentures is necessary to maintain normal facial appearances; angular cheilitis may indicate a *Candida* infection or other systemic disease.
8. Assess intraoral soft tissues for evidence of local or systemic diseases, and record color, texture, size, contour, and presence of pain.	Inflammation, traumatic injury, and chemical irritations may indicate need for referral to dentist for further evaluation.
9. Visually inspect and palpate denture-bearing mucosa.	Determines resilience of overlying mucosa and submucosa; assists in evaluating denture fit and changes produced with increasing age.
10. Assess the structure and form of the alveolar ridges.	Flabby tissue, uneven underlying bone, and bony spikes contribute to poor stability and retention of denture.
11. Document changes in associated structures, including the tongue, floor of the mouth, and oropharynx.	May reveal loose-fitting dentures, lack of wear of the prosthesis, chronic low-grade trauma, systemic conditions, or oral lesions.
12. Assess oral hygiene status.	Improper denture and mouth care potentiates infection and poor adaptation.

Copyright © 2010 by Saunders, an imprint of Elsevier Inc. All rights reserved.

Procedure 55-1	PROFESSIONAL CARE FOR CLIENTS WITH FIXED AND REMOVABLE DENTURES—*cont'd*
STEPS—*cont'd*	**RATIONALES—*cont'd***
13. Ask client to displace the prosthesis away from supporting tissues. The posterior border seal of the maxillary denture is checked by attempting to pull the anterior teeth forward.	Assess retention, which is necessary for satisfactory physiologic performance and appearance of the denture and for proper speaking.
14. Assess stability of the denture with respect to denture position during normal oral functions.	Denture stability is directly associated with retention and fit.
15. Indicate changes in occlusion and articulation.	Freeway space (interocclusal distance) and occlusal vertical dimension are important to client's appearance and comfort.
DENTAL HYGIENE DIAGNOSIS	
16. Analyze objective and subjective assessment data; identify unmet human needs.	Ensures that care will be planned to meet client needs.
17. Present significant findings to dentist.	Collaboration ensures high-quality care and expedites dental care.
PLANNING	
18. Determine a dental hygiene care plan and goals in consultation with client and dentist.	Involvement in decision making increases client motivation, acceptance, and responsibility.
19. Establish with client goals to be achieved.	Ensures client commitment and measure of clinical outcomes.
IMPLEMENTATION	
20. Review self-care and dental care; suggest methods for improvement.	Reinforcement is vital to oral health maintenance.
21. Use disclosing solution to stain plaque and calculus on denture (when appropriate).	Demonstrates need for improved oral and denture care.
22. Counsel client on adequate nutrition.	Corrects nutrient imbalances that compromise integrity of oral tissues.

(Continued)

Copyright © 2010 by Saunders, an imprint of Elsevier Inc. All rights reserved.

Procedure 55-1   PROFESSIONAL CARE FOR CLIENTS WITH FIXED AND REMOVABLE DENTURES—*cont'd*

STEPS—*cont'd*	RATIONALES—*cont'd*
23. Fill a small plastic bag with cleaning solution, submerge the denture in it, and place the bag in an ultrasonic cleaning unit (Figure 55-1).	Provides a safe, effective alternative to manual scaling for removing calculus and extrinsic stain from denture (Table 55-1, see Figure 55-1).

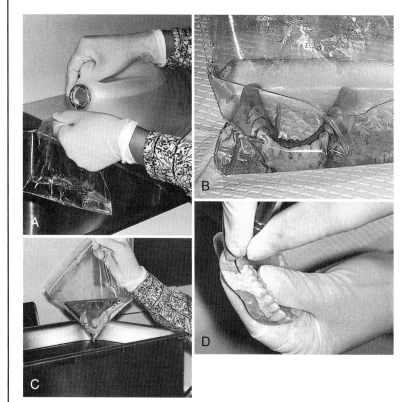

Figure 55-1. Ultrasonic cleaning of denture. **A,** Fill plastic bag with stain and calculus remover solution. **B,** Place denture in bag with solution. **C,** Place bag in ultrasonic cleaner chamber and set for 10 to 14 minutes. **D,** Some dentures may require manual scaling to remove deposits; however, the inner impression is avoided.) (Courtesy Bertha Chan.)

24. Lightly polish the denture with an extremely fine polishing agent (tin oxide) *on external surfaces only,* and thoroughly rinse under warm water (when appropriate).	Restoration of shine may inspire the client to maintain cleanliness of denture. Internal surfaces are avoided to maintain proper fit.

EVALUATION

25. Discuss continued-care interval. Emphasize the importance of regular professional care.	Continued care is essential to maintaining oral health.
26. Measure the achievement of established goals.	Prevents supervised neglect and erroneously dismissing a client who still needs care.
27. Formulate an evaluative statement regarding the level of goal attainment.	Documents client's status for management of legal risks and quality of care.
28. Document service in client's record under "Services Rendered," and date entry.	Ensures integrity of record for both the client's health and legal protection of practitioner.

Copyright © 2010 by Saunders, an imprint of Elsevier Inc. All rights reserved.

TABLE 55-1 Oral Appliance Cleansing Products

Product	Mechanism of Action	Advantages	Disadvantages
Chemical Soak Cleansers			
Alkaline hypochlorite	Dissolves mucins and organic substances of denture plaque matrix	Bactericidal Fungicidal Bleaches stains May inhibit calculus formation	Corrodes metals Odor and taste may be unacceptable May bleach acrylic if used in high concentration or for prolonged periods
Alkaline peroxide	Mechanical cleansing effect caused by the release of oxygen (bubbling)	Some antibacterial effect Removes stain	None
Ultrasonic cleaning devices	Conflicting evidence regarding effectiveness of ultrasonic action per se; chemical solution may provide cleansing action	Removes bacterial plaque Enhances effectiveness of disinfectants	Commonly an in-office procedure Uncertain efficacy of ultrasonic action
Antimicrobial			
Chlorhexidine gluconate 2% solution (not approved for use on dentures in United States)	Antimicrobial action by chemical agent	Antibacterial Antifungal	Only temporary relief of denture stomatitis symptoms Stains denture teeth

Copyright © 2010 by Saunders, an imprint of Elsevier Inc. All rights reserved.

Procedure 55-2	DAILY ORAL AND DENTURE HYGIENE CARE FOR INDIVIDUALS WITH REMOVABLE PROSTHESES

EQUIPMENT

Soft denture brush, tongue cleaner, and a soft intraoral toothbrush; antimicrobial mouth rinse
Basin
Denture cup
Towel
Dilute sodium hypochlorite solution (complete dentures) or commercial denture cleanser (partial dentures)
Warm water
Wall-mounted mirror
Soft nylon toothbrush

STEPS	RATIONALES
1. Explain the importance of daily care for both dentures and soft tissues.	Prolongs life of dentures, promotes healthy oral tissues, and promotes well-being of client.
2. Describe the consequences of oral and denture hygiene neglect.	Augments client awareness of halitosis, inflammation, trauma, or negative bone remodeling on appearance and health.
3. Summarize the client's responsibilities in monitoring oral function and health status.	Client is being taught to recognize early problems may prevent further discomfort and destruction.
4. Advise against the use of denture home-repair kits and encourage the client to return to the dentist for proper care.	Improper denture modification results in further damage to the oral tissues and denture.
5. Discourage use of denture adhesives with a stable and retentive prosthesis. Under dentist supervision, a small amount of adhesive may be evenly applied over the inner surface that directly contacts the oral mucosa. Denture adhesives are not normally used with partial removable dentures.	Dependence on adhesives may indicate need for denture adjustment.
6. Remind the client to brush denture after each meal and before retiring or, at the very least, to rinse it under running water.	Oral biofilm and food debris readily collect on dentures and foster a variety of oral mucosa problems (Table 55-2 on p. 267).
7. Teach self-examination of denture for proper fit, denture deposits, and abraded inner and outer surfaces.	Facilitates self-referral to the dentist to avoid further problems.
8. Teach client that some commercially available denture powders and pastes are too abrasive for dentures and are not recommended for use.	Coarse abrasives alter shine, surface character, and fit of prosthesis.

Copyright © 2010 by Saunders, an imprint of Elsevier Inc. All rights reserved.

Procedure 55-2	DAILY ORAL AND DENTURE HYGIENE CARE FOR INDIVIDUALS WITH REMOVABLE PROSTHESES—*cont'd*

STEPS—*cont'd* | **RATIONALES—*cont'd***

9. Suggest daily use of fresh denture immersion cleansers. Recommend a dilute sodium hypochlorite solution as a cleanser for complete dentures (Figure 55-2; Box 55-1). Soak complete dentures for 5 to 10 minutes, and rinse thoroughly. Partial dentures benefit from alkaline peroxide solutions found in many denture-cleansing products, usually in the form of a tablet. Soak partial denture for 15 minutes or overnight, and rinse thoroughly. Change solutions daily.

Chemical cleansers bathe all denture surfaces, aid clients who lack manual dexterity, minimize accidental breakage of dentures, and can be used while dentures are out of the mouth. Dilute hypochlorite solutions provide nontoxic, bactericidal, and fungicidal actions (see Box 55-1 and Figure 55-2).

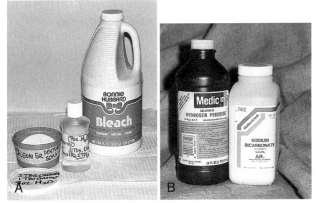

Figure 55-2. Inexpensive denture cleaners. **A,** Combination of sodium hypochlorite, Calgon, and water for denture without metal. **B,** Combination of hydrogen peroxide and sodium bicarbonate forms an alkaline peroxide solution for dentures with metal. (Courtesy Bertha Chan.)

10. Teach the client to remove denture when possible and at night while at rest.

Continuous wearing of dentures inhibits the natural cleansing mechanisms of the tongue and saliva and increases oral biofilm retention.

11. Assemble supplies.

Sets up the necessary materials for proper cleaning technique.

12. Fill basin with water, and line with a small towel.

Prevents breakage of denture should it be accidentally dropped.

13. Gently remove denture, and rinse away saliva and loose debris. In case of complete dentures, remove any denture adhesive material.

Improves ability to assess appliance.

14. Firmly grasp denture in palm of one hand, and hold over water-filled basin.

Prevents accidental breakage of denture.

(Continued)

Copyright © 2010 by Saunders, an imprint of Elsevier Inc. All rights reserved.

Procedure 55-2   DAILY ORAL AND DENTURE HYGIENE CARE FOR INDIVIDUALS WITH REMOVABLE PROSTHESES—*cont'd*

STEPS—*cont'd*	**RATIONALES**—*cont'd*
15. Demonstrate use of soft toothbrush with a mild soap solution or regular toothpaste to remove accumulations on the inner impression and outer polished surfaces, and adapt brush as necessary (Figure 55-3).	Areas difficult to access require special attention. The client must be reminded to access all areas without overexuberant brushing, which may damage the denture or a soft resilient liner (see Figure 55-3).

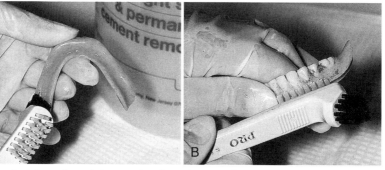

Figure 55-3.   A, Adaptation of denture brush on inner surface of denture. B, Adaptation of denture brush on outer surface of denture. (Courtesy Bertha Chan.)

16. Rinse denture and brush under running water to completely remove all denture cleanser.	Residual cleanser may cause irritation to oral mucosa.
17. Inspect denture for any remaining bacterial plaque biofilm, food debris, or cleanser by visual and tactile examination.	Ensures that all debris has been removed.
18. Place prosthesis in a denture cup filled with room-temperature tap water or denture cleanser, and cover it.	Prevents dehydration and distortion of denture (acrylic resin).
19. On removal of denture, rinse mouth with warm water, antimicrobial mouth rinse, or saline solution.	Removal of large debris from oral cavity is essential to maintaining a healthy oral environment.
20. Teach client to use a soft toothbrush or soft cloth daily to clean edentulous mucosa and tongue by employing long strokes in a posterior to anterior direction.	Maintains sound supporting tissues for dentures. Tongue brushing improves oral malodor.
21. Teach client to use thumb and index finger to massage edentulous tissues daily by applying pressure and then releasing it continually along the ridge. Mechanical, vibratory stimulation with the sides of multitufted soft toothbrush filaments can provide similar results.	Increases keratinization of oral mucosa, circulation, and resistance to denture trauma.

BOX 55-1 Inexpensive, Safe, and Effective Cleaning Solution for Oral Appliances Devoid of Metal

- 1 tablespoon (15 mL) sodium hypochlorite (household bleach)
- 1 teaspoon (4 mL) detergent (e.g., Calgon)
- 4 ounces (114 mL) water

  After soaking, the oral appliance must be rinsed thoroughly with water before reinsertion into the oral cavity.

Copyright © 2010 by Saunders, an imprint of Elsevier Inc. All rights reserved.
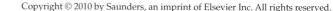

TABLE 55-2 Types of Oral Soft-Tissue Lesions in Denture-Wearing Clients Indicating an Unmet Need for Skin and Mucous Membrane Integrity of the Head and Neck

Oral Manifestation	Due to	As Evidenced by
Reactive Lesions		
Acute ulcers	Ill-fitting dentures Chemical agent irritation: Denture adhesive Denture cleanser Self-medication	Yellow-white exudates Red halo Varying pain and tenderness
Chronic ulcers	Same as above	Yellow membrane Elevated margin Little or no pain
Focal (frictional) hyperkeratosis	Chronic rubbing or friction of dentures	White patch Asymptomatic
Denture-induced fibrous hyperplasia (epulis fissurata, denture hyperplasia)	Ill-fitting denture	Folds of fibrous connective tissue Varying color Asymptomatic Typical on vestibular mucosa at denture flange contact
Infectious Lesions		
Denture stomatitis (denture sore mouth)	Chronic *Candida albicans* infection Poor oral hygiene care Continuous wear of dentures Ill-fitting dentures Systemic factors: anemia, diabetes, immunosuppression, menopause Systemic antibiotics Chemical agent irritation: Denture adhesive Denture cleanser Self-medication Denture base allergy	Generalized redness of mucosa Velvetlike appearance Pain and burning sensations Typical under maxillary denture
Angular cheilitis	Chronic *C. albicans* infection Pooling of saliva in commissural folds Riboflavin deficiency	Fissured at angles of mouth Eroded Encrusted Moderate pain
Mixed Lesions		
Papillary hyperplasia	Chronic *C. albicans* infection Chronic low-grade denture trauma	Multiple round to ovoid nodules: "cobblestone" appearance Generalized red mucosa background Rarely ulcerated Typical under maxillary denture

Copyright © 2010 by Saunders, an imprint of Elsevier Inc. All rights reserved.

Procedure 55-3   DAILY ORAL CARE FOR INDIVIDUALS WITH FIXED PROSTHESES

EQUIPMENT
Soft toothbrush
Interdental cleaners such as variable-diameter floss, dental floss, dental yarn, floss threaders; antimicrobial mouth rinse
Wall-mounted mirror

STEPS	RATIONALES
1. Explain the importance of daily self-care for fixed denture, remaining natural teeth, and periodontal tissues.	Prolongs useful life of fixed denture; promotes healthy tissues and systemic health of client.
2. Describe the consequences of oral and fixed denture hygiene neglect.	Augments client awareness of halitosis and oral disease risk on appearance and health.
3. Summarize the client's responsibilities in monitoring oral function and health status.	Client is being taught to recognize early problems may prevent further discomfort and destruction.
4. Teach the client to brush natural teeth and fixed partial denture after each meal and before retiring. Clients benefit from flossing both remaining natural teeth and fixed denture and using an antimicrobial mouth rinse daily.	Decreases risk of dental caries and periodontal disease.
5. Assemble supplies.	Ensures that materials needed to properly cleanse fixed partial denture and remaining natural teeth are available.
6. Demonstrate use of a soft toothbrush to remove plaque biofilm and gross debris from fixed partial denture and remaining natural teeth (see Chapter 22 in the textbook).	Ensures that plaque-retentive structures are thoroughly cleansed.
7. Demonstrate use of suitable interdental aid to cleanse under the pontic and around abutments and natural teeth (Figure 55-4) (see Chapter 22 in the textbook).	Ensures that all surfaces of the fixed partial denture and natural teeth are cleansed. Shape of pontic determines appropriate floss aid and flossing technique.

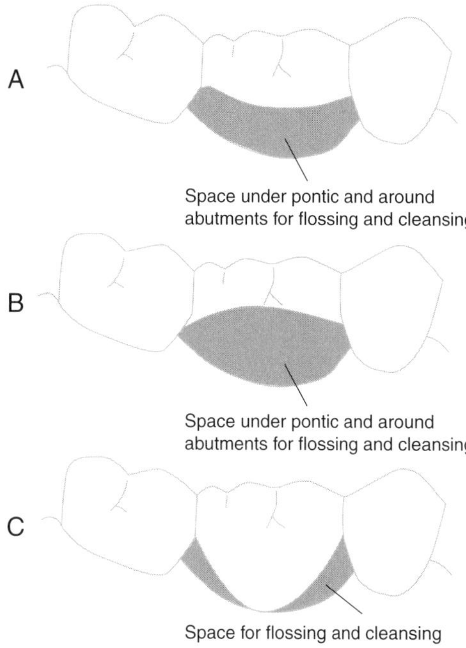

A

Space under pontic and around
abutments for flossing and cleansing

B

Space under pontic and around
abutments for flossing and cleansing

C

Space for flossing and cleansing

Figure 55-4. Fixed partial denture pontics. **A,** Conventional. **B,** Modified. **C,** Conical (bullet). (Courtesy Dr. Joanne Walton, Prosthodontist, Faculty of Dentistry, University of British Columbia, Vancouver, Canada.)

Please refer to the Evolve website (http://evolve.elsevier.com/Darby/hygiene) for competency forms to help evaluate your mastery of each procedure in this chapter.

Copyright © 2010 by Saunders, an imprint of Elsevier Inc. All rights reserved.

PART ▪ II

Client Education Handouts

Handouts, some modified significantly, from Mosby: *Dental practice tool kit*, St Louis, 2004, Author.

Copyright © 2010 by Saunders, an imprint of Elsevier Inc. All rights reserved.

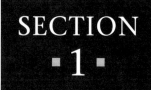

SECTION
▪ 1 ▪

General Dentistry

Copyright © 2010 by Saunders, an imprint of Elsevier Inc. All rights reserved.

PROPHYLACTIC ANTIBIOTICS FOR PREMEDICATION

Patient Name: _____

Date: _____

Reasons for antibiotic premedication are:
- To prevent infective endocarditis
- To prevent infection in a total joint replacement
- To protect persons who are immunocompromised

These conditions might occur following any treatment or activity that causes bacteria to enter the bloodstream (bacteremia). Therefore it is recommended that persons undergoing dental or dental hygiene procedures that cause bacteremia, and who also are at high risk for complication from endocarditis, receive antibiotic premedication before professional care. **For that reason, if you have been diagnosed as having any of the following conditions, you will need to be premedicated before invasive dental or dental hygiene treatment:**

- Prosthetic heart valve or prosthetic material used for cardiac valve repair including bioprosthetic and homograft valves
- Replacement joints such as hips or knees received within the past 2 years
- Congenital heart disease (CHD)
  - Unrepaired cyanotic CHD, including palliative shunts and conduits
  - Repaired CHD with residual defects at the site of or adjacent to the site of a prosthetic patch or prosthetic device (which inhibits endotheliazation)

- Completely repaired CHD with prosthetic material or device during the first 6 months after the procedure
- Previous infective endocarditis
- Intravascular access devices (for chemotherapy, hemodialysis, hyperalimentation)
- Cerebrospinal fluid shunts
- Heart transplant with valvulopathy

Before we can begin treatment in some cases, we must consult with your physician to determine which premedication is recommended for your specific condition. When it has been determined that you need to be premedicated before dental procedures, we will ask you before each dental appointment whether you have taken the premedication.

When your physician, surgeon, or cardiologist determines that it is best for you to be premedicated before certain dental procedures, you must take the premedication. Your physician may prescribe an antibiotic different from those listed in the following table.

If you have not taken the medication as prescribed, we will not be able to perform any dental treatment. There are no exceptions. The result could be a serious illness with a prolonged hospital stay.

Regimens for a Dental Procedure (Single Dose 30 to 60 Minutes before Procedure)

Situation	Agent	Adults	Children
Oral	Amoxicillin	2 g	50 mg/kg
Unable to take oral medication	Ampicillin	2 g IM or IV	50 mg/kg IM or IV
	or		
	Cefazolin or ceftriazone	1 g IM or IV	50 mg/kg IM or IV
Allergic to penicillin or ampicillin oral	Cephalexin*†	2 g	50 mg/kg
	or		
	Clindamycin	600 mg	20 mg/kg
	or		
	Azithromycin or clarithromycin	500 mg	15 mg/kg
Allergic to penicillin or ampicillin and unable to take oral medication	Cefazolin or ceftriaxone†	1 g IM or IV	50 mg/kg IM or IV
	or		
	Clindamycin	600 mg IM or IV	20 mg/kg IM or IV

IM, Intramuscular; *IV,* intravenous.

*Or other first- or second-generation oral cephalosporin in equivalent adult or pediatric dosage.

†Cephalosporins should not be used in a person with a history of anaphylaxis, angioedema, or urticaria with penicillins or ampicillin.

If you have any questions about prophylactic antibiotics for premedication, please feel free to ask us.

Specific Recommendations: _____

_____

_____

Copyright © 2010 by Saunders, an imprint of Elsevier Inc. All rights reserved.

STAYING WELL: HOW TO KEEP YOUR MOUTH HEALTHY

Patient Name: _____   **Date:** _____

Congratulations! You have completed all dental treatment necessary up to this point. If you follow the listed suggestions, you will have the best chance of maintaining that optimum oral health for the longest time. If you are unsure about any aspect of what you should be doing, please ask us for further instruction.

- Brush, floss, and use recommended dental cleaning aids correctly, at least once each day.
- Brushing and flossing cleans only about 20% of the mouth. To reach the other 80%, we recommend that you rinse twice daily for 30 seconds with an ADA-accepted antimicrobial mouth rinse. If you experience dry mouth symptoms, we recommend that you:

  _____
  _____
  _____

- Given your unique oral care needs, we also recommend the following oral care products and/or devices for your use:_____

  _____
  _____

- Come to the office for recare hygiene appointments at the specific intervals we recommend. This is very important. Every mouth is different. Based on the number of dental restorations you have, the number and alignment of your teeth, your apparent ability at this time to keep your teeth clean, and your medical history, we recommend that the interval be no longer than _____ months. With this interval, there is the best opportunity to prevent gum disease or correct problems found early when they are small, easier, and less expensive to treat.
- Each time you come in for procedural dental hygiene care, make your next hygiene recare appointment before you leave the office. But please try to remember when you are due for an appointment. No matter how attractive we make our reminder cards, they seem to have a habit of getting mixed up in junk mail and being discarded without being noticed.

- If you have followed our advice, you should receive years of successful service from your teeth. Natural teeth and restorative materials are subjected to great stress on a daily basis. Please do not put things in your mouth that do not belong there. This will tremendously shorten the effective life span of your teeth and restorations.
- Do not chew on ice or frozen candy bars, bite on hard candy, or keep hard candy or breath mints in your mouth on a routine basis. Any sugary food that you keep in your mouth for a long time (as it dissolves) can easily and quickly cause tooth decay. You can use sugar-free candy and mints that contain xylitol.
- If you smoke, stop. Remember that smoking has a negative effect on your gum tissue and on your general health.
- Smoking and drinking coffee, tea, and cola beverages will have a tendency to stain or darken your teeth over time. This can be reversed with your regular recare dental hygiene and, if necessary, noninvasive tooth whitening procedures.
- If you are having your dental treatment scheduled for time or financial reasons, please continue at the time we have discussed.
- If you have had a protective mouth guard made (to protect your teeth and new restorations or reduce the effects of a bruxing or grinding habit), please wear it as instructed.

We have used the most appropriate diagnostic and treatment knowledge, procedures, and materials available for your treatment. Teeth and restorations can break from excessive force or trauma. If you take care of your car, it will last longer than if you never change the oil, fluids, and so on, and it will cost you much less to keep in operation. Your teeth and gums need regular maintenance care, too. No individual treatment you received costs as much as your car, but with adequate care you probably will have your restorations longer than your car.

Thank you for giving us the opportunity to serve you, and we hope to see you soon.

Specific Recommendations: _____

_____
_____

Copyright © 2010 by Saunders, an imprint of Elsevier Inc. All rights reserved.

HOW TO BRUSH! HOW TO FLOSS!

Patient Name: _____   **Date:** _____

An old humorous expression says, "You don't have to brush all your teeth every day. Only the ones you want to keep!" And while we laugh at these words, the message could not be more correct. To maintain good oral health, teeth must be thoroughly cleaned each and every day. One good method of brushing is called the *modified Bass technique.* It is quite effective. We can instruct you on how to brush properly. It is certainly easier to see it done than to read and imagine. But this will help you get started.

Use a multitufted, soft, nylon-bristled toothbrush. Hard-bristled toothbrushes can easily damage your teeth and gums. Soft-bristled toothbrushes last about 3 months before they need to be replaced. When the toothbrush bristles become worn, they will not give you the best possible performance. Medium- and hard-bristled brushes will last longer, but almost everyone brushes too hard to use these brushes. If you use medium- and hard-bristled brushes or brush improperly with any toothbrush, you can cause permanent damage to your gum tissue, causing it to wear away. This can also wear notches into the tooth itself, exposing the dentin. In both cases, severe tooth sensitivity could develop.

THE MODIFIED BASS METHOD

- The bristles of the brush should be angled toward the area where the tooth meets the gum, approximately a 45-degree angle.
- The bristles of the brush should be able to gently slide under the gum tissue. Gently move the brush back and forth so that there is a vibrating motion, **not a scrubbing motion.** The brush head should be able to cover and clean about two teeth at a time.
- Brush each area for about 10 seconds, then roll the bristles to the biting surface. Move the brush head so that it overlaps a small portion of the tooth just brushed and the next teeth. Repeat until all teeth have been brushed.

Brush all teeth. Start on the cheek side of the back teeth, at one corner of your mouth, brushing as you move across to the opposite corner. Then switch to the inside (tongue or palate side), and again brush from one corner to the other. Brush both upper and lower teeth using the vibrating back-and-forth motion.

Some areas will require you to switch the brush to a different angle such as the inside (tongue and palate side) of the top and bottom front teeth. Using the tip or small end of the brush will help clean around this curved area. Use the same type of vibrating motion with the brush, moving up and down against the tooth.

If you see blood on your toothbrush, try to clean the gum area more thoroughly for several days until the bleeding stops. If you continue to see bleeding, contact your dental hygienist.

Brushing the biting surfaces of the teeth is easy. Place the bristles on the biting surface of the teeth into the grooves, and brush back and forth. Be sure to brush the biting surfaces of left side and right side, upper and lower teeth.

The tooth surfaces should feel smooth and free of any fur-like coatings when your tongue is rubbed over them. Lastly, brush the tongue gently from back to front to remove any coating that has accumulated. You will find that your food will taste better too when your tongue is kept clean.

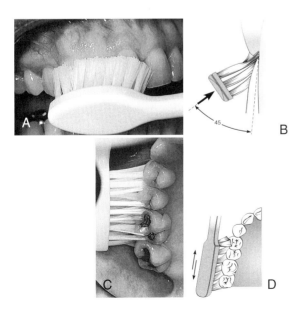

The Bass toothbrushing method. **A,** Proper intrasulcular position of brush in the mouth aims the filaments toward and into the gingival sulcus. **B,** Diagram shows the ideal placement with slight subgingival penetration of the filament tips. **C,** Place toothbrush so that filaments are angled approximately 45 degrees from the long axis of the tooth. **D,** Start at the most distal tooth in the arch and use a vibrating, back-and-forth motion to brush. (**B** and **D,** From Newman MG, Takei HH, Klokkevold PR, Carranza FA, eds: *Carranza's clinical periodontology,* ed 10, St Louis, 2006, Saunders.)

(Continued)

Copyright © 2010 by Saunders, an imprint of Elsevier Inc. All rights reserved.

HOW TO BRUSH! HOW TO FLOSS!—cont'd

USE OF DENTAL FLOSS

Start with a 14- to 16-inch piece of floss. Any type of floss is okay to use. Most people find nonshredding floss, which is thinner, easiest to use.

- Lightly wrap the floss around the forefingers of each hand until there is a length of about 1 to 1½ inches available between the fingers. Don't wrap it so tightly that you cut off circulation and your fingers turn blue!
- Using your thumbs and forefingers, position the floss over the spot where two teeth meet.
- With a **gentle** buffing motion, back and forth, move the floss between the teeth and slide it first under the gum around one of the teeth in a U shape.
- Move the floss up and down a few times, then reverse the U and floss the other tooth. The floss needs to get under the gum.
- Then remove the floss and place it between the next two teeth. Holding the floss taut between your fingers will give you more control, and flossing will be easier. If you see blood on the floss, try to clean the gum area more

thoroughly for several days until the bleeding stops. If you continue to see bleeding, contact your dental hygienist.

- Note that some people benefit from other types of interdental cleaning aids such as interdental brushes and sponges, wooden piks, and end-tufted brushes. Ask your dental hygienist if these oral care devices are appropriate for you.
- Remember, brushing and flossing cleans only about 20% of the mouth. To reach the other 80%, we recommend that you rinse twice daily for 30 seconds with an ADA-accepted antimicrobial mouth rinse.

When you are able to perform these daily procedures effectively, you will significantly reduce your risk of gum disease and decay and the associated expenses of treatment. There are other flossing aids available if you have problems using your hands. Let us know about these problems. Power toothbrushes can also be used. Again, talk to us about these devices. Keeping your teeth healthy for the rest of your life can be accomplished—one day at a time.

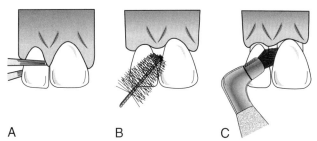

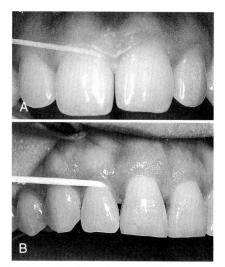

Use of interdental plaque control devices. **A,** Dental floss. **B,** Interdental brush. **C,** End-tuft brush.

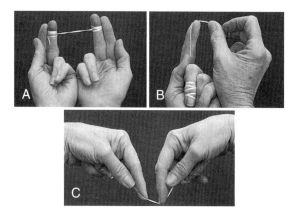

A, Dental floss. **B,** Dental tape. (**A,** From Perry DA, Beemsterboer PL: *Periodontology for the dental hygienist,* St Louis, 2007, Saunders. **B,** From Newman MG, Takei HH, Klokkevold PR, Carranza FA: *Carranza's clinical periodontology,* ed 10, St Louis, 2006, Saunders.)

If you have any questions about how to brush or floss, please feel free to ask us.

Specific Recommendations: _____

_____

_____

Copyright © 2010 by Saunders, an imprint of Elsevier Inc. All rights reserved.

ENERGY DRINK ALERT

Patient Name: _____   **Date:** _____

We have recently noticed a developing and serious tooth decay problem in some of our patients. What we are seeing is tooth decay that progresses much more quickly than usual. This decay is seen on root surfaces and around the margins of restorations (fillings) and crowns (caps) where the tooth and restorative material meet. In some individuals these restorations were placed only a short time ago. From discussion with the patients who exhibit this extreme and unusual type of decay, there seem to be common factors (e.g., they drink diet beverages, soda, sports drinks, energy drinks, and bottled iced tea). Their brushing and flossing habits appear to be adequate. They are taking no special medication. All seem to be concerned with their weight.

Years ago this type of decay was seen in patients who kept candy, mints, or other edible breath fresheners in their mouths for hours, causing tooth decay. Although other factors may be the actual or contributing causes of this problem, the only currently detected causes are the beverages—soda and artificially sweetened bottled iced tea.

Sugar in food and drink feeds the bacteria present in dental plaque, allowing the bacteria to produce lactic acid. The lactic acid breaks down the minerals in the tooth enamel, which causes white spot lesions and cavities. Although diet drinks are sugar-free, they are also very acidic. This acid also breaks down the minerals in the tooth enamel, causing cavities. By the time the saliva dilutes these acids enough to bring the mouth back to its proper pH balance, new or additional decay may already be in progress. Frequently, before the mouth reaches its proper pH balance, the patient is already uncapping another bottle or can of that drink!

Suggestions for the reduction or elimination of this type of decay include:

- Reduction or cessation of the drinking of these drinks and substituting plain water
- Rinsing your mouth with water as soon as possible after beverage contact
- Use of fluoride mouth rinses, and stronger prescription topical fluoride treatments both in the office (two to four times each year) and at your home. We may even need to recommend the use of special fluoride delivery trays to increase the time that fluoride can remain in contact with the teeth. This will help make the enamel of the teeth stronger to resist the acid attack that starts decay. It will also promote a better equilibrium in the constant enamel demineralization-remineralization process that occurs in everyone's mouth. Decay lesions in the very beginning stages can be stopped and even reversed in this way.
- Use products that contain xylitol. Xylitol has been shown to decrease the number of tooth decay producing bacteria in the mouth if used in therapeutic doses. Look for sugarless breath mints and sugarless gum that contain xylitol. Use these products about 4 to 5 times daily to control the growth of decay-causing bacteria. Use of these products can also help prevent the transmission of these decay-causing bacteria among family members and significant others.
- Chewing gum with Recaldent may also help remineralize your teeth.

Be aware that some of the things you put in your mouth in the hope of losing weight may actually have the adverse effect of causing you to lose teeth.

If you have any questions about this accelerated decay, please feel free to ask us.

Specific Recommendations: _____

_____

_____

Copyright © 2010 by Saunders, an imprint of Elsevier Inc. All rights reserved.

REDUCING YOUR RISK OF TOOTH DECAY (DEMINERALIZATION)

Patient Name: _____   Date: _____

DENTAL DECAY

Dental caries (decay) is a chronic bacterial infection of the enamel, dentin, and/or pulp of the tooth. The tradition in dentistry has been to surgically remove the diseased portion of the tooth by "drilling" out the decay and then filling the resulting hole in the tooth with some inert material. As most adults know, this procedure will be performed over and over again when new decay begins or when the filling breaks or the tooth fractures.

Would it not be better to eliminate the cause of the infection and thus not be forced to have decayed areas and some healthy tooth structure drilled from the teeth? We believe the bacterial cause of the infection should be eliminated to prevent future decay.

REDUCING THE RISK OF DENTAL DECAY

There are several positive steps that you can take to reduce your risk of dental decay. First, all the active decay in your mouth should be treated immediately. Next, all teeth that would benefit from **sealants** (see additional handout) should be treated. This will prevent bacteria from reaching into the pits, fissures, and grooves that normally exist on the occlusal (biting) surfaces of teeth. Any stray bacteria that may still be in the sealed area are effectively cut off from their source of food and become inactive. Although sealants are most effective on teeth that have not been previously restored, they can be successfully placed on teeth filled with bonded fillings.

The infection can be treated with antimicrobials. We believe that the use of a fluoridated mouth rinse twice daily or use of a prescription fluoridated dentifrice as directed provides a great advantage. Not only is fluoride effective against bacteria, it also creates an environment that promotes remineralization of slightly damaged enamel. The decay process is reversed, and the tooth may not have to be drilled. We may also prescribe a chlorhexidine mouth rinse, a prescription-only antimicrobial oral rinse that kills *Streptococcus mutans.*

Over-the-counter products that contain therapeutic doses of xylitol are also effective in controlling *S. mutans.* For example, sugarless mints and gums that contain xylitol should be used about 4 to 5 times daily to decrease *S. mutans.* Chewing gum with Recaldent may also help remineralize your teeth.

Your diet and oral self-care are important in dental decay prevention. When you eat junk food and drink sugary liquids, your teeth are more prone to decay. The more frequently you snack, the more prone your teeth will be to decay. If your brushing and flossing are not effective, your teeth will be more prone to decay. When you can't brush after a meal, at least rinse your mouth with water within 15 minutes to dilute the acids forming from the ingested food or drink. If you have a diminished salivary flow, take frequents sips of water during the day to help dilute the acids produced by the bacteria.

If you have a continuing problem with active decay, we recommend more frequent preventive recare appointments. It has been repeatedly shown that patients who have good oral self-care and maintain a recare interval of 3 to 4 months have many fewer dental problems (cavities or gum disease).

The routine 6-month recare interval is rarely our recommended schedule. You might need to have your teeth cleaned by the hygienist twice each year, or you may need to be seen more frequently.

For certain individuals, we also suggest testing the oral bacterial levels to determine the magnitude and presence of *S. mutans* infection and to determine your risk level for future dental disease.

(Continued)

Copyright © 2010 by Saunders, an imprint of Elsevier Inc. All rights reserved.

REDUCING YOUR RISK OF TOOTH DECAY
(DEMINERALIZATION)—cont'd

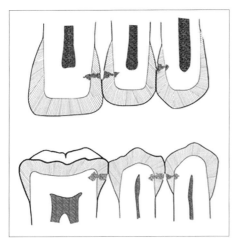

Decay between the teeth

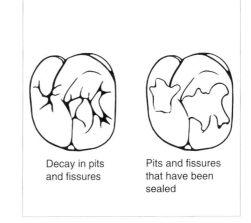

Decay in pits and fissures

Pits and fissures that have been sealed

If you have any questions about reducing your risk for dental decay, please feel free to ask us.

Specific Recommendations: _____

_____

_____

Copyright © 2010 by Saunders, an imprint of Elsevier Inc. All rights reserved.

WHEN RADIOGRAPHS ARE NECESSARY

Patient Name: _____   **Date:** _____

We take only necessary radiographs. A necessary radiograph is one that is used to diagnose the extent of a dental problem that we already know exists, such as a broken tooth, a cavity, a periodontal pocket, or an abscess. We also must use radiographs as part of an initial or periodic oral examination. In these examinations, radiographs are used to determine whether there are problems in a beginning stage that cannot be seen merely by looking at the tooth or area.

We can see only about 50% of your oral conditions without radiographs. Radiographs allow us to see, among other things, the areas between the teeth and at and below the margins of fillings and crowns and the location and density of bone that supports your teeth. With this information we can make a full diagnosis, treating small or hidden problems before they become really big problems. Radiographs are **not** considered a preventive measure. However, they do allow us

to diagnose and treat a problem early, thus preventing it from becoming worse.

Sometimes we must take several radiographs of one particular area. Radiographs are only a two-dimensional, black-and-white representation of three-dimensional, colored tooth and bone. Radiographs taken from different angles give a more three-dimensional and therefore truer look at various anatomic features. We will have a much clearer picture of type, size, and location of any problems.

The healthier your mouth is, the fewer radiographs we need to recommend. The more dental problems you have had, the more monitoring and therefore the more radiographs we may need. However, if we don't take the radiographs, the problem may grow, undetected, and even more radiographs than originally recommended may be necessary.

RADIATION SAFETY

We are very concerned with radiation safety. Appropriate protective lead shields are **always** provided to you. We work in the office around the radiographic units every day. We have a vested interest in taking only necessary radiographs for both

your health and ours. Be assured that the only radiographs we recommend are those we need in order to accurately diagnose and provide quality care.

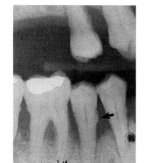

Radiograph showing vertical bone destruction, furcation involvement, and subgingival calculus *(arrow).*

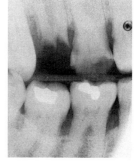

Radiograph showing vertical bone loss and furcation involvement on tooth 30.

If you have any questions about radiographs, please feel free to ask us.

Specific Recommendations: _____

_____

Copyright © 2010 by Saunders, an imprint of Elsevier Inc. All rights reserved.

REVERSING TOOTH DECAY

Patient Name: _____   Date: _____

If you were asked to describe a cavity, you would probably say that the process is similar to rusting—something that happens on the outside of the tooth that makes the tooth soft and creates a hole that will eventually be visible. You might even have the notion that bacteria are involved. You would be right in both cases.

The process of decay is a complicated interplay between acidic and basic chemical states in the mouth. The salivary flow and content, presence of decay-causing bacteria, age of the teeth, diet, and level of plaque all play a role in the decay (demineralization) as well as the rebuilding (remineralization) process involved in tooth decay.

DEMINERALIZATION

At the very earliest stage of the decay process, there is not an actual "hole" in the tooth. There is, however, an alteration of the mineral content of the enamel. This stage of decay is completely invisible to the eye. It cannot be detected by an x-ray examination. It is a microscopic change in which, owing to the level of acid in the immediate area, the building blocks of enamel (calcium and phosphate) begin to dissolve on a microscopic level. When the acid environment is left unchecked (plaque is allowed to accumulate undisturbed against the tooth surface), more and more of the bonds between calcium and phosphate dissolve. This is a process called *demineralization*. If the acid challenge becomes severe and more of the underlying structure of the tooth begins to dissolve, the outer surface becomes unsupported. It is at this time that the actual hole, or what you call a *cavity*, appears.

REMINERALIZATION

When the outer surface of the enamel is still intact, with no break detectable, there is an opportunity for the bonds between calcium and phosphate to become relinked through a process termed *remineralization*. The great news is that dental science discovered that in the presence of fluoride these bonds actually become stronger than they were initially. It is in this way that an early cavity can be reversed.

When this happens, the tooth does not need to be drilled and filled.

The process of demineralization and remineralization can be seen as a tug of war on the molecular level of all surfaces of all your teeth, all the time! Using a low-concentration sodium fluoride mouth rinse for 1 minute daily helps to tilt the balance in favor of mineralization.

HOW YOU CAN PROMOTE REMINERALIZATION

There are several steps you can take on a daily basis to help ensure that you are promoting remineralization. These are as follows:

- Control your diet: watch the types of decay-promoting foods and beverages you eat and drink and their frequencies.
- Improve your oral self-care by brushing with a fluoride toothpaste and flossing daily.
- Use a low-concentration topical fluoride on a daily basis (e.g., 0.05% NaF mouth rinse).
- Use an ADA-accepted 0.05% sodium fluoride mouth rinse and other anticaries agents such as xylitol, Novamin, and Recaldent as directed on a regular basis. Look for products that carry the ADA Seal of Approval.
- Maintain your dental hygiene recare schedule.

The early stages of dental decay can be reversed with no loss of tooth structure, and you can help promote a healthy mouth by following just a few simple rules.

(Continued)

Copyright © 2010 by Saunders, an imprint of Elsevier Inc. All rights reserved.

REVERSING TOOTH DECAY—cont'd

Parent/Caregiver Recommendations For Caries Prevention: Ages 0 to 5 Years

Daily Oral Hygiene
- Small amount of fluoride-containing toothpaste by cloth or brush twice daily
- Selective daily flossing

Diet
- Elimination of bottles with sugared fluids or juices
- Limited between-meal snacks, limited sodas; substitution of non–caries-causing snacks

Sugar-Free Gum
- For parent or caregiver of high-risk infant, use of xylitol-containing gum four to five times daily

Antibacterial Rinse
- For parent or caregiver, use of chlorhexidine gluconate (0.12%) once daily for 2 weeks every 2 to 3 months and use of fluoride rinse (0.05% NaF) daily in intervening weeks

Evidence-Based Therapy for High–Caries-Risk Individuals

- Fluoride toothpaste at least two times daily
- Increase of fluoride to 5000 ppm toothpaste for age 6 years through adult
- Fluoride varnish two or three times annually
- Xylitol for mothers and caregivers of 0- to 5-year-olds
- Chlorhexidine (once daily 1 week each month) and xylitol for age 6 years through adult
- Calcium phosphopeptide paste with fluoride (MI Paste Plus)
- Sealants
- Glass ionomer restorations and sealant
- Minimally invasive restorations

If you have any questions about the process of decay, please feel free to ask us.

Specific Recommendations: _____

_____

_____

Copyright © 2010 by Saunders, an imprint of Elsevier Inc. All rights reserved.

TOPICAL FLUORIDE: AT HOME AND IN THE DENTAL OFFICE

Patient Name: _____   Date: _____

WHY TOPICAL FLUORIDE?

The use of fluoride to reduce and eliminate decay is one of the most highly studied and documented public health measures yet. We will use a 4-minute tray-type fluoride delivery or a fluoride varnish at least twice a year, usually after your dental hygiene recare appointment. We have found that this type of preventive agent does the following:

- Reduces the solubility of enamel to acid attack, making the teeth more resistant to decay
- Aids in remineralizing the tooth enamel where decay has just begun

Research has also shown that you can benefit from a nonprescription 0.05% sodium fluoride mouth rinse, especially if you use it faithfully every day.

- When used daily on a longer-term basis, it reduces tooth decay and sensitivity to temperature changes
- Reduces the surface tension of the enamel so that plaque does not easily adhere to the tooth

For over-the-counter fluoride toothpastes and mouth rinses, look for those that carry the ADA Seal of Acceptance or CDA Seal of Recognition. If you have had recent active decay, no matter what your age, we will recommend fluoride therapy for you.

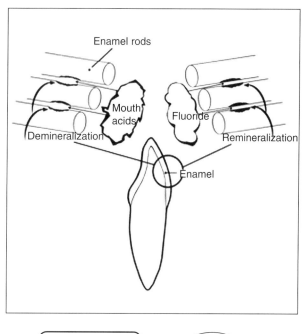

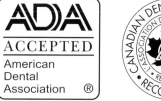

SPECIAL FLUORIDE APPLICATIONS

Another option for topical fluoride is available to patients with tooth or root sensitivity, high decay risk, root decay, or dry mouth (xerostomia). If you have been diagnosed as having any of these dental problems, we will make custom fluoride trays for you. We will then either prescribe or dispense a high-concentration fluoride gel product for you to use nightly in the tray.

The instructions are simple.

- Dry your teeth as much as possible, either with a gauze square or washcloth or by sucking air through your teeth. The fluoride will work better if the teeth are not quite so wet.
- Because trays fit closely to the teeth, place a small amount of fluoride gel into the tray every few teeth, and then place the trays into your mouth.

- Spit out the excess. If you notice an excess of fluoride, place a smaller amount in the trays at your next application.
- Leave the trays in place for ____ minutes. Then take the trays out. Spit out the saliva and fluoride that remain.
- **Do not eat or drink for ____ minutes.**

The number of weeks that you will need to apply tray fluoride in this manner depends on your decay risk. If diminished salivary flow has caused an increase in your decay rate, you will need to follow this procedure until saliva flow returns to normal. In the case of sensitive teeth, you will need to follow this procedure until the sensitivity is reduced. However, please note that sensitivity reduction is usually a gradual process; do not expect overnight improvement. Root desensitization may also require that additional products be placed over the area as an adjunct procedure.

If you have any questions about the use of topical fluorides in the home or dental office, please feel free to ask us.

Specific Recommendations: _____

_____

_____

Copyright © 2010 by Saunders, an imprint of Elsevier Inc. All rights reserved.

ATTRITION, ABRASION, AND ABFRACTION

Patient Name: _____   **Date:** _____

WHY TEETH WEAR

The natural friction of teeth moving against one another produces wear of the enamel. It is considered a natural process and happens over many years, so the changes are very gradual. Attrition (wear or loss of tooth substance) of the biting surfaces of teeth occurs in one out of every four adults in the United States, or approximately 25% of the population.

You may notice these types of changes by observing that your front teeth appear to be chipping. These teeth might look shorter and the biting edges may appear flat and discolored, especially on the lower front teeth. This process can occur more rapidly when you have a nonpurposeful biting, grinding, or clenching habit that can cause teeth to be in contact longer and more forcefully, either during waking hours or when sleeping.

GRINDING AND CLENCHING HABITS

Grinding and clenching habits are usually a physical expression of psychologic or emotional stress. Many times, patients are completely unaware of their clenching, grinding, or biting habits. Most typically this destructive habit occurs during sleep, and patients commonly deny knowing that it occurs.

These habits can occur during periods of high stress or at times of high personal demand. Whenever nonfunctional wear of the teeth occurs, the enamel will wear more quickly than normally expected. When this happens, the underlying dentin of the tooth is exposed, and this creates a problem.

DENTIN ATTRITION

Enamel is quite hard and resistant to wear. Dentin, on the other hand, has a higher organic component and does not handle the frictional forces of grinding, biting, and clenching very well. Consequently, once the outer covering of the tooth (enamel) is worn away, the underlying dentin will begin to wear faster, exposing even more of the dentin to the oral cavity. The tooth can chip and fracture. The dentin also has a tendency to show more stain from smoking, food, and drink. Coffee, tea, cola drinks, and red wine are noted for causing unsightly brown or orange stain on the dentin.

Even when you eliminate the offending habit, once the dentin is exposed it will continue to wear more quickly than the surrounding enamel. This will cause a dish- or donut-shaped area that progresses into a larger defect. It is best to restore the areas as soon as possible (even if they are not yet cosmetic problems) to prevent further deterioration of the tooth structure.

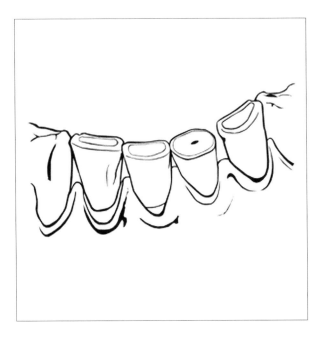

(Continued)

Copyright © 2010 by Saunders, an imprint of Elsevier Inc. All rights reserved.

ATTRITION, ABRASION, AND ABFRACTION—cont'd

ABFRACTION

Loss of tooth structure right above the crown of the tooth was once thought to be due solely to over-rigorous toothbrushing with a medium or hard toothbrush (abrasion). Although over-rigorous toothbrushing can cause some loss of tooth structure, evidence suggests that the torque on the tooth causes a weakening and loss of the tooth structure that is called *abfraction.*

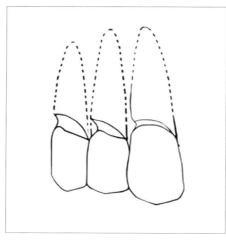

TREATMENT OPTIONS

There are several possible solutions to attrition, abrasion, and abfraction problems, depending on the level of tooth wear.
- You can elect to do nothing. Your teeth will probably continue to wear down, stain, and become increasingly unsightly as they lose their proper shape, break, chip, and/or discolor. They may become more sensitive to temperature changes and acidic and sweet foods. Excessive wear may even require endodontic treatment (root canal therapy). In the most advanced cases the back teeth are actually worn flat and the jaw relationships change to the extent that the jaw joint (temporomandibular joint [TMJ]) does not function properly, resulting in pain.
- A mouth guard or bite guard can be made, which prevents your teeth from coming into contact when you clench or grind. It is worn at times of high stress when you are most prone to clenching and grinding.

- Fractured and worn posterior (back) teeth can be restored. Cast restorations can be used to restore and maintain a proper jaw relationship. Cast gold is usually the material of choice for patients who have clenching and grinding habits. The final decision on materials will be based on an evaluation of each individual situation.
- Exposed dentin on front teeth can be restored with a tooth-colored resin material bonded directly to the areas.
- Identify, manage, and eliminate the cause of your stress.

Unfortunately, once the tooth has been worn away, it will not grow back. It can only be repaired. It is much better to stop the progression of attrition, abrasion, and abfraction. When is the best time to begin treatment for the bruxing and grinding habit? As soon as the problem is diagnosed.

If you have any questions about attrition or abrasion, please feel free to ask us.

Specific Recommendations: _____

_____

_____

Copyright © 2010 by Saunders, an imprint of Elsevier Inc. All rights reserved.

ORAL MALODOR

Patient Name: _____

Date: _____

Periodically, everyone experiences bad breath. The occasional meal—heavy with garlic, onions, or spices—may leave a lingering odor, but it is a temporary problem. Chronic bad breath is another problem entirely. It can be caused by periodontal disease, dry mouth, oral biofilm, decay in teeth, or decay under fillings or crowns, as well as by digestive system or sinus problems. Foul breath odor caused by any of these conditions needs to be corrected by your dentist or physician.

Although there can be medical and/or systemic problems that cause the breath odor, most of the time bad breath is the result of things left on and around your teeth. Your mouth is warm, moist, and dark—the perfect place for bacteria to grow and decompose. When this happens and the teeth and tongue are not cleaned properly on a daily basis, a chronic odor can result. Bad breath can be eliminated, or at least controlled, by removal of food debris, plaque, or calculus; replacement of broken fillings causing a food trap; restoration of areas of decay; and/or elimination of gum disease. Plaque that accumulates at or along the gum line can also find its way into the deep recesses on the top surface of your tongue, contributing to mouth odor.

Toothbrushing, tongue cleaning, and cleaning between the teeth correctly, at least once a day, are the best prevention and cure for bad breath. Twice daily use of an ADA-accepted antibacterial mouth rinse is also recommended to control bacteria throughout the mouth. Not only will these procedures prevent periodontal disease and decay by removal of bacteria, they will also remove all food debris. Manufacturers of toothpastes, toothbrushes, floss, tongue scrapers, and antimicrobial mouth rinses make claims that their products help prevent bad breath, and they may provide temporary relief of that symptom. For over-the-counter products select those that carry the ADA Seal of Acceptance or the CDA Seal of Recognition.

- To keep the saliva flowing and to reduce bacteria in the mouth, you can use chewing gum or mints that contain xylitol.

No matter which product you use, be sure to thoroughly remove the bacterial plaque (oral biofilm) on a daily basis.

The key to preventing dental problems and preventing bad breath odor is to clean your teeth and tongue properly every day. The best way to learn how to clean your mouth is by visiting us. You have the ability to take good care of your mouth; it is just a matter of using the products, devices, and personal skills best suited to your unique oral conditions. Whether you have many fillings, crowns or bridges, removable partial or full dentures, implants, braces, or other appliances in your mouth, there is a product, method, or tool that will work for you.

Also, to ensure fresh breath, have your teeth professionally treated by the dental hygienist on a regular basis. The goal here is not only to correct any disease-related problems but also to prevent any problems from beginning.

Your oral malodor problem does not have to be a chronic source of embarrassment. Most often it is a sign of a dental or medical problem. The sooner it is treated, the easier and less expensive it will be to fix.

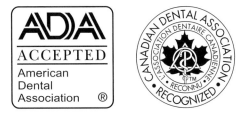

If you have any questions about bad breath, please feel free to ask us.

Specific Recommendations: _____

_____

_____

Copyright © 2010 by Saunders, an imprint of Elsevier Inc. All rights reserved.

SENSITIVE TEETH

Patient Name: _____ **Date:** _____

Teeth can become sensitive for many reasons. Sometimes the sensitivity is an indication of a potentially serious problem. Other times the dentally related problem may be small but the effects (the sensitivity) are extremely uncomfortable. A tooth can become sensitive after it has been prepared (drilled) for a restoration (filling). You may have been anesthetized during the procedure, so you did not feel any discomfort when the nerve in the tooth reacted to the heat generated by the drill. The closer the drill comes to the nerve, the more likely it is to cause a sensitivity problem. The high-speed rotation of the bur in the drill generates heat, and the response of the nerve to heat is inflammation. This inflammation is felt by you as "sensitivity." If the decay, fracture, or drilling was not too deep, this sensitivity will decrease over time. A week to a month or two is not an unusual length of time for the sensitivity to disappear. A good sign is the continued decrease of sensitivity. However, if the occlusion (bite) is off after the restoration has been placed, the tooth may either become sensitive or may stay sensitive. Once the bite is adjusted, though, the sensitivity should disappear.

Additional reasons for single tooth sensitivity are gum recession, decay, a defective restoration, or a fractured tooth. Given any of these conditions, temperature changes, mouth acids, and sweets will make it sensitive. If a filling is defective or failing, leakage around the filling may cause the tooth to become sensitive. In these cases the solution can be removing the decay or defective filling and placing an appropriate restoration. If the tooth is fractured, you may be sensitive to temperature changes or when chewing food. This fracture condition may be a hairline crack that is hard to diagnose. If you think you might have this type of sensitivity, please ask for the separate handout that explains the "cracked tooth syndrome" in much greater detail.

Tooth sensitivity can also be caused by a dying nerve. This can be the result of a deep cavity or an unknown injury. Commonly the sensitive tooth holds an old large filling. The nerve may have been damaged during drilling, and the nerve has been dying gradually ever since. If this is the problem, the tooth will need endodontic treatment.

Two other reasons for tooth sensitivity are related. One is loss of tooth structure that looks like notching of the tooth surface and/or recession of the gum tissue (exposing the root surface of the tooth) caused by gum disease; improper brushing (either brushing too hard, brushing with a toothbrush that is too hard, or using a toothpaste that is too abrasive); or using an improper brushing technique. This sensitivity can range from mild to extreme; the degree of sensitivity does not appear to be related to the size of the root exposure or notch. Finally, purposeful repositioning of the gum tissue during gum surgery can also lead to tooth sensitivity. While recession from brushing is slow, gum recession after gum repositioning occurs very quickly. The portion of the tooth once covered with gum and bone may now be exposed. Root sensitivity in these instances can be quite severe and immediate. It can sometimes last for months or years if not treated.

TREATMENT OPTIONS

Treatment in these last two instances is similar.

- If there is a notch in the tooth or the shape of the defect is appropriate, the defect is restored (filled in) with a bonded, tooth-colored material. This can give immediate relief—sometimes partially, sometimes fully.
- When there is no defect to be restored, the exposed and sensitive root surfaces are covered with a dentin bonding, 5% sodium fluoride varnish, or material containing Nova-Min. This material is invisible and has very little thickness, so you do not notice any change in the appearance of the tooth, but it works. It may have to be reapplied because the material has been worn away by toothbrushing.

- One self-care treatment is the use of a sensitivity toothpaste that will block the sensation of pain or coat the exposed nerve endings on the tooth surface. Select an over-the-counter sensitivity toothpaste that carries the ADA Seal of Acceptance or the CDA Seal of Recognition. A small amount of sensitivity toothpaste can be dabbed onto the sensitive tooth areas and left there overnight.
- One self-care treatment is the daily use of a 0.4% stannous fluoride gel. Fluoride mouth rinse used daily may also be effective.

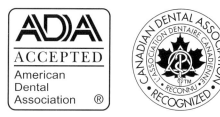

If you have any questions about tooth sensitivity, please feel free to ask us.

Specific Recommendations: _____

_____

_____

Copyright © 2010 by Saunders, an imprint of Elsevier Inc. All rights reserved.

XEROSTOMIA: DRY MOUTH

Patient Name: _____   **Date:** _____

Xerostomia (dry mouth) is not a condition everyone should expect. You may notice it as you age, because of a change in hormones, or it may occur as a result of medication and/or radiation therapy in the head and neck region.

WHY XEROSTOMIA IS A PROBLEM

Saliva is important to oral health for several reasons. The flow of saliva helps clear debris from the oral cavity. It provides minerals necessary to support the process of remineralization. Tooth enamel daily undergoes acid attack that removes inorganic minerals from teeth. This is called *demineralization*. Remineralization is the opposite of demineralization. It occurs when inorganic molecules flow into a region of weakened enamel and make it stronger.

When the salivary flow is reduced, a chain of problematic events occurs. The natural cleansing action is diminished, as are the buffering action and remineralization properties of saliva. People with diminished salivary flow experience a very fast rate of decay, many times faster than normal and occurring over several teeth. This type of dental decay is typically noted along the gum line, around existing dental work, and on exposed root surfaces.

PREVENTION

You can help prevent the dental decay that can result from xerostomia.

- Brushing and flossing correctly at least once each day becomes very important.
- Frequent sips of water or sucking on ice chips during the day can help moisten the mouth and help clear debris.
- Daily use of a ADA-accepted or CDA-accepted mouth rinse containing fluoride can help remineralize the teeth.
- Use a toothpaste containing fluoride that carries the ADA Seal of Acceptance or CDA Seal of Recognition.
- We recommend a daily brushing with a prescription, high-concentration sodium fluoride gel or paste. We will either dispense this or give you a prescription for it.
- Chew sugarless gum that contains xylitol, suck on sugarless candy or mints that contain xylitol, or chew a rubber band to help stimulate salivary flow.

- In moderate to severe cases, custom-made delivery trays can be made for you to use at home. These will keep the high-concentration fluoride in a position to "soak" your teeth with fluoride for several minutes at a time.
- Use a line of over-the-counter products especially formulated for dry mouth: mouth rinse, dentifrice, artificial saliva, and mouth moisturizer.
- If dry mouth continues to be a problem for you, the dentist can write you a prescription for a medication that can increase saliva production.
- We recommend that you have professional dental hygiene care and receive an office-applied topical fluoride treatment every 3 months while the condition persists.

Dry mouth can have serious dental consequences and must be treated accordingly.

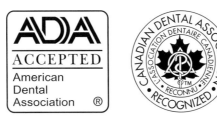

If you have any questions about xerostomia, please feel free to ask us.

Specific Recommendations: _____

_____

Copyright © 2010 by Saunders, an imprint of Elsevier Inc. All rights reserved.

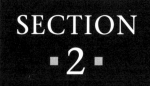

Copyright © 2010 by Saunders, an imprint of Elsevier Inc. All rights reserved.

CONGENITALLY MISSING TEETH

Patient Name: _____

Date: _____

Most of us will have 32 permanent teeth develop during our lifetime. This has been considered a normal complement of teeth. Some people, however, do not develop a full set of 32 teeth. It is quite common for people to be missing one or more of the third molars (wisdom teeth). And as the jaw dimension of modern human beings has decreased in size, there is no room for the proper placement of the third molars in a mouth, and they must be extracted.

Not as common, but not at all unusual, is a condition in which certain permanent front teeth never develop. When permanent teeth do not develop, they are considered to be congenitally missing. The term for this condition is *congenitally missing teeth.* When this happens, it is frequently one or both of the upper lateral incisors, which are the smaller teeth on either side of the two top front teeth. Less often the permanent canines or premolars do not develop.

The problem that results from congenitally missing teeth involves the space where the tooth (teeth) should have been. The teeth nearest the space shift into different positions to fill in the gap, often resulting in a crowded smile—when in fact, some teeth are missing!

The problems resulting from missing permanent teeth can be reduced or eliminated with early detection and a plan for future treatment. The usual treatment involves orthodontics to move the permanent teeth into better position or keep the permanent teeth in the correct location. Because we treat missing lateral incisors so often, the treatment routine is well established. The best esthetics, the most natural look, will be achieved by leaving the adjacent permanent central incisors and canine teeth in their customary places.

When there are missing lateral incisors, it is likely that we will recommend a bridge, a dental implant, or moving the canines into their positions. This will keep the bone in the missing tooth space at the proper level. We will then recommend moving the canines back into their proper positions. This may sound like extra treatment, but it is needed to keep the bone at the proper height for future tooth replacement treatment.

The sequence of treatment is orthodontics as early as necessary to maintain the space. The further the teeth have shifted from this original position, the more orthodontic treatment will be necessary. Then, while the child and mouth are growing, a removable replacement tooth is made. This appliance is worn until the teeth are ready to receive the implant or bridge, after age 18 or so when the mouth and dental structures are more mature.

When the permanent teeth further back in the mouth are missing, it is common for baby teeth to be retained in these spaces. Sometimes the baby teeth can last for years, but they do not have the root structure to remain stable over a lifetime. Because the retained baby teeth are meant for a small mouth, they do not have the right size, shape, or function as the permanent teeth. When lost, they can be replaced with implants or a bridge. Your own particular situation will determine the best course of treatment.

If you have any questions about congenitally missing teeth, please feel free to ask us.

Specific Recommendations: _____

_____

_____

Copyright © 2010 by Saunders, an imprint of Elsevier Inc. All rights reserved.

FLUOROSIS, MOTTLED ENAMEL, AND WHITE SPOTS

Patient Name: _____   Date: _____

FLUOROSIS AND MOTTLED ENAMEL

Fluoride is the dental marvel of our lifetime and a definite benefit to the oral health of our nation. But too much of a good thing can cause problems! Fluorosis of the teeth and mottled enamel can occur when there is too much fluoride ingestion while the teeth are forming. Prescription fluoride supplements of the proper dose are normally given to children who have less than the desired level in their diets. A child can get too much fluoride if it's available from multiple sources. Children with access to a public water system containing fluoride may also be prescribed fluoride supplements, or they may swallow fluoride-containing toothpastes, mouth rinses, or certain fruit drinks, which may increase their fluoride intake above recommended levels. Fluorosis is a condition in which teeth form with unsightly dark spots on them. Some medications and illnesses can cause a similar problem. These dark spots, most often seen on the permanent teeth, are not more prone to decay, just unattractive. Several or all of the teeth can be affected. The color change (usually brown-orange or flat or opaque white) can be mild, moderate, or severe.

TREATMENT OPTIONS

Generally speaking, three solutions are possible. Sometimes the stain is very superficial and can be merely polished off. It does not return. There is no pain involved in this procedure. The enamel is simply polished and made smooth again.

Many times it is quite easy to whiten the brown spots to match the surrounding tooth color. This is most often an in-office procedure (as opposed to whitening yellow teeth, which can be done at home with custom-made tooth-whitening trays). Strong whitening chemicals are placed on the dark area and activated by light or heat or both. Several applications (in the same visit) are done, and the stain usually disappears in one visit!

If the stain is very dark or goes deep into the enamel, the whitening may work, but not enough to remove the total discoloration. In this instance a combination of whitening and a bonded composite tooth-colored restoration will solve the problem. The tooth is whitened, and then the remaining dark area is prepared (drilled) to receive a bonded-type filling. The natural color of the tooth is matched, and a resin is bonded onto the prepared section. The color match can be nearly perfect, and patients see a big improvement over what was there before.

WHITE SPOTS

White spots on teeth can also be caused by too much fluoride, illness, medication, or an interruption of the proper enamel formation. The spots may be barely visible, or they may contrast with the surrounding tooth. If the teeth dry out, as in the case of a patient who routinely breathes through his or her mouth, the white spots become quite prominent. If they go too deep into the tooth, however, they must be restored with tooth preparation and bonding of a tooth-colored material. White spots affect the permanent teeth more often than baby teeth. Although these spots cannot be bleached out, as can fluorosis discolorations, whitening of all the teeth may make the spots less noticeable.

The best solution to your problem will be discussed with you during your examination.

Note: White spots associated with ingesting too much fluoride during tooth development must be differentiated from white spot lesions, which are precursors of tooth decay.

If you have any questions about fluorosis, mottled enamel, or white spots, please feel free to ask us.

Specific Recommendations: _____

_____

_____

Copyright © 2010 by Saunders, an imprint of Elsevier Inc. All rights reserved.

YOU CAN HAVE WHITER TEETH!

Patient Name: _____   Date: _____

The least damaging and most conservative way of making your teeth lighter is with the use of a whitening solution. Contrary to what you might think, brushing your teeth harder with an abrasive toothpaste will not make your teeth whiter, but rather may darken them faster. The tooth-whitening con-cept has been around for many years, and the techniques have become easier and less expensive to accomplish. Today, there are two convenient methods to whiten dark teeth: at-home whitening and in-office whitening.

WHY DO TEETH GET YELLOW?

The intrinsic (normal) color of your teeth is related to the color and thickness of the enamel and dentin, as well as the types of foods and liquids you ingest. The thinner the enamel, the darker the underlying dentin; the more coffee, tea, cola beverages, and red wine you drink, the darker your teeth will be. Cracks that are commonly found in the enamel of your teeth may provide a pathway for discoloring fluids to reach the underlying dentin.

If you have a yellow, brown, or orange shade to your teeth, in most cases it can be made lighter by the whitening pro-cedure. Whitening works very well in removing age-related darkening of your teeth. This age-related darkening is most likely due to years of stain accumulation or other environ-mental factors, rather than genetics. No drilling or anesthesia is required for whitening. Your teeth will not become weaker. Because the mineralization of teeth varies so much from person to person, there is no way to determine how many office visits it will take to effect the color change or how white the teeth will get. The darker your teeth are, the more time required for the change and the more distinctive the color change will be.

The whitening procedure will also work to a lesser degree on teeth with tetracycline discoloration. It does take more time to achieve good results on this type of stain, and, unfortunately, sometimes the change is minor. We have seen several fair to good results from both in-office and at-home whitening.

TWO AVAILABLE TECHNIQUES

There are two types of whitening available. One is done by the patient at home, and the other is done by us during an office visit. They can be done separately or in conjunction with each other. The at-home technique involves using a soft, thin, comfortable, custom-made mouth tray. An impression is made of your teeth, and custom whitening trays are fabri-cated. Then at home you place the whitening solution in the trays and wear them for several hours each day or sleep with them in place all night. For in-office whitening, you come to the office for 1 or 2 hours, and a stronger whitening solution is applied by us and activated for that time. Usually only one visit is required.

Please check with the dentist or dental hygienist before you purchase over-the-counter whitening products. We can best advise you about product effectiveness and safety.

The color change should last for 3 to 7 years in most peo-ple. The color change you see immediately after the whiten-ing is completed will regress one shade over the course of 1 to 3 months, with most of the change taking place in the first week. If you drink a lot of coffee, tea, cola beverages, or red wine or if you smoke or eat pigmented foods like blueberries, the teeth may begin to turn darker again. When this happens, the whitening process can be repeated.

Possible side effects of tooth whitening include temporary discoloration of the gum tissue if the office whitening solution comes into contact with the gum. This goes away quickly. The teeth may become slightly sensitive to temperature changes for a short time. This also goes away quickly. There is **no** dam-age to the tooth enamel, dentin, or pulp from the whitening process. Fillings and crowns do not whiten. When your teeth change to a lighter color, you may need to have those fillings and/or crowns redone. We will let you know whether this is a possibility before we whiten your teeth. There are no other adverse effects known.

The teeth that show when you talk, smile, or eat are the teeth that would benefit your appearance most if whitened. Usually the top teeth are whitened because they are much more visible than the bottom teeth, but both arches can be successfully whitened. The lower teeth take about three times as long to reach the color change of the top teeth.

If you have any questions about whiter teeth, please feel free to ask us.

Specific Recommendations: _____

_____

_____

Copyright © 2010 by Saunders, an imprint of Elsevier Inc. All rights reserved.

AT-HOME TRAY SYSTEM: TOOTH WHITENING INSTRUCTIONS

Patient Name: _____   Date: _____

A technique is now available for whitening your teeth at home. The whitening procedure works best for teeth that have a yellow shade, although it can work to a lesser extent with teeth that have a gray shade or tetracycline discoloration. A mouth guard will be constructed from an impression that is taken of your teeth. This will hold the whitening solution against your teeth. The general instructions for mouth guard tooth whitening are as follows. They may be slightly modified by us to suit your particular needs.

1. Before using the tooth whitening gel, brush and floss your teeth. Rinse your mouth.
2. As demonstrated, place a small amount of whitening gel into the mouth guard in each tooth to be whitened.
3. Insert the mouth guard as instructed, allowing the excess material to extrude. Spit out the excess solution. If there is much to spit out, place less bleach in the tray at the next application.
4. Wear the mouth guard as instructed. Keep the mouth guard in place for _____ hours. Follow this routine each day until the whitening gel we supply is finished. You may wear the trays with the whitening solution during the day, or you may choose to wear the trays while you sleep. Diminished salivary flow while sleeping will keep the whitening gel active for a longer period. How long or how much you can wear the tray depends entirely on your comfort. If there is no tooth sensitivity, you can wear the trays as often as you want. If you start to develop tooth sensitivity, **stop** wearing the trays until the sensitivity is gone (a day or two at most), and then begin again.
5. Do not eat or drink for 30 minutes after you have removed the mouth guard and finished the whitening session. After each use, rinse the mouth guard out with water, dry it, and store it in a safe place.
6. Return to the office to have the whitening progress evaluated after _____ days of whitening.
7. Note any changes you might see in your gums, and be sure to bring such changes immediately to our attention. Any sensitivity or alteration in the appearance of the gums is temporary.

8. **Home mouth guard whitening must be done only under the supervision of a dentist.**
9. Because the mineralization of teeth is so variable from person to person, there is absolutely no way to determine how much color change can be expected or how long it may take to achieve the color change. Expect that it can take as long as several weeks for teeth that are especially dark. This time frame, of course, depends on how often you wear the trays filled with whitening gel. If you do the procedure every other day, it will take twice as long to finish than if you do it every day. If you skip a few days, it will not affect the final result. The ultimate color change will be the same whether you take 1 week or 1 month or longer. The important aspect in this is the contact time of the tray and gel with the teeth to be lightened.
10. The lighter tooth color you see immediately after the whitening process is finished will regress one shade darker over 1 to 3 months, with most of the regression evident after the first week. Lower teeth may take longer to whiten than top teeth.
11. Your eating and drinking habits and resident chromogenic bacteria will determine the duration of the whitening effect. Most patients maintain a satisfactory result for 3 to 7 years. If you smoke or drink a lot of tea, coffee, colas, or red wine, your teeth will, over extended time, darken again.
12. **Keep your whitening trays in a safe place.** At some point you may decide to "touch up" your teeth by whitening for a short duration. Touch-ups do not take as long or require as much whitening product.
13. To prolong the effectiveness of your whitening treatment, you can use an over-the-counter whitening product. Please check with the dentist or dental hygienist before you purchase over-the-counter whitening products. We can best advise you about product effectiveness and safety.
14. If you are going to have fillings replaced, you should wait at least 2 weeks after the whitening is completed for the tooth color to stabilize before new restorations are placed.

If you have any questions about mouth guard tooth whitening, please feel free to ask us.

Specific Recommendations: _____

_____

_____

Copyright © 2010 by Saunders, an imprint of Elsevier Inc. All rights reserved.

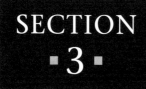

SECTION ·3·

Pediatric Dentistry

Copyright © 2010 by Saunders, an imprint of Elsevier Inc. All rights reserved.

A CHILD'S FIRST VISIT TO THE DENTIST AND DENTAL HYGIENIST

Patient Name: _____   Date: _____

GETTING READY

A child's first visit to the dentist should be at a much earlier age than most parents think. The first dental visit should occur by age 1 or when the first teeth erupt. During this visit we will teach you how to care for your child's teeth and what preventive measures you should be taking for your infant at this early stage. Many dental problems can be prevented when we have the opportunity to examine your child and visit with you in the early developmental stages. For example, early childhood tooth decay can be prevented by applying fluoride varnish to the baby teeth when they erupt.

The first cleaning for your child (pedodontic prophylaxis) should be done at about 1 year of age. At about 2 to 2 ½ years of age, depending on the child's behavior, your child can sit in the dental chair for teeth cleaning and fluoride application. It is important to note that this should not be the first time the child visits our office. Before this visit we would like the child to come in with a parent or caregiver who is receiving professional dental hygiene care. We have many toys, books, and children's movies that can be fun. In this way children come to know the dental office as a very pleasant, nonthreatening place. It is hoped that by the time they come for their own care they have been to the office several times. They know the dentist, the dental hygienist, and the way the office and dental equipment looks. They will have a good idea of what will be expected of them. They will have had only good experiences with people at this location.

Usually, infants and toddlers introduced to dentistry in this manner are very excited about having their own dental appointments.

It is important for parents and caregivers to always talk positively about going to a dental appointment as well as about the appointment after it has occurred. Children are very smart. They may not know what some of the words mean, but they can understand how you feel about it. You should try not to use any words around them that might have an unpleasant connotation: toothache, drill, pull, hurt, pain, unhappy, and so on. Always talk about how happy you are to go to the dentist and what a great experience it was. If your appointment was stressful, talk about it in private where children cannot overhear. If necessary, and if your child asks, tell him or her about how glad you are that the dentist or dental hygienist is making your mouth feel good again, without mentioning any of the discomfort.

It is also important to ensure that the children are not threatened by the dentist or dental hygienist and to avoid making the dentist or dental hygienist appear to be the "heavy." Don't tell children, for example, that if they eat candy, they will have to go to the dentist to get their teeth drilled and filled. Children will then think of the dentist's office as a place where you get punished for doing something bad. We want children to be completely comfortable and to not worry when it is time for a dental appointment.

THE VISIT

By the time the child has a dental procedure performed, at the age of 2 to 2½ years, it will usually be very simple, quick, and entirely painless. Of course, we assume you have followed all the preventive suggestions we have given you: using fluoride supplements, if appropriate; brushing the child's teeth with a fluoride toothpaste; having fluoride varnish "painted" on the teeth twice a year; putting nothing in a night bottle but water; and so forth.

First, we will spend time with the child in a show-and-tell mode. We will show the child the various instruments: polishers, mirrors, "Mr. Thirsty" (saliva ejector), the wind and water jet (air-water syringe), and so on. The dental hygienist will also begin to instruct the child in proper brushing techniques. At this young age, children do not manipulate dental floss and a brush properly. This is a responsibility for the parent or caregiver. Because children admire and try to imitate

adults, your good example of brushing and flossing each day will help tremendously in this area. Children will see that it is something you do, which they will then try to imitate.

Also during this visit, the dentist or dental hygienist will "count" the child's teeth while looking for decay or other problems. Then the dental hygienist will "tickle" (clean and polish) the teeth. Stains and plaque that might have accumulated will be removed. It is very unusual for a child to have periodontal problems.

If the child is prepared correctly, the first treatment visit at the dentist will be anticipated with no anxiety, proceed smoothly, and make the child excited about coming again. What you do at home in preparation for this first visit is most important to its success. There are children's books that can be borrowed from the public library that can also help the child understand. Good luck!

If you have any questions about your child's first visit to the dentist, please feel free to ask us.

Specific Recommendations: _____

_____

_____

Copyright © 2010 by Saunders, an imprint of Elsevier Inc. All rights reserved.

EARLY CHILDHOOD CARIES

Patient Name: _____   Date: _____

WHAT IS EARLY CHILDHOOD CARIES?

Early childhood caries, which used to be called "baby bottle tooth decay" and "nursing caries," is a severe form of dental decay found in very young children who presumably are put to sleep with any liquid other than water in a bottle. Children who have experienced prolonged breast-feeding will have the same type of tooth decay patterns. Many times, the decay is very advanced before the parent notices the problem. This is another reason that we want to see your child for his or her first dental visit while those new teeth are still in the eruption phase and before the child's first birthday.

HOW DOES EARLY CHILDHOOD CARIES DEVELOP?

The teeth most affected by early childhood caries are the upper front teeth. As the child falls asleep with a bottle containing any liquid other than water (or at the breast), pools of the liquid collect against the tooth surfaces. Sugars in the liquid feed the bacteria found in bacterial plaque to produce an acid, which starts the decay process. When the demineralization process is not stopped through proper prevention, the crowns of the teeth can be destroyed to the gum line; abscesses can develop, and the child can experience severe pain, discomfort, and dental disability.

WHAT IS THE BEST PREVENTION?

When children are given acidic and sugary drinks for a prolonged period of time, the result can be very damaging to tooth structure. Similarly, when oral bacteria are fed small amounts of sugared or acidic beverages nonstop over a day's time, the results can be quite damaging to tooth structure.

We believe the best prevention for this type of problem begins with an understanding of the decay process and how you can prevent it before it even starts. We recommend that you bring your children to the dentist before the first birthday so that we can perform an infant oral examination and discuss oral care, including the following points:

- Children should not be put to sleep with a sugared or acidic liquid in a bottle. No milk. No juice. No soda. Plain water only.
- Children, including infants, require daily oral cleansing. If no teeth are present, the gums should be gently wiped with a wet cloth, gauze, or baby toothbrush.
- When teeth are present, they should be brushed. By about age 2 to 3, teeth should be brushed with fluoridated toothpaste, but only with a very small amount—about the size of a pea or less.
- Liquid sugars and other easily fermentable carbohydrates such as white bread, cakes, cookies, or crackers should be given with meals and not as "snacks."
- The proper level of systemic fluoride should be ingested daily by the time your child is 6 months of age. We will discuss with you the fluoride supplementation regimen specific to your geographic location and the age of your children.

- Dental decay is an infectious disease that can be transmitted from parent to infant, or sibling to sibling. Persons with dental decay are infected with *Streptococcus mutans*. Parents and caregivers need to eliminate caries infection in their own mouth so that it is not transmitted to infants and children. The infection can be controlled by the following recommendation: Use 10 mL of 0.12% chlorhexidine gluconate prescription mouth rinse at bedtime for 1 minute once daily for a 1-to 2-week period every 2 to 3 months for approximately 1 year. Because chlorhexidine loses its effectiveness in the presence of sodium lauryl sulfate or fluoride, this regimen should be performed about 30 minutes after toothbrushing with a dentifrice that contains these two ingredients.
- The use of 0.12% chlorhexidine gluconate gel can be used in infants and children for early childhood caries.
- Xylitol-containing gum and mints used at least 5 times daily can inhibit the growth of bacteria that cause tooth decay.
- Fluoride varnish can be used 2 to 3 times annually on very small children who are at moderate to high risk of early childhood caries.

If you have any questions about early childhood caries, please feel free to ask us.

Specific Recommendations: _____

_____

Copyright © 2010 by Saunders, an imprint of Elsevier Inc. All rights reserved.

ERUPTION PATTERNS OF TEETH

Patient Name: _____   **Date:** _____

Teeth begin forming very early in life, as early as the second trimester of pregnancy. That is why it is so important for pregnant women to follow a proper diet: not only to have a healthy baby, but to ensure the proper formation of the teeth. When the hard tissue (the future enamel) of the tooth is forming, minerals and nutrients are taken up by the teeth and incorporated into the structure of the enamel. Good nutrition makes the teeth stronger. Poor nutrition can interfere with proper enamel formation. Eat wisely. Consult your physician about needed vitamin supplements and before taking any medications.

This reference will help you know when baby teeth, also called *primary teeth,* are due to come in and eventually fall out as the permanent teeth erupt. Girls' teeth usually come in before boys' teeth. There is a 6- to 8-month leeway that is considered a normal variation on either side of the average age teeth come into the mouth. Some children might get teeth even earlier or later than that. It depends on their growth patterns. We hope to see teeth come in later, rather than earlier. If the teeth come in later, there is a good chance the mouth will be bigger so the teeth have the necessary room to grow straight. The older a child is when he or she gets a tooth, the more manual skill the child will have for brushing and flossing the tooth. However, it must be the parent's or caregiver's responsibility to clean the child's teeth and mouth daily.

The primary dentition consists of 20 teeth. Adults typically have 32 permanent teeth, although there is evidence that many adults do not have tooth buds for the four wisdom teeth.

PRIMARY TEETH

Primary teeth start forming at 4 to 6 months in utero, the second trimester of pregnancy. After the baby is born, the teeth continue to grow and erupt into the mouth. The teeth erupt at the following ages:

- Lower central incisors: 6 months
- Lower lateral incisors: 7 months
- Upper central incisors: 7.5 months
- Upper lateral incisors: 9 months
- Lower canines and eyeteeth: 16 months
- Lower second molars: 20 months
- Upper second molars: 24 months

PERMANENT TEETH

The enamel of the permanent teeth actually begins forming at 3 to 4 months of age. If your drinking water is not fluoridated, make sure your baby receives the necessary fluoride supplements. Permanent teeth develop under the baby teeth. Pressure from the upward movement of the permanent tooth causes a resorption of the root of the baby tooth. When the root disappears, the tooth loosens and eventually falls out. If the permanent tooth does not come in directly under the baby tooth, the baby tooth root will not resorb and not loosen. The second tooth will come in either in front of or behind the baby tooth. This is common. When it happens, see the dentist to determine whether the baby tooth should be removed to permit the proper positioning of the permanent tooth. The teeth erupt at the following ages:

- Lower central incisors: 6 to 7 years
- Lower first molar: 6 to 7 years
- Upper first molar: 6 to 7 years
- Upper central incisors: 7 to 8 years
- Lower lateral incisors: 7 to 8 years
- Upper lateral incisors: 8 to 9 years
- Lower canines: 9 to 10 years
- Upper first premolars: 10 to 11 years
- Lower first premolars: 10 to 12 years
- Upper canines: 11 to 12 years
- Lower second premolars: 11 to 12 years
- Lower second molar: 11 to 13 years
- Upper second molar: 12 to 13 years
- Wisdom teeth: 17 to 22 years

Be sure to obtain dental sealants for your child's molars and premolars!

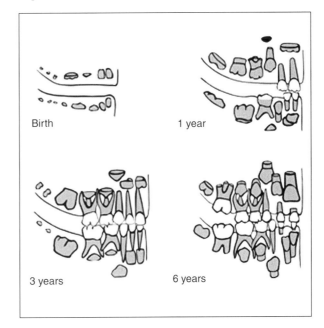

Birth   1 year

3 years   6 years

If you have any questions about the formation of teeth, please feel free to ask us.

Specific Recommendations: _____

Copyright © 2010 by Saunders, an imprint of Elsevier Inc. All rights reserved.

PREVENTION OF DENTAL DISEASE IN INFANTS AND CHILDREN

Patient Name: _____   Date: _____

There are a number of positive steps that you can take to ensure that your child has few, if any, cavities and dental-related problems. A daily routine of proper and effective oral self-care (toothbrushing and dental flossing) is the most important part of prevention. Scheduled visits with the dentist and dental hygienist for examinations and prophylaxis (cleaning) procedures are also very important for your child's dental well-being. These suggestions will help keep your child's teeth and gums disease-free.

1. Clean your infant's teeth daily with a wet washcloth, baby toothbrush, or wet 2-inch-square gauze pad. A smear or pea size of fluoridated toothpaste should be used to brush teeth at age 1 year, especially if the child has a moderate to high risk of tooth decay.
2. Floss your child's teeth daily until the child can develop the ability to do it alone. This may not be an easy transition, but it is well worth the effort.
3. Once the teeth can be seen breaking through the gum tissue, night bottles should contain only water. Fluids from night bottles pool around the teeth while the infant sleeps. Night bottles containing milk, juice, punch, soda, and sports drinks can cause **extensive** tooth decay (early childhood caries).
4. If you do not live in an area with fluoridated drinking water, the infant may be given a fluoride supplement. Dosage will depend on the age, diet, and weight of the infant. Your pediatrician or your dentist can write a prescription for fluoride supplements.
5. Children do not develop the dexterity to properly brush and floss their own teeth until about age 7 or 8. You must make sure that the job is done well, even if it means doing this oral care for them. Your own good example of brushing and flossing your teeth daily will greatly enhance your child's willingness and abilities in this area.
6. Your child's first visit to the dentist should be as an infant, as teeth are just beginning to erupt but before the first birthday. During this visit we will give you guidelines as to what you can expect in terms of oral development and what type of nutrition and oral care tips are appropriate for your child.
7. Your child's first treatment visit to the dentist should take place at 1 year of age. An examination, cleaning, and fluoride varnish treatment will be completed at this time.
8. The topical fluoride treatment given at the time of the child's regular cleaning appointment is important.

It helps make the teeth that are already in the mouth stronger and more resistant to decay and plaque accumulation. Systemic fluoride supplements strengthen the enamel of unerupted teeth. Topical fluoride adds to the benefit.

9. A plastic coating known as a *sealant* can be placed on the chewing surfaces of the back teeth. Sealants can reduce the incidence of decay on the treated surfaces by 90%. It should be placed on back teeth, both premolars and molars. It is sometimes placed on baby teeth. Sealants are usually applied when children are about 6 years old as the permanent teeth erupt. The dentist or hygienist will advise you as to when he or she believes the sealant can be successfully placed.
10. When your child can understand and perform the "rinse and spit" routine, it is time to begin using a nonprescription fluoridated mouth rinse. This is not a mouthwash used to cover bad breath. It is actually a nightly supplement to the topical fluoride treatments your child receives at the dentist's office. However, it is not nearly as strong as the office version. This is not a prescription medication.
11. Until about age 7 or 8, the parent or caregiver should still supervise the child's oral hygiene self-care.
12. Thumb sucking should be discouraged after age 4.
13. All children should be supervised when using fluoridated toothpaste and oral rinses. If not monitored they may swallow more than the recommended daily amounts of fluoride.
14. Keep dentifrices and oral rinses away from children to avoid accidental ingestion.
15. Fluoride varnish can be used on very small children who are at risk of dental decay.
16. Xylitol-containing gum and mints can be used as treats to inhibit the growth of bacteria that cause tooth decay.

If these suggestions are followed, your child may never develop any tooth decay. If decay should begin, it will be easy to treat. Nothing replaces thorough daily brushing and flossing or good eating habits. Regular dental examination and dental hygiene appointments are vital. You will find that following these instructions will prove to be very effective in helping your child to maintain optimal dental health.

If you have any questions about dental disease prevention, please feel free to ask us.

Specific Recommendations: _____

_____

_____

Copyright © 2010 by Saunders, an imprint of Elsevier Inc. All rights reserved.

DENTAL SEALANTS

Patient Name: _____   Date: _____

WHY SEALANTS?

Decay on back teeth, premolars, and molars usually begins in the grooves and fissures that normally exist on the biting surfaces of the back teeth. Dental sealants are clear plastic coatings that can be placed on the biting and grinding surfaces of posterior teeth. These sealants prevent the formation of decay on the treated surfaces. Sealants can even be placed on teeth with small areas of decay known as *incipient carious lesions.* The sealants will stop the customary progress of tooth destruction. The sealant can remain on the tooth from 3 to more than 20 years, depending on the tooth, the type of sealant used, and the eating habits of the patient. Sealants are placed only on teeth that have not been previously restored.

The sealant is placed on the tooth through a chemical-mechanical bonding procedure. There is no drilling or local anesthesia required for sealant application. It is entirely painless and noninvasive.

We are dedicated to the prevention of oral disease. It is clear that if decay is prevented from the beginning or is small enough that a sealant can be used, there is a great savings in time, money, discomfort, and tooth structure. Decayed teeth must have the decay removed by drilling, then they must be filled. This drill and fill may have to be done several times over the patient's lifetime as the filling ages and needs replacement. We strongly suggest that patients who have teeth that can be successfully protected with a sealant material consider having this procedure performed as soon as possible after tooth eruption.

SEALANTS AND PREVENTION

We especially advise that children have the sealant applied to their teeth as soon as the teeth break through the gum and the biting surfaces of the teeth are exposed. If the teeth cannot be totally isolated from the moisture in the mouth during the bonding process, it is likely that the sealant will not remain on the tooth for as long a period of time as expected. Some newer sealant systems can be placed in the presence of moisture. The sealant is most often applied to permanent teeth, but sometimes a situation arises in which it would be beneficial to have the sealant applied to a primary tooth.

A study found that one application of sealant reduced biting surface decay 52% over a 15-year period. Another study showed that decay on biting surfaces could be reduced 95% over 10 years if 2% to 4% of the sealants were routinely repaired each year. We expect sealants to last many years. Replacing or repairing sealants, as needed, on an ongoing basis will give the best protection.

A sealant is not meant as a substitute for proper brushing and flossing habits. The effectiveness of the sealant is reduced if oral self-care is neglected. Also, cavities can still form on untreated surfaces. Therefore a topical fluoride treatment remains an essential and necessary preventive intervention.

Sealants are recommended by the U.S. Public Health Service, the Surgeon General of the United States, the American Dental Association, the American Academy of Pediatric Dentistry, the Canadian Dental Association, and the American Dental Hygienists' Association. We know that sealants are one of the most important treatments available for prevention of dental decay.

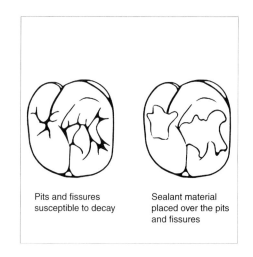

Pits and fissures
susceptible to decay

Sealant material
placed over the pits
and fissures

If you have any questions about sealants, please feel free to ask us.

Specific Recommendations: _____

_____

_____

Copyright © 2010 by Saunders, an imprint of Elsevier Inc. All rights reserved.

SUPPLEMENTAL FLUORIDE

Patient Name: _____

There are several methods by which you or your child can receive fluoride. The most common method is a topical application. This includes fluoride contained in drinking water, mouth rinses, toothpastes, and gels and professionally applied fluoride treatments (tray delivery or painted on) in the dental office. Each of these fluoride-containing vehicles is meant to work on the exposed surface enamel of the tooth that is in the mouth. The fluoride makes the enamel harder and provides the building blocks for remineralization. Fluoride can also inhibit the growth of bacteria. In topical oral self-care products, the fluoride concentration is low, but the repeated and daily application of the fluoride can help ensure that your teeth have fewer cavities.

Before teeth can be seen, while they are still developing under the gums, the teeth can also be made stronger and more resistant to decay with the use of fluoride. Systemic fluorides are found in the diet, dispensed by prescription, and swallowed. We strongly recommend that your children receive the benefits of this proven decay fighter if you live in an area where the water has little or no fluoride in it.

The overuse of fluoride supplements (systemic), in conjunction with the swallowing of fluoride toothpastes and mouth rinses by young patients, proved to be too much of a good thing. Many dentists noticed a higher incidence of small white spots forming on front teeth suggestive of mild fluorosis. Although not a dental disease, these white spots can be unsightly.

The recommendations for the use of prescription fluoride tablets are as follows:

If your children fall into the age groups in this table, **and if you do not have a fluoridated water supply and if they are not ingesting fluoride in their diets,** they should be taking supplemental fluoride. Systemic fluoride, which also has a topical effect, makes the enamel stronger and better able to resist acid attack from bacteria and less susceptible to decay. It is one of the most important preventive actions you can take for your children. In our opinion, even one cavity is too many. The best way to preserve teeth is to keep them undrilled and unfilled. This requires serious preventive measures: brushing, flossing, good diet, and fluoride supplements when necessary. It is good practice to keep flouride away from children to prevent accidental ingestion.

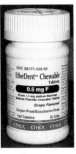

Example of a fluoride supplement available by prescription.

	Less Than		More Than
Age	0.3 ppm	0.3-0.6 ppm	6 ppm
Birth–6 months	None	None	None
6 mo–3 yr	0.25 mg/day	None	None
3 yr–6 yr	0.50 mg/day	0.25 mg/day	None
6 yr–16 yr	1.0 mg/day	0.50 mg/day	None

Fluoride Concentration in Drinking Water (Parts per Million [ppm])

If you have any questions about supplemental fluoride, please feel free to ask us.

Specific Recommendations: _____

_____

_____

Copyright © 2010 by Saunders, an imprint of Elsevier Inc. All rights reserved.

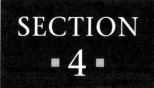

Copyright © 2010 by Saunders, an imprint of Elsevier Inc. All rights reserved.

FURCATION INVOLVEMENT

Patient Name: _____   **Date:** _____

The roots of the teeth are covered and surrounded by bone and gum tissues when they are in their normal, disease-free state. Only the crown portion is visible. Some teeth toward the back portion of your mouth have two or three roots extending into the jaw bone from the crowns of the tooth. This V-shaped area where the tooth branches or forks into two or three roots is called the *furcation* or *furca*. Normally the furca is also covered with bone and is attached to the tooth by periodontal ligament fibers.

As long as the furcation of a multirooted tooth is covered with the normal amount of bone and gum, everything is fine and the furca holds no exceptional interest for the dentist or dental hygienist. When there is pocket formation, an alteration in the density of the furca bone, or if bone actually starts to resorb (to disappear owing to some type of dental pathology), the furca area becomes difficult to clean and maintain. Continued loss of bone would lead to loss of the tooth.

The loss of the bone in the furca area is caused by periodontal disease (gum disease). The periodontal pathology in the furca could be part of a localized problem—only present at that one site—or a sign that there is a more widespread problem that needs attention. The breakdown of bone in the furcation could also indicate that the nerve inside the tooth is dying, and the tooth will need a root canal (endodontic treatment).

If the breakdown is specific to the site on that one tooth, treatment would be localized. The type of therapy recommended would depend on the severity of the breakdown. Minimal disease might be treated by scaling and root debridement and reinforcement of personal oral self-care. Treatment of a more extensive breakdown could involve aggressive periodontal procedures including but not limited to scaling and debridement, periodontal surgery, and bone augmentation. You may be referred to a periodontist for these procedures.

If the furca breakdown is a sign of more widespread periodontal disease, the whole mouth will be evaluated and specific treatment recommendations will be made.

You may think that teeth are difficult to floss and brush when tooth alignment and gum position are ideal. When there is bone loss in a furca, daily oral self-care becomes more complicated. A furca is a difficult area to clean—the more bone loss, the more difficult. In extreme cases there is no bone or gum left in the furca, and a patient could actually place an interdental cleaning aid completely between the roots of a two-rooted tooth. For a three-rooted tooth with a furcation involvement, the cleaning process is even more of a challenge.

You have been diagnosed as having a furcation involvement problem. After careful examination, a treatment recommendation will be made. Our recommendation will be based on not only treating your furcation problem but also preventing further bone loss.

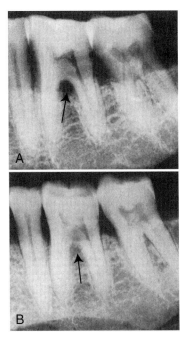

Furcation involvement. **A,** Triangular radiolucency in bifurcation area of mandibular first molar indicates furcation involvement. **B,** Same area, different angulation. The triangular radiolucency in the bifurcation of the first molar is obliterated, and involvement of the second bifurcation is apparent. (**A,** From Newman MG, Takei HH, Klokkevold PR, Carranza FA, eds: *Carranza's clinical periodontology,* ed 10, St Louis, 2006, Saunders.)

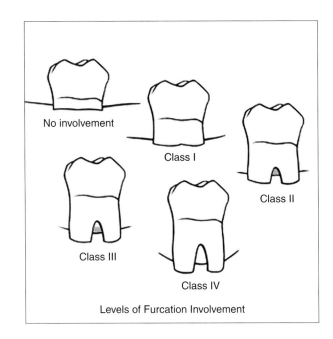

If you have any questions about a furcation involvement, please feel free to ask us.

Specific Recommendations: _____

_____

Copyright © 2010 by Saunders, an imprint of Elsevier Inc. All rights reserved.

GINGIVAL ENLARGEMENT

Patient Name: _____   Date: _____

PREDISPOSING FACTORS

Gingival enlargement is an increase in the size of the gum tissues. It is characterized by inflammation of the soft tissues surrounding the teeth. The gum tissues will appear shiny and swollen and dark red to bluish purple in color. The predisposing factors in this inflammation can include but are not limited to systemic factors (diabetes mellitus), antiepileptic medications (such as Dilantin, Mysoline, and Depakene), immunosuppressant drugs (cyclosporine), calcium channel blockers (Procardia, Calan, Cardizem, and Bayotensin), select other medications, hormonal changes associated with pregnancy, oral contraceptives, and the

types of hormonal changes younger teenagers experience during puberty, hence the term "drug-influenced gingival enlargement." We can see gingival enlargement associated with pregnancy, oral contraception, hormone replacement therapy, and puberty.

These conditions **do not** necessarily cause the gums to become inflamed or enlarged, but rather in the presence of plaque and an increase in blood hormone levels, the response of the gum tissues can be out of the ordinary. Gingival enlargement can also occur just because of a large presence of bacterial plaque in the absence of any of these factors.

INDICATIONS

If you have any of these predisposing factors or take certain drugs, there is a potential for gingival enlargement. If you have gingival enlargement, you will probably notice that your

gums bleed when you brush and floss. Bleeding is always a sign of disease, inflamation, or infection.

ELIMINATION AND/OR PREVENTION

To eliminate or prevent these problems, your oral self-care must be thorough. You must brush and floss and do whatever other oral self-care procedures you have been instructed to do every day. This may clear up the problem entirely. If not, you will need to adjust the interval between recare appointments with the dental hygienist. A time frame of 2, 3, or 4 months between professional dental hygiene care, depending on the severity of the problem, may be appropriate for prevention of gum enlargement. This maintenance interval will be necessary for as long as the predisposing factors exist. If medication is the factor, you will need to see the hygienist at the interval recommended.

If you are pregnant, gingival enlargement could persist until the hormonal changes associated with pregnancy revert back to normal. Until then, you need to schedule your oral recare appointments with the dental hygienist as recommended. Similarly, if you take oral contraceptives and notice signs of recurring gum inflammation (bleeding when brushing and flossing), assuming that your oral self-care is thorough, a more regular recare schedule may be necessary.

Gingival enlargement in young teens is generally seen where oral self-care in not adequate. A 3-month professional care interval is best in this circumstance. Some teenagers have inadequate oral self-care habits. Junk food and sugary, acidic drinks (even juice) coupled with almost nonexistent brushing and flossing cause serious gum disease, bad breath, and decay. Generally the hormonal change stabilizes and the acute problem resolves. For this age group, social issues of wanting to be more attractive many times will influence oral self-care habits when all the dental attention in the world cannot!

These recommendations are designed to prevent gum problems. Prevention is better and much less expensive than any cure. If you have dental insurance, it will probably **not** cover the additional necessary dental hygiene care. Although you do need these procedures to maintain your oral health, these situations are considered unusual by the carrier and are not generally covered.

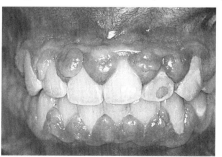

Severe cyclosporine-associated gingival enlargement.

If you have any questions about gingival hyperplasia, please feel free to ask us.

Specific Recommendations: _____

_____

Copyright © 2010 by Saunders, an imprint of Elsevier Inc. All rights reserved.

GINGIVITIS

Patient Name: _____   **Date:** _____

Almost everyone knows what a cavity is. Because of the far-reaching effects of advertising by multipurpose toothpaste and antimicrobial oral rinse manufacturers, almost everyone has heard of **gingivitis.** What may not be quite clear to you, however, is exactly what gingivitis is. You may recognize it as a problem but not know why and how serious it might be. You may even know that it is a type of gum (periodontal) disease. You may also know that it is somehow related to plaque (oral biofilm) and tartar (calculus) on teeth. But why should you be concerned about having it?

WHAT IS GINGIVITIS?

Gingivitis is an infection of the gum tissues surrounding the teeth. It is a very common infection and affects almost 95% of the world's population. This infection can be characterized by redness, swelling, and bleeding of the gums around the teeth. This gum infection absolutely needs to be treated as soon as possible. Gum infections are almost always preventable with sound daily oral self-care.

Gingivitis is the mildest form of periodontal disease and is reversible. By definition, with gingivitis there is no loss of bone that supports the tooth. If treated early, gingivitis can be eliminated. If left untreated, it can progress into the more serious form of periodontal disease called *periodontitis.* In the more serious form of disease, the bone and gum tissues can be permanently affected. Bleeding gums, one of the signs of gingivitis, are a sign of inflammation and infection in the mouth. Your gum tissues should never bleed. It is not normal for blood to appear on your toothbrush when you have finished brushing. Gingivitis does not generally hurt, so you may not even know that you have it. It can be localized (around a few teeth) or generalized (around most or all of the teeth). Gingivitis is seen most often in patients who do not brush and floss well daily, but it can also be related to medication or certain systemic diseases. Bad breath can be another sign of gingivitis. If you are using a mouthwash to control bad breath, you may need professional dental attention. Although bad breath can be related to some medical problems, most often it is just a result of debris that is not cleaned properly from your teeth, gums, and tongue and that is decomposing in the dark, warm, and moist environment of your mouth—a perfect place to breed disease-causing bacteria.

HOW IS GINGIVITIS TREATED?

If you have bleeding gums, you should be concerned to take action. Healthy tissue anywhere in our bodies does not bleed. So what can you do to stop the bleeding?

We can help you eliminate the gingivitis. It involves a good professional scaling and good oral self-care habits. Plaque (soft debris made up of bacteria) and tartar (calculus or hardened plaque) must be removed before the gum tissues can heal and the infection can be eliminated. If it has been some time since you had your teeth cleaned properly, it may take more than one appointment to get you back in health.

Get your teeth and gums professionally scaled on a regular basis. Keep them clean with daily brushing and flossing. The infection you have will be eliminated. Twice daily, brush with a multipurpose dentifrice that carries the ADA Seal or CDA Seal to control gingivitis and plaque. The twice daily use of an ADA-approved antimicrobial mouth rinse is also affective against gingivitis. If this does not achieve the desired outcome, then the prescription rinse of 0.12% chlorhexidine gluconate can be used. If you keep your teeth and gums clean, they can be healthy for your whole life.

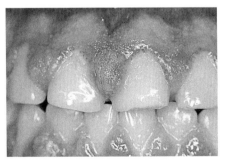

Gingival enlargement, particularly on interdental papillae.

If you have any questions about gingivitis, please feel free to ask us.

Specific Recommendations: _____

_____

Copyright © 2010 by Saunders, an imprint of Elsevier Inc. All rights reserved.

INSUFFICIENT ATTACHED GINGIVA

Patient Name: _____   Date: _____

If you were to view a cross-section of the tooth and jaw, you would see, from the tip of the tooth toward the coral pink to brown pigmented gingiva (gum), the following:

- The enamel-covered portion of the tooth gently constricting as it approaches the gingival area
- The margin of the gingival tissue (which just abuts the tooth)
- The gingival tissue that is firmly bound down to the underlying bone and cannot be moved, perhaps with a pebbly appearance
- Reddish smoother-looking mucosal tissue, which is very movable and not tightly bound to the underlying bone. This area is called *oral mucosa* and may be redder in color than the other described gingival tissue and covers the inside of the mouth (cheeks, lips, floor of the mouth).

The focus of this topic is on the zone of attached gingiva. As part of your oral examination, we use a periodontal probe to measure and record the depth of the sulcus around your teeth. The sulcular depth is the depth of the space between the marginal gingiva and the attached gingiva. The periodontal probe used to measure this sulcus is gently inserted under the margin of the gingiva and placed into the sulcus until it is stopped by the gingival tissue attachment, which is tightly bound to the bone. This measurement helps to determine your periodontal health. In health, the sulcular depths measured are 3 millimeters or less. This tightly attached zone of gingival tissue surrounding the tooth is quite important.

This zone of attached gingiva needs to be intact and of adequate width to protect the tissue around the tooth. Periodontal disease can cause gingival tissue, gingival attachment, and bone to break down. If attached gingiva is diseased, improper (too hard) brushing or a strong muscle attachment can pull on the attached gingival tissue, further contributing to its breakdown. The 1- to 3-millimeter normal depth can increase to 4 millimeters, or even more. The normal gingival margin (gum line) is scalloped (like small, regular waves). If there is insufficient attached gingiva, the scalloping will be altered, and the receding gingiva will turn red and bleed easily. The receded area will be more prone to trapping bacterial plaque and food debris, will be harder to clean, and will continue to be inflamed and infected. The gum recession can extend close to or into the mucosa. You might have seen this condition in your own mouth. Insufficient attached gingiva needs to be corrected or it can lead to tooth loss.

Once the condition has been diagnosed, the correction requires periodontal surgery. Usually a periodontist (gum specialist) will perform this procedure. You will receive a local anesthetic to numb the area; tissue may be harvested from the hard palate and then repositioned over the problem area to re-establish the correct width of attached gingival tissue.

Although this is a relatively common problem, patients do not recognize it. If you have insufficient attached gingiva, get it treated as soon as possible.

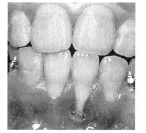

Irregular gingival contours and recession with severe gingival inflammation. (Courtesy Dr. Kenneth Marinak, Adjunct Clinical Instructor, Gene W. Hirschfeld School of Dental Hygiene, Old Dominion University, Norfolk, Virginia.)

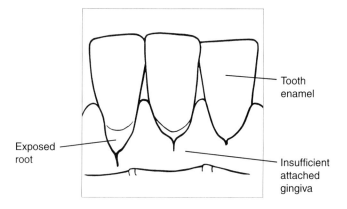

If you have any questions about insufficient attached gingiva, please feel free to ask us.

Specific Recommendations: _____

_____

_____

Copyright © 2010 by Saunders, an imprint of Elsevier Inc. All rights reserved.

NECROTIZING ULCERATIVE GINGIVITIS

Patient Name: _____   **Date:** _____

Necrotizing ulcerative gingivitis is an acute inflammatory destructive disease of the gum tissues. Other names that have been used to describe this disease process are *trench mouth* and *Vincent's disease or infection.*

SYMPTOMS

Necrotizing ulcerative gingivitis can occur at any age. However, it is usually seen in young people between the ages of 15 and 30. Often, it occurs in high school or college students under stress (e.g., studying for examinations) or soldiers going into battle. Poor dietary habits, poor oral hygiene, inadequate sleep, and lowered resistance to infection are significant risk factors. Signs of necrotizing gingival disease may include the following:

- Sudden onset
- Pain and soreness to the extent that normal chewing is difficult
- Bleeding that is spontaneous on even the slightest of pressure
- Metallic or unpleasant taste
- Slight fever
- Swollen lymph glands
- Feted mouth odor
- Sloughing of gingival tissue
- Blunted, necrosed tissue between the teeth

CAUSES

Necrotizing ulcerative gingivitis is an infectious disease caused by a specific complex of disease-causing microbes that develop and increase once the body's defenses have been lowered. Major predisposing factors are smoking, stress, very poor oral self-care, inadequate sleep, and poor nutrition.

TREATMENT

Treatment for necrotizing ulcerative gingivitis involves both our dental team and you. Treatment consists of careful evaluation of your personal habits: what you eat and how you care for your mouth. We will remove the accumulated oral biofilm, dental calculus, dead bacterial cells, and decomposing food from those infected areas and instruct you in oral self-care habits that will help eliminate the disease and prevent its return. Your job is to make certain that you follow these instructions:

1. **Carefully follow all oral self-care tips.** Do not allow anyone to use your toothbrush. Use only the softest toothbrush possible to gently but thoroughly clean your teeth. Allow your brush to dry between uses.
2. **Follow through with all your appointments.** Because you are no longer in severe pain does not mean the infection is gone. The underlying periodontal infection can recur if it is not completely treated.
3. **Frequent rinsing** with a mixture of warm water and 3% hydrogen peroxide for the first three days while the symptom are acute.
4. **Twice-daily rinses** with 0.12% chlorhexidine gluconate is advised for about three weeks.
5. **Avoid using tobacco** products in any form.
6. **Balance your diet** with whole grains, green vegetables, proteins, and fruits. Avoid highly seasoned food and alcoholic beverages. We may prescribe a vitamin for you during this time as well.
7. **Get adequate rest.** The body will heal much faster when well rested.
8. If you have been prescribed any rinse or antibiotic, be sure to use it, following the instructions carefully.

Necrotizing ulcerative gingivitis can be a serious medical condition that will need to be closely monitored. Because necrotizing ulcerative gingival can recur, it is essential that we have your full cooperation and understanding of the treatment from the start.

If you have any questions about necrotizing periodontal disease, please feel free to ask us.

Specific Recommendations: _____

_____

_____

Copyright © 2010 by Saunders, an imprint of Elsevier Inc. All rights reserved.

PERIODONTAL DISEASE

Patient Name: _____   **Date:** _____

Periodontitis is an infectious, inflammatory disease classified according to how much damage has been done to the soft and hard tissue structures surrounding the teeth, namely the gingiva (gums) and bone. **It is an infection in your mouth.** It can affect some or all of your teeth to varying degrees. Some risk factors for periodontal disease include smoking, diabetes mellitus, specific bacteria, poor oral hygiene, stress, bleeding gums, age, gender, and race, and our immune systems, but the condition is usually related to how well you are able to keep your teeth clean through proper oral self-care. The better you clean your teeth to remove all the plaque bacteria, the less likely you will develop periodontal disease.

PROGRESS OF THE DISEASE

The bacteria that cause this disease first cause the gum tissue to become inflamed, bleed, and pull away from the teeth. As the problem becomes more serious, the bone that supports the teeth also becomes infected and begins to break down and resorb. The teeth then become loose. Once the bone disappears, it is extremely hard for new bone to be rebuilt. The damage is permanent, and your teeth, the surrounding bone, and your general health will be compromised.

Periodontal disease is classified into several types. The mildest form of this infection is signaled by red and swollen gum tissue that bleeds easily. There is seldom any pain involved at this stage. You may notice also that your breath becomes offensive and you feel the need to use mouthwash. Our sense of smell adjusts to the same odors, so we lose our ability to detect our own offensive, bad breath. As the disease progresses, the gum tissue becomes more red and swollen, more bleeding can be seen on the toothbrush and floss, and the teeth begin to become loose. This tooth mobility is a sign that there is a severe problem. There may still be no pain at this advanced stage. At this point, the management of your problem may involve periodontal surgical procedures. If this is the case, you may be referred to a periodontist (gum specialist) for further treatment. Most of the time, periodontal disease starts and continues because risk factors have not been controlled. Once we have diagnosed this disease, we will inform you of the problem, work to modify your risk factors, and suggest treatment options. If treatment is not completed, however, the disease will continue to progress. Unfortunately the disease is quite invisible to most people until severe and possibly irreversible damage has occurred.

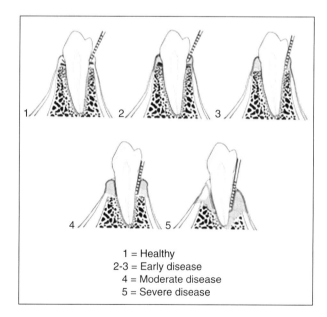

1 = Healthy
2-3 = Early disease
4 = Moderate disease
5 = Severe disease

(Continued)

Copyright © 2010 by Saunders, an imprint of Elsevier Inc. All rights reserved.

PERIODONTAL DISEASE—cont'd

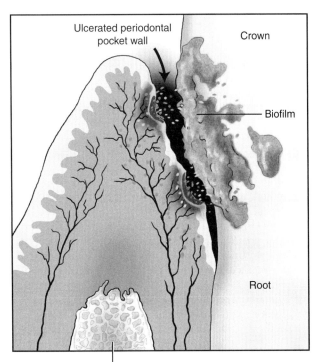

Drawing of the interface between the gingiva and tooth in a case of periodontal disease. The epithelium of the pocket wall is ulcerated. These ulcerations allow subgingival bacteria in the adjacent periodontal pocket access to the systemic circulation.

SOLUTION

If the disease has been diagnosed in the early stages and has not progressed to bone loss, scaling and root planing over multiple appointments supplemented with antimicrobial therapies may be needed. In the most advanced cases, periodontal surgery and tooth loss are inevitable. You will receive a plan of care, an estimate of the number of appointments required, and the fees for the recommended treatment.

Periodontal disease is a condition that must be treated quickly and then controlled over the lifetime. We believe that if the infection is aggressively treated in its early stages,

nonsurgical periodontal treatment may be possible and effective. Although we do not automatically rule out periodontal surgical intervention, we hope you can either avoid it or reduce the amount you will need.

Successful treatment of your periodontal problem will depend on several factors. But the most important of these is your ability to perform excellent oral self-care—brushing, flossing, and using periodontal aids—on a routine, daily basis. In addition, smokers should stop smoking. Without this, periodontal treatment will fail and the disease will return.

If you have any questions about periodontal disease, please feel free to ask us.

Specific Recommendations: _____

_____

Copyright © 2010 by Saunders, an imprint of Elsevier Inc. All rights reserved.

PERIODONTAL DISEASE AND SYSTEMIC HEALTH

Patient Name: _____

Date: _____

Research suggests a strong correlation between oral (peri-odontal) infections and generalized (systemic) medical problems. There are over 500 different types of bacteria normally found in the mouth, and infections in the mouth can affect the entire body.

A gum infection is similar to an infection that might occur elsewhere in your body. When the body recognizes bacterial invaders, the immune system initiates a response to fight off the invader. If disease-causing bacteria multiply past a critical number and the body's immune system can no longer keep the infection in check, problems begin. Poor oral self-care, genetics, prescription medication, smoking, illness, systemic problems, and/or diminished salivary flow might further overcome the body's immune system.

You might say, "My gums have always bled like this," and not seek treatment. Imagine seeing blood seeping from your eyes when you washed your face. You would seek immediate medical attention and perhaps even go to an emergency room! Yet blood seeping from the gums during toothbrushing or flossing is equally indicative of a health problem that needs professional attention from the dentist and dental hygienist.

Gum disease is an infection in your mouth, no different from an infection elsewhere in your body. The bacteria invade the soft tissues and the bone and enter the bloodstream. In this way they are able to circulate throughout the entire body. Along with the bacteria are dead cells (pus), metabolic by-products, and toxins from the bacteria, food debris, and viruses.

Researchers are examining a link between periodonlal disease and systemic conditions such as cardiovascular disease, pneumonia, chronic obstructive pulmonary disease, premature birth and low birthweight, stroke, diabetes mellitus, obesity, and rheumatoid arthritis. Although the scientific data have yet to confirm that oral disease causes these systemic conditions, it is important for us to recognize the possible implications. The oral cavity is part of the human biology linked to all other body systems and is a portal of entry for disease-causing organisms. It makes sense to keep the mouth as clean as possible to reduce the risk of not only oral infection but possibly systemic inflammation as well, the common denomenator in many chronic diseases.

Thorough oral self-care need not be difficult or time-consuming. The benefits are more than just fresh breath and an attractive smile. Investing just a few minutes a day caring for your teeth and gums and scheduling professional dental hygiene visits at regular intervals as advised can make the difference between whole body health and disease.

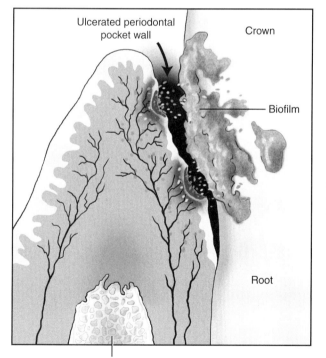

Drawing of the interface between the gingiva and tooth in a case of periodontal disease. The epithelium of the pocket wall is ulcerated. These ulcerations allow subgingival bacteria in the adjacent periodontal pocket access to the systemic circulation.

If you have any questions about periodontal disease and general health, please feel free to ask us.

Specific Recommendations: _____

_____

Copyright © 2010 by Saunders, an imprint of Elsevier Inc. All rights reserved.

POCKET DEPTH MEASUREMENT

Patient Name: _____   **Date:** _____

When a dentist or physician is preparing a treatment plan, clinical and radiographic data are collected and results are analyzed. Treatment decisions depend on information gathered, the evidence-based treatments available, and the values of the patient. The more accurate the diagnostic information, the better the diagnosis and treatment. In the realm of periodontal disease, diagnosis is based in part on the collection and analysis of numbers, specifically, measurements of the depth of the sulcus (pocket) under the gum tissue that surrounds each tooth.

A periodontal examination generally consists of taking at least six measurements around every tooth. Areas of gum recession, pus, tooth mobility, and bleeding are also recorded. The evidence of bleeding is significant. Healthy gum tissue does not bleed when gently probed. Factors such as smoking restrict bleeding, so lack of bleeding alone does not signify a healthy site.

These measurements (in millimeters) are one of the key diagnostic tools (along with tissue color, position, and shape) a dentist and dental hygienist use to determine the severity of periodontal (gum) disease. Measurements generally range from 0 (best) to 12 (worst) mm. Probing of the sulcus (space in between the gum and the tooth) around the tooth often shows normal depths of 1 to 3 mm when there is no gingival recession with greater depths between the teeth where they touch as opposed to the direct cheek side or tongue side. The numbers will vary from position to position and tooth to tooth. Measurements are rarely uniform throughout the entire mouth. The higher numbers indicate more severe soft- and hard-tissue involvement, and the greater the number of higher readings, the more likely that surgical intervention is needed. In general:

- 0 to 3 mm with **no bleeding:** Great numbers. No periodontal disease present.
- 1 to 3 mm **with bleeding:** Gingivitis (the mildest form of gum disease) present. Probably no bone loss unless there is gingival recession. Usually treated with a professional oral prophylaxis (cleaning) and improved oral self-care.
- 3 to 5 mm with **no bleeding:** Smoking may be a factor in lack of bleeding. Because a patient cannot reliably clean deeper than 3 mm on a routine basis, there is high potential for gum disease to begin. Recommend nonsurgical periodontal care, then periodontal maintenance care three or four times a year.
- 3 to 5 mm **with bleeding:** Early to moderate periodontal disease. Treatment is nonsurgical periodontal therapy consisting of scaling and root planing, ADA-accepted antimicrobial mouthrinses, and/or site-specific antimicrobials and other medications. Supporting bone may be involved. More frequent and extensive periodontal maintenance appointments are required. Some surgical intervention is possible. Recommend non-surgical periodontal care, then periodontal maintenance care three to four times a year.
- 5 to 7 mm **with bleeding:** Soft- and hard-tissue damage and bone loss. Treatment will involve nonsurgical periodontal therapy—scaling and root planing. Multiple appointments will be needed. Localized surgical intervention probable. Systemic submicrobial antibiotics and site-specific antimicrobials commonly used. Teeth may have started to become loose. Referral to a periodontist is common.
- 7 mm and above **with bleeding:** Advanced periodontal disease. Aggressive nonsurgical and surgical treatment required if teeth are to be saved. Surgery almost always required. Referral to periodontist is common. Systemic submicrobial antibiotics and site-specific antimicrobials commonly used.

In summary, low pocket depth measurements are good and high measurements are bad. The presence of deep periodontal pockets corresponds to more extensive periodontal disease and the need for more advanced periodontal treatment.

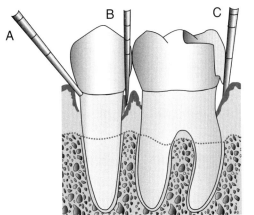

Periodontal probing limitations. **A,** Wrong angulation of probe. **B,** Probe blocked by calculus. **C,** Probe blocked by overhanging restoration. (From Newman MG, Takei HH, Klokkevold PR, Carranza FA, eds: *Carranza's clinical periodontology,* ed 10, St Louis, 2006, Saunders.)

If you have any questions about pocket depth, please feel free to ask us.

Specific Recommendations: _____

Copyright © 2010 by Saunders, an imprint of Elsevier Inc. All rights reserved.

SMOKING AND CHRONIC PERIODONTITIS

Patient Name: _____

Date: _____

If you are a smoker, you are at a higher risk for lung cancer, cardiovascular disease, stroke, and oral disease. Smoking weakens the immune system, causes cell death, and may be responsible for more than 50% of cases of chronic periodontitis. It has been reported that more than 85% of all periodontal cases are present in people who smoke. More than 90% of periodontal infections that appear to be resistant to treatment (refractory disease) are found among smokers. Smokers are 2.6 to 6 times more likely to have periodontal disease; former smokers also are more likely to have periodontal disease than persons who never smoked. A person who smokes will have poor healing and does not respond as well to periodontal therapy as a nonsmoker.

Cancer-causing chemicals are released during smoking; this causes a profound challenge to the immune system, which, when working properly, is responsible for helping us ward off infections. Because periodontal disease is an infection, it is easy to see how a weakened immune system further contributes to the disease process. Many smokers show few areas of bleeding during a periodontal charting because one of the effects of smoking is reduced circulation.

If you are reading this, you are most likely a smoker who has periodontal disease. Many smokers would like to stop this addictive habit. Quitting is difficult, but it can be done. The decision to quit is the first step. There really are many aids today to help you quit. Our office can be a great source to help you stop smoking. If you would like us to make suggestions for a healthier lifestyle, do not hesitate to ask!

Some suggestions for quiting include:
- Establish a quit date.
- Join a support group through the American Cancer Society or American Lung Association, or at a local hospital.
- Use a QUITLINE: 1-800-QUIT-NOW (1-800-784-8669).
- Use an over-the-counter nicotine replacement therapy (nicotine patch, nicotine gum, or nicotine lozenge) or a prescription non-nicotine agent.
- Plan ahead when the environment will increase your desire to smoke. Think about how you will avoid a relapse.
- Obtain more suggestions to help you quit at www. smokefree.gov.

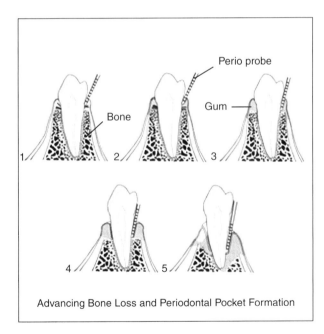

Advancing Bone Loss and Periodontal Pocket Formation

Benefits of Stopping Tobacco Use

- I won't have the smell of tobacco on my breath or stains on my teeth.
- I will save money.
- It will reduce my chances of getting mouth cancer.
- My friends and family want me to quit.
- I'll be setting a good example for my children.
- I'll feel more in control of my life.
- I'll feel more liberated and self-assured that I can set goals and accomplish them.
- It will reduce my chances of heart trouble.
- It will reduce my chances of gum disease.
- It will reduce my chances of hypertension and circulatory problems.
- It will increase my chances of being around to support my family and of seeing my children grown up.
- Two weeks to 3 months after quitting smoking, circulation improves, walking becomes easier, and lung function increases up to 30%.
- One year after quitting smoking, the risk of coronary heart disease decreases to half that of a smoker.
- Five years after quitting smoking, the risk of stroke is reduced to that of people who have never smoked.
- Fifteen years after quitting smoking, the risk of coronary heart disease is similar to that of people who have never smoked.

Adapted from U.S. Department of Health and Human Services: *Surgeon General report on the health benefits of smoking cessation,* 1990.

If you have any questions about smoking and oral health, please feel free to ask us.

Specific Recommendations: _____

_____

_____

Copyright © 2010 by Saunders, an imprint of Elsevier Inc. All rights reserved.

ORAL PROPHYLAXIS

Patient Name: _____

There is nothing more important to your dental health than maintaining a clean mouth. Prevention of oral infection optimizes our general health. A clean mouth will be disease-, infection-, and trouble-free. A clean mouth will not be predisposed to developing either decay or periodontal (gum) disease. Very important functions of the dental hygienist include teaching you how to keep your teeth and gums healthy and regularly providing an oral prophylaxis. The oral prophylaxis involves the scaling of the teeth to remove oral biofilm, dental calculus,

Date: _____

and extrinsic, tooth stain to promote a healthy oral environment. This procedure is accomplished in one appointment that occurs every 3 months to 1 year to prevent or control gingivitis. It is not a procedure to treat periodontal disease.

The theory and practice of oral disease prevention and oral health promotion have undergone revolutionary changes based on research evidence. The preventive needs of every individual differ. The old adage "See your dentist every 6 months" is not necessarily valid today.

YOUR PERSONAL PLAN

The recare and examination interval that we have recommended for you is designed for your unique oral care needs. And your needs, too, can change. The interval between oral prophylaxis appointments that is established for you is a function of many things. These include the following:

- General health status/presence of systemic disease
- Pharmacologic history
- Dexterity and hand-eye coordination
- Age
- Diet
- Stress levels
- Oral habits
- Position and alignment of the teeth
- Number, type, size, and location of restorations
- Restorative materials used
- Periodontal and dental history
- Location of bone and periodontal tissues
- Risk factors for dental decay

- Risk factors for periodontal disease
- Risk factors for oral cancer
- Motivation to perform oral self-care effectively
- Ability to perform oral self-care effectively

Simply stated, the more complex your dental situation and the more your tooth position and alignment deviate from the normal, the harder you will find it to keep your teeth clean and your gums healthy.

Recent studies have identified many of the microorganisms that cause gum disease and decay. They can be controlled if we work together. These studies also show that a prophylaxis every 6 months may not be adequate for some individuals. In order to prevent destructive oral disease, prophylaxis appointments in intervals of anywhere from 3 months to a year may be recommended.

You don't have to let periodontal disease develop! We are here to be your guide to good health.

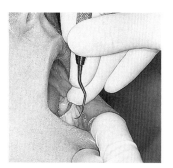

Same arch fulcrum positioned near area being scaled.

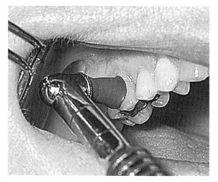

Polishing the buccal surfaces of the maxillary right posterior quadrant.

If you have any questions about your oral prophylaxis intervals, please feel free to ask us.

Specific Recommendations: _____

_____

Copyright © 2010 by Saunders, an imprint of Elsevier Inc. All rights reserved.

SCALING, ROOT DEBRIDEMENT, AND ROOT PLANING

Patient Name: _____   Date: _____

THE PROCEDURE

Scaling is a periodontal dental procedure in which plaque and calculus are removed from the tooth both above (supra-gingival) and below (subgingival) the gum (gingiva). Root debridement is the mechanical treatment of periodontitis by the removal of tooth and root surface irregularities (including plaque, clinically detectable calculus, and all plaque-retentive factors) so that the adjacent soft tissues in the periodontal pocket can heal. Root planing is a procedure in which diseased or altered portions of the root surface, the cementum, and dentin are removed and the resulting new surface is made smooth and clean. The more altered and damaged the root surface has been from calculus (tartar) and plaque accumulation, the greater the need for root planing.

The purpose of scaling, root debridement, and root planing is to eliminate microorganisms, endotoxins, and calculus to reduce inflammation, promote tissue regeneration, and make root surfaces biologically acceptable to gingival tissues. Any tooth deposits that can cause inflammation of the gum tissue must be eliminated. The root surface must be made as smooth as possible. Irregularities in the root surface can accumulate bacteria and contribute to gum inflammation. Irregularities are sites for bacteria and plaque buildup. The bacteria and the toxins they produce in the plaque are held against the tooth by the calculus. In this way, plaque and calculus on the teeth are risk factors to gum disease.

Depending on the severity of your particular periodontal problem, scaling and root planing may be the definitive treatment and no further procedures will be required. In many cases scaling and root planing are only part of the overall therapy. They are demanding procedures. They require much more time than the familiar oral prophylaxis. Scaling and root planing are usually performed in multiple appointments, with a quarter of the mouth or half the mouth treated at each appointment. In this office we find that most patients are most comfortable if the area to be treated during the root planing procedure is anesthetized with a local anesthetic agent.

The scaling and root planing may have to be repeated in the future. It is customary to place the patient on a 3- to 4-month periodontal maintenance schedule. Scientific evidence clearly shows that for individuals who have periodontal disease, an interval of 6 months is too long. We are familiar with your particular periodontal situation and will determine the appropriate interval for you. As your situation changes, there may be changes in the length of this interval.

Other than the teeth being somewhat sensitive after scaling, root debridement, and root planing, there is some postoperative discomfort. The sensitivity will diminish with time and meticulous oral hygiene. If you have been diagnosed as having severe periodontal infection, the sensitivity may remain for quite some time, and further at-home and in-office procedures may be needed to eliminate sensitivity. Although many dental procedures can be considered elective, we consider scaling, oral debridement, and root planing to be necessity for your oral health.

PREVENTING RECURRENCE OF DISEASE

Once scaling, root debridement, and root planing have been completed, it is most important for you to practice the brushing and interdental cleaning techniques in which you were instructed. If we have recommended any additional oral care products and devices, you must use them, too. Your cooperation is vital if the procedures are to be successful. To remain disease-free, you will need to remain constant in your oral self-care regimen.

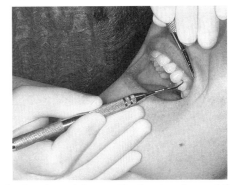

Extraoral palm-down fulcrum. The front surfaces of the fingers rest on the left lateral aspect of the mandible while the maxillary left posterior teeth are instrumented. (From Newman MG, Takei HH, Klokkevold PR, Carranza FA: *Carranza's clinical periodontology,* ed 10, St Louis, 2006, Saunders.)

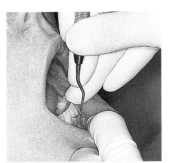

Same arch fulcrum positioned near area being scaled.

If you have any questions about scaling, oral debridement, and root planing, please feel free to ask us.

Specific Recommendations: _____

Copyright © 2010 by Saunders, an imprint of Elsevier Inc. All rights reserved.

SCALING, ROOT DEBRIDEMENT, AND ROOT PLANING: POSTPROCEDURAL INSTRUCTIONS

Patient Name: _____

Date: _____

- The oral prophylaxis just completed has been preventive in nature because of your thorough oral self-care. That means that there was no periodontal disease evident. The prophylaxis was completed with the minimum of trauma to your teeth and soft tissues. In this event, you should have insignificant postoperative discomfort in your mouth. Congratulations on a job well done. Keep up the good work. We would rather assist you in preventing periodontal disease than in controlling the problems periodontal disease causes.

- A therapeutic scaling, root debridement, and root planing has been completed. In this case, the gingival (gum) tissue showed signs of infection and inflammation and you may have had significant calculus (tartar) buildup. You may notice that your teeth feel different where the calculus was removed. The soft tissues may be sensitive or sore for approximately 1 day as they begin to heal. You may find that taking an over-the-counter pain reliever (aspirin, ibuprofen, and so on) will help during this 24-hour period. You may also rinse your mouth every few hours with warm saltwater. Make sure that you brush and floss your teeth during this time as you have been instructed. Be gentle, because the brushed areas may be sore, but be thorough! You do not want to have the periodontal infection begin again.

  - When you have had scaling, root debridement, and root planing, or other more involved periodontal procedures, you can expect your gingival (gum) tissues to be sore. This is normal when the gum tissues have been infected and inflamed for some time. The more severely they have been affected, the more discomfort you can expect. This soreness should resolve. You may clean your teeth with a soft bristled toothbrush and a multipurpose dentifrice that carries the ADA Seal of Acceptance and rinse with an ADA-accepted antimicrobial mouth rinse.

- You may also notice that the teeth have become sensitive to temperature and chemical changes after the scaling, root debridement, and root planing. This sensation frequently occurs when the surfaces of the roots of your teeth have been cleaned and are exposed. Removal of the debris covering the roots leaves the roots open to temperature and chemical stimulus. If the problem persists, please let us know.

- When you examine your gums closely in a mirror, you will also observe that the color, texture, and position of your periodontal tissues will undergo a change as the healing takes place. The swollen, reddened gum tissue will shrink, become more firm, and return to a healthy contour and color. Watch for these welcome signs of improvement, and be encouraged by the healing process.

- Please do not forget to brush, floss, and use other periodontal cleaning aids as you have been taught. We also recommend that you rinse twice daily for 30 seconds with an ADA-accepted antimicrobial mouth rinse to control bacterial growth in the entire mouth. It is important that you begin establishing proper oral self-care habits immediately. If you find that the recently treated areas are sensitive to the brushing and interdental cleaning, be gentle—**but be thorough!** With proper technique you cannot damage the teeth or gingival tissues.

- Brush 2 to 3 times daily with a fluoride-containing toothpaste. Rinse with a fluoride-containing mouth rinse once each day. Consider multipurpose toothpaste, too.

- Use the oral irrigator with the periodontal attachment as instructed. Fill the reservoir with the following:
  ❑ water   ❑ chlorhexidinegluconate0.12%   ❑ other _____

- Use the periodontal cleaning aids as you have been shown _____.

- Please return in _____ weeks for a _____-minute appointment. During this time, your periodontal tissues will be evaluated for the expected improvement and to determine the effectiveness of your oral self-care and the possible necessity of further periodontal treatment. This appointment will include reprobing the periodontal tissues.

- Because of your periodontal condition, we strongly recommend that you return for your next examination and preventive prophylaxis or periodontal maintenance appointment in _____ months.

If you have any questions about these instructions, please feel free to ask us.

Specific Recommendations: _____

_____

_____

Copyright © 2010 by Saunders, an imprint of Elsevier Inc. All rights reserved.

SCALING, ROOT DEBRIDEMENT, AND ROOT PLANING: RE-EVALUATION

Patient Name: _____   **Date:** _____

The goal of scaling, root debridement, and root planing is to remove all plaque, toxins, and calculus both above and below the gum line; reduce inflammation; promote tissue regeneration; and make the tooth surface biologically acceptable to the gingival tissues. After healing has occurred, the tissues will shrink, and a re-evaluation of the condition of the gum and supporting structures will reveal any areas that may need re-treatment. Your oral self-care habits will be re-evaluated at the same time, and any revisions to our recommendations will be made. If we have not yet removed tooth stain, we will be selectively polishing your teeth at this appointment to remove tooth stain. Once all tissues have responded, the goals of scaling, root debridement, and root planing have been met, and your self-care is effective, a periodontal maintenance interval will be established for you.

At the periodontal maintenance appointment, we will once again be evaluating your oral self-care to determine whether we need to recommend different procedures to keep your oral health at its best. We will re-examine your periodontal tissues for evidence of healing by remeasuring the probing depths around each tooth. Any areas of bleeding will be noted and treated; your teeth will then be selectively polished, and a topical fluoride treatment or desensitizing treatment may be performed.

Topical fluoride prevents tooth decay and has a bacteriostatic effect on the oral bacteria during treatment and for several hours afterward. It appears to be harder for the bacteria that cause gum disease to multiply and cause problems when topical fluoride is used.

If the goals of scaling, root debridement, and root planing have not been met, we will either re-treat those areas that have become reinfected or refer you to a periodontist for specific diagnosis and perhaps periodontal surgery. The periodontal surgery will correct some of the hard-tissue (bone) and soft-tissue defects that were caused by the periodontal infection.

At this time we may also consider using one or more of the newer nonsurgical therapies available for localized deep periodontal pocket sites that have not healed as much as we would like. The site-specific therapy may be recommended for the first time or as a re-treatment. We will then monitor the results to determine whether a referral to a periodontist is appropriate.

A final word about how often you should have your teeth maintained. Modern dentistry considers a patient who has had periodontal disease to be never completely "cured." If you do not take care of your teeth and gums, the problem can come back. It is in the best interest of your oral health to have your teeth examined and maintained at an interval of _____ months in most cases, not every 6 months as you have heard for years.

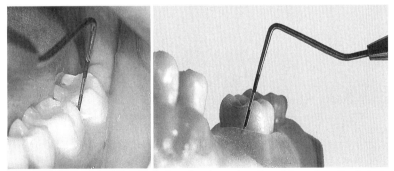

For proximal readings, periodontal probe is slightly angled under the col and positioned vertically to touch contact area between adjacent teeth.

If you have any questions about the re-evaluation appointment, please feel free to ask us.

Specific Recommendations: _____

_____

_____

Copyright © 2010 by Saunders, an imprint of Elsevier Inc. All rights reserved.

CHLORHEXIDINE GLUCONATE ORAL RINSE 0.12%

Patient Name: _____   **Date:** _____

Chlorhexidine gluconate oral rinse 0.12% provides long-term antimicrobial benefits. It is effective in reducing the redness, swelling, and bleeding of gum tissue that are present in gingivitis. This is not a cure for periodontal disease and should not be considered a major treatment for this type of infection. Use of this rinse for up to 6 months does not appear to cause any significant changes in bacterial resistance or overgrowth of opportunistic bacteria or other organisms. It does not appear to cause any adverse changes in the normal microbial system that exists in the mouth.

The normal dosage is ½ fluid ounce (10 mL) per use. (Use measuring cup provided, or see markings inside cap.)

USE DURING PERIODONTAL THERAPY OR DENTAL IMPLANT TREATMENT

If you are currently undergoing periodontal therapy or dental implant treatment, rinse as we have directed. Rinse twice a day, for 30 seconds each time, morning and evening about 30 minutes after brushing and interdental cleaning. Do not eat, drink, or rinse with water for 30 minutes after rinsing. Continue this routine until all phases of your periodontal or implant therapy are complete. If you are instructed to do so, you can also use this rinse in your oral irrigator (e.g., Waterpik).

USE DURING CROWN AND BRIDGE PROCEDURES

If you are having a crown, inlay, onlay, or bridge procedure, please rinse with chlorhexidine gluconate 0.12% for 2 weeks before the tooth preparation appointment through 2 weeks after the final restoration is cemented or bonded into place. Dental research has shown that the use of this rinse will help to make gum tissue tight and healthy. The preparation and impression appointment will be easier and faster with less bleeding. The tissue also returns to normal faster after these procedures. For this use, rinse only once each day about 30 minutes after brushing and interdental cleaning, before you go to bed.

USE TO CONTROL THE BACTERIAL INFECTION THAT CAUSES TOOTH DECAY

Dental decay is an infectious disease that can be transmitted from parent to infant, or sibling to sibling. Persons who have dental decay are infected with *Streptococcus mutans*. People need to eliminate caries infection in their own mouth so that it is not transmitted to others and so they can prevent tooth decay. The infection can be controlled by the following recommendation:

- Use 10 mL of 0.12% chlorhexidine gluconate prescription mouth rinse at bedtime for 1 minute once daily for a 2-week period every 2 to 3 months for approximately 1 year. Because chlorhexidine loses its effectiveness in the presence of sodium lauryl sulfate or fluoride, this regimen should be performed about 30 minutes after toothbrushing with a dentifrice that contains these two ingredients.

PRECAUTIONS

Use of this rinse can cause brown staining of the teeth, tongue, and some types of restorations. The stain can be easily removed by a professional polishing. If you brush and floss your teeth thoroughly, this will be much less of a problem. Some patients may notice a slight change in taste sensations while using the rinse. This taste alteration will return to normal after the rinse is discontinued. Rinsing with water makes the taste worse.

Do not use this product if you are pregnant (or are currently trying to conceive).

If you have any questions about the use of this rinse, please ask us.

Specific Recommendations: _____

_____

_____

Copyright © 2010 by Saunders, an imprint of Elsevier Inc. All rights reserved.

PERIOSTAT: SYSTEMIC SUBMICROBIAL DOSE OF DOXYCYCLINE

Patient Name: _____

Date: _____

You have been diagnosed as having periodontal disease. Up until now, the treatment for periodontitis has included debriding the area of plaque, calculus, damaged tooth surfaces, and bacterial toxins; performing proper oral self-care; using antiplaque and antigingivitis oral care products; and, when necessary, surgically correcting the defects caused by the disease.

It was discovered that the antibiotic tetracycline used in daily small doses is useful in inhibiting the destructive enzymes that your body produces that break down gum and bone tissues and cause periodontal diseases.

Periostat is a doxycycline (20 mg, twice daily systemically) that is used to reduce the number of destructive enzymes in your body. Side effects are minimal. It cannot be given to people who are allergic to tetracycline or who are pregnant. It has been shown to improve the attachment of fibers to teeth and reduce pocket depth. It is not to be considered a cure for the disease. It is an adjunctive procedure to root planing, root debridement, and scaling. It is taken orally twice a day for at least 3 to 9 months. Please take this prescription as directed: Do not skip a day. Research has shown that the use of this medication along with the treatment of scaling and root planing has a more positive outcome than when root planing and scaling are done alone.

This medication works more effectively in severely diseased teeth than in moderately diseased sites. The use of this medication as directed can reduce or eliminate the need for certain periodontal surgical procedures, or at least place a "hold" on the destructive process for a limited time until the corrective and definitive surgery can be accomplished.

Periostat is a nonsurgical or presurgical modality that helps in the long-term management of chronic periodontal disease. You can benefit from this prescription if it is used in conjunction with root planing and scaling. It is not a "magic bullet" that will cure your periodontal disease: It does not replace your daily oral self-care regimen, and you must take it twice a day for an extended period of time.

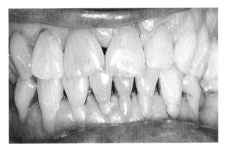

Significant recession of varying degrees throughout the mouth. Note composite restorations at cervical areas on the teeth along with the tobacco stain in mandibular interproximal areas.

If you have any questions about Periostat, please feel free to ask us.

Specific Recommendations: _____

_____

Copyright © 2010 by Saunders, an imprint of Elsevier Inc. All rights reserved.

SITE-SPECIFIC CONTROLLED RELEASE DRUG THERAPY

Patient Name: _____

Date: _____

Oral bacteria are a major risk factor in periodontal disease. Periodontal disease is an infection in the gum and bone tissues around a tooth or teeth, and often there are no symptoms. You may find out that you have periodontal disease when you have your mouth examined by a dentist or dental hygienist.

For many years physicians have been treating infections in our bodies with antimicrobial agents and antibiotics. We now have the ability to treat individual infected areas in our mouths with a site-specific drug. It does not have to be taken orally and then carried by the bloodstream throughout the entire body. Rather, it is placed at the site where treatment is needed. There are several types of medications that can be placed directly into the site of the infection. The material is placed exactly where it is needed; therefore only a very small amount of the drug needs to be administered.

A site-specific drug is generally used where a 5-mm or deeper periodontal pocket is present after other treatments have been performed successfully and the infection persists. It is a very conservative treatment and not a surgical procedure.

THE PROCEDURE

This procedere is done at the re-evaluation appointment:

The selected drug material is placed in the affected site. Multiple sites may be treated at the same time. You should not brush or floss the area where the drug has been placed as instructed. You may not notice an immediate improvement in the area. The area might feel a bit uncomfortable, like a popcorn kernal is caught under your gum. The healing process may take several months, during which the placement of the drug may need to be repeated. This is not unusual. During every periodontal maintenance appointment, we will evaluate your total periodontal health status.

These are several site-specific periodontal therapies that have evolved over time. Although the dental insurance industry and the American Dental Association years ago agreed on an assigned procedure code for site-specific antibiotic therapy, it may not yet be a payable benefit with your particular dental insurance plan. Don't let possible insurance coverage (or lack of it) dictate your needed treatment.

We will select the most appropriate site-specific drug therapy for your periodontal condition.

❏ Atridox—A doxycycline hyclate gel is placed into the diseased pocket, where it will dissolve in 7 to 10 days.

❏ Arestin—A minocycline hyclate powder is placed into the diseased pocket, where it will dissolve in 7 to 10 days.

❏ PerioChip—A chlorhexidine gluconate gelatin disk is placed into the diseased pocket, where it will dissolve in 7 to 10 days.

❏ Other _____

You should not brush or floss the area for _____ days. Avoid vigorous chewing in the treated area. You will need to return to our office in _____ days for evaluation of this site.

Until site-specific drug therapy became available, a regular scaling and root planing, systemic antibiotic therapy, excellent oral self-care, and periodontal surgery were your only options. We can now offer a comfortable, nonsurgical treatment option for difficult-to-treat areas.

The other option you have is no treatment of the problem or a referral to a periodontist for possible surgical correction. Site-specific drug treatment is a much more conservative approach than surgery. The site-specific drug treatment has the potential to reduce periodontal pocket depth and need for surgical corrective procedures.

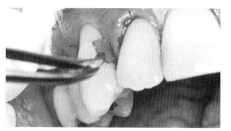

Chlorhexidine chip being inserted into periodontal pocket.

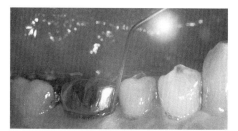

Doxycycline gel being administered subgingivally.

If you have any questions about site-specific antibiotic therapy, please feel free to ask us.

Specific Recommendations: _____

_____

Copyright © 2010 by Saunders, an imprint of Elsevier Inc. All rights reserved.

SUBGINGIVAL IRRIGATION

Patient Name: _____

Date: _____

Subgingival irrigation (flushing) of the periodontal pocket tissues is a nonsurgical, adjunctive treatment for periodontal disease.

In a healthy mouth, there is a crevice or ditchlike space around every tooth, called a *sulcus*. We have an instrument called a *periodontal probe* to gently measure this sulcus space. The healthy sulcus should measure between 1 and 3 millimeters, and no bleeding or pain should occur during probing. Gum tissue should be tightly attached to the bone surrounding each tooth. When the gum tissue is infected and periodontal disease is present, the tissues become red and swollen, and the sulcus depth increases to form a periodontal pocket. When the sulcus is over 3 millimeters deep, it is difficult, if not impossible, to keep the bacteria levels under control with normal oral self-care. The pocket depth can continue to increase.

Subgingival irrigation may aid in the removal of debris, bacteria, and toxins that cannot be routinely removed with normal oral self-care. A stream of fluid under slight pressure is delivered under the gum tissue to the appropriate site(s). The area is flushed out. The irrigation in the office is usually done with an antimicrobial agent that has a substantive effect: The molecules of the antimicrobial cling to your teeth

and tissues and keep working for hours after the subgingival irrigation is completed. Water or other chemicals can also be used. If you are told that subgingival irrigation should be part of your daily oral self-care routine, you will be instructed in the proper solution and technique to use.

If the subgingival irrigation is properly accomplished, you can remove from the sulcus a high percentage of problem bacteria and toxins that cannot be reached with normal care efforts. The flushed and disturbed area should show a reduced level of bacteria with a reduced potential to cause periodontal disease. It may take some time for the bacteria and debris to build up to a level where they can again cause further or continued problems.

Subgingival irrigation is not a substitute for excellent oral self-care or for periodontal surgery, but it is another modality we can use in the treatment of periodontal disease and in the maintenance of periodontal health. If you are in active initial periodontal therapy, the subgingival irrigation may be a part of your treatment. If you are in maintenance, it may be part of your periodontal maintenance care at home. If we recommend that you perform this procedure daily as part of your normal oral self-care, you will receive further instructions.

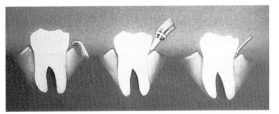

Three standard jet tips for home irrigation systems.

If you have any questions about subgingival irrigation, please feel free to ask us.

Specific Recommendations: _____

_____

_____

Copyright © 2010 by Saunders, an imprint of Elsevier Inc. All rights reserved.

Copyright © 2010 by Saunders, an imprint of Elsevier Inc. All rights reserved.

Copyright © 2010 by Saunders, an imprint of Elsevier Inc. All rights reserved.

Steps of the Dental Hygiene Process of Care

Steps	Definition
Assessment	The systematic collection of data to identify client problems, needs, and strengths
Diagnosis	The use of critical decision-making skills to reach conclusions about the client's dental hygiene needs based on all available assessment data and evidence in the literature*
Planning	The establishment of realistic goals and dental hygiene interventions to facilitate† optimal oral health
Implementation	The process of carrying out the dental hygiene care plan designed to meet the assessed needs of the client
Evaluation	The measurement of the extent to which the client has achieved the goals specified in the plan of care

Note: Documentation occurs throughout each step of the process to ensure quality care and protection of practitioner's legal risks.
*Reference: American Dental Hygienists' Association (ADHA): *Educational standards position paper*, 2001, ADHA.
†Reference: Fones AC: *Mouth hygiene*, ed 4, Philadelphia, 1994, Lea and Febiger.

Copyright © 2010 by Saunders, an imprint of Elsevier Inc. All rights reserved.

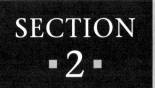

Communication and Culture

Checklist of Interpersonal Attending

Skill Area	Criterion
Eye contact	Listener consistently focuses on the face and eyes of the speaker
Body orientation	Listener orients shoulders and legs toward the speaker
Posture	Listener maintains slight forward lean, arms maintained in a relaxed position
Silence	Listener avoids interrupting the speaker and uses periods of silence to facilitate communication
Following cues	Listener uses verbal and nonverbal cues to facilitate communication and indicate interest and attention
Distance	Listener maintains distance of 3-4 feet from speaker
Distractions	Listener avoids distracting behaviors such as pencil tapping, looking at a clock, and extraneous movements

Adapted from Geboy MJ: *Communications and behavior management in dentistry*, Baltimore, 1985, Williams and Wilkins.

Techniques for Communicating with Clients through the Life Span

Level	Developmental Characteristics	Communication Techniques
Preschoolers	Beginning use of symbols and language; egocentric, focused on self; concrete in thinking and language	Allow child to use his or her five senses to explore oral healthcare environment (handle a mirror, feel a prophy cup, taste and smell fluoride, etc.) Use simple language and concrete, thorough explanations of exactly what is going to happen Let child see and feel cup "going around" or compressed air before putting in his or her mouth
School-age children	Less egocentric; shift to abstract thought emerges, but much thought still concrete	Demonstrate equipment, allow child to question, give simple explanations of procedures
Adolescents	Concrete thinking evolves to more complex abstraction; can formulate alternative hypotheses in problem solving; may revert to childish manner at times; usually enjoy adult attention	Allow self-expression and avoid being judgmental Give thorough, detailed answers to questions Be attentive
Adults	Broad individual differences in values, experiences, and attitudes; self-directed and independent in comparison with children; have assumed certain family and social roles; periods of stability and change	Appropriately applied therapeutic communication techniques: maintaining silence, listening attentively, conveying acceptance, asking related questions, paraphrasing, clarifying, focusing, stating observations, offering information, summarizing, reflective responding
Older adults	May have sensory loss of hearing, vision; may have high level of anxiety; may be willing to comply with recommendations, but forgetful	Approach with respect, speak clearly and slowly Give time for client to formulate answers to questions and to elaborate Be attentive to nonverbal communication

Adapted from Potter PA, Perry AG: *Fundamentals of nursing: concepts, process, and practice*, ed 3, St Louis, 1993, Mosby.

Copyright © 2010 by Saunders, an imprint of Elsevier Inc. All rights reserved.

Guide to Working with People of Various Religious Groups*

Religious Group	Basic Beliefs and Concepts	Healthcare Practices and Beliefs
Christian Scientists	Metaphysical approach to religion, sickness, and healing Prayer and religious counsel will heal the sick Sickness is mentally originated and can be cured through proper mental processes Body is its own laboratory Healing is private, abstract, and highly intellectual	Healing done by certified practitioner employing three dimensions of therapeutic treatment: Affirmation/denial/argument tries to destroy sick person's belief in suffering Absolute consciousness of good tries to convince sick person that he or she is well Impersonal treatment practitioner focuses on own thoughts to free afflicted person Accept drugless practices, e.g., osteopaths and chiropractors, and natural methods, such as dietary regulation and manipulation of the body
Eastern Orthodox	God did not create humans in God's image; however, humans have the potential to become like God in terms of goodness Do not believe in original sin of Adam; rather, humans choose to imitate Adam	Humans need the spirit of God for healing to occur Caring for the sick has a special place in the church Praying for the sick is a very involved process Sick are encouraged to seek scientific medical cures
Evangelists	Authentic and authoritative Holy Scriptures The life, teachings, death, and resurrection of Christ and eternal life *Deliverance Evangelists:* Believe Holy Spirit has given them power of divine healing	Healing occurs by God in only some situations; God heals all through different people, modalities, and techniques
Jews	Ten Commandments are a holy contract Modern contracts govern areas of personal and human behavior in an attempt to embody the spirit of Ten Commandments Reverence for life Emphasis on family and education Traditional Jewish kosher diet	Emphasis on cleanliness Circumcision performed to prevent disease Person responsible for avoiding threats to personal health
Mormons (similar to conservative Protestants)	Two personages of God (Father and Son) have flesh-and-bone bodies; Holy Spirit does not Salvation comes through atonement of Christ and obedience of laws of Gospel	Holy handkerchief (faith-healing method and laying on of hands) Seek scientific relief for illness and poverty
Native American Church or Peyotists (Native Americans)	Belief in Great Spirit and Christian Trinity Earth is our mother to be treated with respect All people are brothers and sisters Abstinence from alcohol Peyote is consumed to have closer contact with God; ritual is performed under guidance of "road chief"	Peyote is medicine Through prayer and communion with God, sins are forgiven and illness is cured
Pentecostalism (composed of Evangelists and Fundamentalists)	Concerned with holiness (state of mind and spiritual purity), literal interpretation of the Bible, and renewal of Pentecostal experiences, e.g., speaking in tongues	Divine healing, prophecy, and working miracles

Copyright © 2010 by Saunders, an imprint of Elsevier Inc. All rights reserved.

Spiritualism (Hispanics, Africans, African Americans, Native Americans)	Visible world includes invisible world inhabited by good and evil spirits that influence human behaviors Spirits become visible through mediums Mediums share same ethnicity, cultural language, and social class as their followers	Mediums treat emotional and physical illness, whole person concept Powers of mediums derived from supernatural
Protestantism	Four principles of Protestantism Resolution to live by faith Freedom to initiate new life Openness to truth revealed in scientific and nonscientific ways	Four principles of Protestantism lend themselves to faith healing as well as modern Western medicine
Islam (some people from Middle East, Northern Africa, Pakistan, India, Bosnia, Macedonia, Montenegro, Serbia, Micronesia)	Vocation in the world (caring for sick and poor) Five obligations of all Muslims: Profess of faith in Allah Pray five times daily in the direction of Mecca Give alms to the poor Fast during the holy month of Ramadan Once in a lifetime, make a pilgrimage to Mecca (*Hajj*) Faith in the will of Allah *Qur'an* and its verses (*hadith*) provide a guide to living Life is lived in harmony with the commands of Allah Pork and alcohol are forbidden; *Halal* meat can be consumed Traditional Muslims may follow: *Purdah*: women are covered from head to foot in a *bur-qua* which includes a face cover (*niqab*). Some women may simply wear a head cover (*hijab*).	Science of modern medicine Emphasizes cleanliness, including mouth cleanliness Sewak or miswak from a plant (*Salvadore persica*) may be used to clean mouth Sewak is part of a religious ritual Prayer and recitation stimulate the body Ramadan is a way of reducing stress on the digestive system Healthcare sought primarily from the mullah or imam Hakim is a Muslim practitioner who combines religious rituals for health Uses herbs and natural religious ritual for treating illness Man knows Allah through illness Mohammed wrote about the process of cleaning one's teeth as an act that is pleasing to Allah May be treated by a same-gender healthcare provider; may require a same gender interpreter

*Religion affects healthcare practices, beliefs, and interactions with healthcare providers. It is important to remember that not all people from a given religious group will act in a standard manner. Great variability exists within cultural groups based on socioeconomic status, level of education, and overall life experiences. This chart is not meant to be generalized to all people within a specific religion, but rather to serve as a beginning guide.

Copyright © 2010 by Saunders, an imprint of Elsevier Inc. All rights reserved.

Guide to Working with People of Various Cultural Groups*

Cultural Group	Basic Beliefs and Concepts	Healthcare Practices, Beliefs, Common Health Problems, and Remedies
African/African American	Life is a process rather than a state No division among physical, emotional, and spiritual needs Present oriented Strong religious and community group support networks	Health occurs when there is harmony with nature; illness is disharmony Belief in both white magic and black magic Living and dead things influence health Employ faith healers, root doctors, and spiritualists to cast out evil spirits and demons Voodoo can cause or prevent malevolent forces Illness can be preventive by avoiding people who carry evil spirits, eating a good diet, and prayer **Common health problems:** Hypertension, cardiovascular disease, sickle cell disease, lactose-enzyme deficiency, obesity, diabetes, chemical and alcohol abuse, human immunodeficiency virus (HIV) infection May use home remedies or folk healing **Remedies:** Bangles: thin silver bracelets that let evil out and prevent it from entering the body; sound of bangles frightens evil spirits Talismans: drawn symbols that are worn or carried to ward off sickness Asafetida: known as "incense of the devil"; rubbed on to ward off colds and evil Snake: dehydrated, ground to a powder, and mixed with water; applied to skin lesions
Hispanics or Latin Americans (Spaniards, Cubans, Mexicans, Central and South Americans)	*Curanderos, espiritista, partera, senora:* folk healers, some of whom use the premise of humoral pathology *Humoral pathology:* Basic functions of body are regulated by body fluids (humors) defined by temperature and wetness: Blood (hot and wet) Phlegm (cold and wet) Black bile (cold and dry) Yellow bile (hot and dry) "Evil eye" is harmful magic Strong influence of Catholic Church and family Flexible sense of time Respect for tradition Belief in bad magic, spells, and other harmful magic	Good health means balance among four humors Health is the result of good luck or rewards from God Can maintain health and avoid disease via a balance among four humors Foods are classified as hot or cold unrelated to their temperature; hot and cold food must be eaten or avoided at certain times Illness is caused by an improper diet of hot and cold foods, dislocation of body parts, the supernatural, or envy *(envidia)* from others Illness can be prevented by proper diet, wearing of amulets, use of candles, prayer, avoiding too much success and harmful people Illness is the result of bad luck, punishment from God, or an imbalance among four humors **Common health problems:** Diabetes, poor nutrition, obesity, oral disease, hypertension, cardiovascular disease, hepatitis C, parasites, lactose-enzyme deficiency, HIV, coccidioidomycosis Expectations of the family to care for the young and the elderly **Remedies:** Burning candles to ward off evil spirits Amulets worn to ward off evil and as a protection against the evil eye *Manzanilla* (chamomile), an herb used to treat stomach disorders, anxiety, and insomnia

Copyright © 2010 by Saunders, an imprint of Elsevier Inc. All rights reserved.

Group		
Asian or Pacific Islanders (Chinese, Hawaiians, Filipinos, Koreans, Japanese, Southeast Asians, e.g., Laotians, Cambodians, Hmong, Vietnamese)	The body is a gift that must be cared for and maintained Seldom complain about pain Strong family ties Preference for humility, modesty, self-control Respect for authority and tradition	Health is a state of harmony among body, mind, spirit, and nature (Taoism) Illness is caused by an upset in the balance (among body, mind, spirit, and nature) or by the weather, overexertion, or prolonged sitting Illness can be prevented by proper diet, exercise, avoiding temperature changes, and taking certain remedies May be disturbed by loss of blood, because they consider it to be body's life force May refuse surgery because they believe the body should remain intact **Common health problems:** Diabetes, tuberculosis, lactose-enzyme deficiency, malnutrition, hypertension, communicable diseases, cancer (esophageal, stomach, liver) coccidioidomycosis, and suicide May use acumassage, acupressure, and acupuncture (see Figure 5-5) Use of soy sauce may be a concern during nutritional counseling for individuals with high blood pressure **Remedies:** Jen Shen Lu Jung Wan: tonic taken to strengthen the entire system Thousand-year eggs: old uncooked eggs eaten daily for good health Huo Li Jian Mei Su: pills taken to maintain youth, health, and beauty Tiger balm: all-purpose salve to relieve minor aches and pain Ginseng root: most famous all-purpose Chinese and Korean medicine Acupuncture: use of metal needles at certain points in the body to treat and control pain
Native Americans and Alaskan Natives	Both nature and the body must be treated with respect Great respect for elders Value placed on working together Present-oriented Accumulation of wealth and goods is frowned on	Health is the result of total harmony with nature Prevention of illness is achieved through harmony of the body, mind, and spirit Illness can be associated with evil spirits, displeasing the holy people, disturbing nature, misusing a sacred ceremony Illness is the result of disharmony among the body, mind, spirit, and nature Large extended families who expect to be included in the healthcare process **Common health problems:** Alcoholism, suicide, obesity, tuberculosis, poor nutrition, oral disease, diabetes, hypertension, sexually transmitted diseases, accidents, and gallbladder disease **Remedies:** Sandpainting by medicine man Mask: to hide from evil spirits Sweet grass: burned as a rite of purification Thunderbird: a charm worn for protection and good luck Estafiata: leaves used to treat stomach ailments
Whites	Youth valued over age Punctuality, physical attractiveness, competitiveness, cleanliness, achievement valued Control of emotion Emphasis on the nuclear family versus the extended family	Use of herbs, ceremonies, fasting, meditation, heat, and massage Health is viewed as freedom from illness and disease; illness is the presence of disease symptoms, pain, disability, malformations Illness may be the result of punishment from God, breaking religious rules, drafts, climate **Remedies:** Varied because of the influence of multiple European cultures, e.g., malocchio—horn-shaped amulet used by Italians to ward off the "evil eye"

(Continued)

Copyright © 2010 by Saunders, an imprint of Elsevier Inc. All rights reserved.

Guide to Working with People of Various Cultural Groups*—*cont'd*

Cultural Group	Basic Beliefs and Concepts	Healthcare Practices, Beliefs, Common Health Problems, and Remedies
South Asian	May follow Hinduism, Christianity, Sikhism, Islam, Zoroastrianism Modesty is highly valued Arranged marriages still common Elders and education highly valued Primary body forces (dosha): Vata, Pitta, Kapha	Balance of the dosha yields health May prefer same-gender healthcare provider Indian system of medicine known as Ayurveda emphasizes prevention and herbs The belief that pain and suffering are the result of karma may make symptom control difficult **Common health problems:** Malaria (in South India), cardiovascular disease, tuberculosis, pneumonia, rheumatic heart disease, nutritional deficits, cigarette smoking, dental caries, periodontal disease, sickle cell anemia, and infectious diseases **Remedies:** Herbal remedies of Ayurveda Yoga
Developing countries	Use of "magic" for good and evil throughout culture Believe in the "here" world and "nether" world Avoid certain people, cold air, and evil eyes Distrust in nature Faithful to punitive god Suspicious of other people Distrust friends, relatives, and strangers	Protective and evil magic determine illness, come from supernatural Spells and sacrifices will bring back health Will use healers from more than one healthcare system Good health centers on personal rather than scientific behaviors Explain emotional and physical illness in terms of imbalance between individual and physical, social, and spiritual life **Common health problems:** Malnutrition, high maternal and infant mortality, parasitic and infectious diseases **Remedies:** Herbs and home remedies
West Indies	Little value placed on time Present-oriented Belief in voodoo	Obeah (witchcraft, black magic) power is very strong: scientific proof of sticking needles into people with bleeding or pain and frightening victims to death **Common health problems:** Malnutrition, hypertension, lactose intolerance, high maternal and infant mortality, parasitic and infectious diseases, sickle cell anemia, cancer (esophageal and stomach), coccidioidomycoses **Remedies:** Folk medicine, traditional healer (rootworker)

*It is important to remember that not all people from a given culture will act in a standard manner. Great variability exists within cultural groups based on socioeconomic status, level of education, and overall life experiences. This chart is not meant to be generalized to all people within a specific culture, but rather to serve as a beginning guide.

Copyright © 2010 by Saunders, an imprint of Elsevier Inc. All rights reserved.

Dental Hygiene Cultural Assessment

Culturally Relevant Categories	Key Questions to Ask the Client or to Consider
Ethnic origin	Ethnic identification of the client?
	Place of birth?
	Place of childhood?
Race or racial mix	Racial background?
Domiciliary history	Where the client lived and where the client now lives?
	Years in this country?
Valued habits, customs, behavior	Behaviors, customs, values, and beliefs about health, oral health, healthcare providers, and the healthcare system?
	How the client values courtesy, family, work, gender roles?
	How the client expresses emotion, stress, pain, spirituality, fear?
Communication	Communication style, e.g., manner of speaking, language spoken, need for interpreter, reading skill, method of showing respect or deference, eye contact, gesticulations, zone of territory?
Health beliefs and practices	Healing systems and practices used by the client (wearing of charms, using herbs or potions, voodoo, prayer, curandero, herbalist, etc.)?
	Explanation of disease and illness (fatalism, punishment from God, germ theory, evil spirits, imbalance between yin and yang, curse, etc.)?
	How the client determines seriousness of a health problem; when to seek care and from whom?
Nutritional factors	Culturally or religiously determined food preferences? Restrictions?
	Foods used to treat illness or to achieve a desired characteristic?
Sociologic factors	Impact of socioeconomic status and environment on health and disease, living conditions, lifestyle, access to healthcare?
	Family's (or significant others') role in dental hygiene care?
	Key people or institutions that influence client's health behavior (family, school, mosque, church, synogogue, NAACP, Tribal Council, etc.)?
Psychologic factors	Client's response to the healthcare system (e.g., anxiety, distrust, fear, loss of dignity, nonadherence, avoidance)?
	Client's relationship to people, institutions, and environments from other cultures?
Physical characteristics	Normal limits for individuals within this ethnic group (e.g., skin color, gingival color, facial characteristics)?
	Growth and development pattern variations within the cultural groups?
	Disease risk factors prevalent within client's cultural, racial, or ethnic group?
	Protective factors present?

Adapted from Bloch B: Bloch's ethnic/cultural assessment guide. In Orgue MS, Bloch B, Monroy LA, eds: *Ethnic nursing care: a multicultural approach,* St Louis, 1983, Mosby; U.S. Department of Health and Human Services: *Oral health in America: a report of the Surgeon General,* Rockville, Md, 2000, U.S. Department of Health and Human Services, National Institute of Dental and Craniofacial Research, National Institutes of Health.

Copyright © 2010 by Saunders, an imprint of Elsevier Inc. All rights reserved.

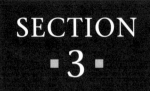

Infection Control

Types of Hand Hygiene

Methods	Agent	Purpose	Area	Duration (Minimum)
Routine handwash	Water and nonantimicrobial soap (i.e., plain soap[a])	Remove soil[b] and transient microorganisms	All surfaces of hands and fingers	15 seconds[c]
Antiseptic handwash	Water and antimicrobial soap (e.g., chlorhexidine, iodine and iodophors, chloroxylenol [PCMX], triclosan)	Remove or destroy transient microorganisms and reduce resident[d] flora (persistent activity)[e]	All surfaces of hands and fingers	15 seconds[c]
Antiseptic handrub	Alcohol-based handrub[f]	Remove or destroy transient microorganisms and reduce resident[d] flora (persistent activity)[e]	All surfaces of hands and fingers	Until hands are dry
Surgical antisepsis	Water and antimicrobial soap (e.g., chlorhexidine, iodine and iodophors, chloroxylenol [PCMX], triclosan)	Remove or destroy transient microorganisms and reduce resident flora (persistent activity)	Hands and forearms[g]	2-6 minutes
	Water and nonantimicrobial soap (i.e., plain soap[a]) followed by an alcohol-based surgical hand scrub product with persistent activity			Follow manufacturer's instructions for surgical hand scrub product with persistent activity[h]

From Centers for Disease Control and Prevention (CDC): *Frequently asked questions. Hand hygiene.* Available at: www.cdc.gov/oralhealth/infec-tioncontrol/faq/hand.htm. Accessed February 2008.

[a]Pathogenic organisms have been found on or around bar soap during and after use. Using liquid soap with hands-free controls for dispensing is preferable.

[b]Transient microorganisms often acquired by healthcare personnel during direct contact with patients or contaminated environmental surfaces. Transient microorganisms most frequently associated with healthcare-associated infections and are more amenable to removal by routine hand washing than resident flora.

[c]Time reported as effective in removing most transient flora from the skin. For most procedures a vigorous, brief (at least 15 seconds) rubbing together of all surfaces of premoistened lathered hands and fingers followed by rinsing under a stream of cool or tepid water is recommended. Hands should always be dried thoroughly before gloves are donned.

[d]Waterless products (e.g., alcohol-based hand rub) are especially useful when water facilities are unavailable (e.g., during dental screenings in schools) or during boil-water advisories. Alcohol-based hand rubs should not be used in the presence of visible soil or organic material.

[e]Persistent activity. Prolonged or extended activity that prevents or inhibits proliferation or survival of microorganisms after application of a product. Previously, this property was sometimes termed *residual activity.*

[f]Resident flora are species of microorganisms that are always present on or in the body; not easily removed by mechanical friction; and less likely to be associated with healthcare-associated infections.

[g]Removal of all jewelry, washing as described above, holding the hands above the elbows during final rinsing, and drying the hands with sterile towels.

[h]Before beginning surgical hand scrub, remove all arm jewelry and any hand jewelry that may make donning gloves more difficult, cause gloves to tear more readily, or interfere with glove usage (e.g., ability to wear the correct-sized glove or altered glove integrity).

Infection-Control Management of Instruments and Devices Based on Classification

Category	Definition	Process	Examples
Critical	Penetrate soft tissue or bone	Sterilization	Surgical instruments, periodontal scalers, surgical dental burs
Semicritical	Contact mucous membranes or nonintact skin	Sterilization or high-level disinfection	Dental mouth mirrors, amalgam condensers, dental handpieces, most hand instruments
Noncritical	Contact intact skin	Low- to intermediate-level disinfection	X-ray head or cone, blood-pressure cuff, facebow

Copyright © 2010 by Saunders, an imprint of Elsevier Inc. All rights reserved.

Immunizations Strongly Recommended for Healthcare Personnel (HCP)

Vaccine	Dose Schedule	Indications	Major Precautions and Contraindications	Special Considerations
Hepatitis B recombinant vaccine*	Three-dose schedule administered intramuscularly (IM) in the deltoid; 0, 1, 6-second dose administered 1 month after first dose; third dose administered 4 months after second. Booster doses are not necessary for persons who have developed adequate antibodies to hepatitis B surface antigen (anti-HBs).	Healthcare personnel (HCP) at risk for exposure to blood and body fluids.	History of anaphylactic reaction to common baker's yeast. Pregnancy is not a contraindication.	No therapeutic or adverse effects on hepatitis B virus (HBV)-infected person; cost effectiveness of prevaccination screening for susceptibility to HBV depends on costs of vaccination and antibody testing and prevalence of immunity in the group of potential vaccines; healthcare personnel who have ongoing contact with patients or blood should be tested 1-2 months after completing the vaccination series to determine serologic response. If vaccination does not induce adequate anti-HBs (>10 mIU/mL), a second vaccine series should be administered.
Influenza vaccine (inactivated)[†]	Annual single-dose vaccination IM with current vaccine.	HCP who have contact with patients at high risk or who work in chronic-care facilities; HCP aged ≥50 years or who have high-risk medical conditions.	History of anaphylactic hypersensitivity to eggs or to other components of the vaccine.	Recommended for women who will be in the second or third trimesters of pregnancy during the influenza season and women in any stage of pregnancy who have chronic medical conditions that are associated with an increased risk of influenza.[‡]

Adapted from Bolyard EA: Hospital Infection Control Practices Advisory Committee. Guidelines for infection control in health care personnel, 1998, *Am J Infect Control* 26:289, 1998; CDC: Immunization of health-care workers: recommendations of the Advisory Committee on Immunization Practices (ACIP) and the Hospital Infection Control Practices Advisory Committee (HICPAC), *MMWR* 46(No. RR-18), 1997; CDC: Prevention and control of influenza: recommendations of the Advisory Committee on Immunization Practices (ACIP), *MMWR* 52:1, 2003; and CDC: Using live, attenuated influenza vaccine for prevention and control of influenza: supplemental recommendations of the Advisory Committee on Immunization Practices (ACIP), *MMWR* 52(No. RR-13), 2003.

*A federal standard issued in December 1991 under the Occupational Safety and Health Act mandates that hepatitis B vaccine be made available at the employer's expense to all HCP occupationally exposed to blood or other potentially infectious materials. The Occupational Safety and Health Administration requires that employers make available hepatitis B vaccinations, evaluations, and follow-up procedures in accordance with current CDC recommendations.

[†]A live attenuated influenza vaccine (LAIV) is FDA-approved for healthy persons aged 5-49 years. Because of the possibility of transmission of vaccine viruses from recipients of LAIV to other persons and in the absence of data on the risk of illness and among immunocompromised persons infected with LAIV viruses, the inactivated influenza vaccine is preferred for HCP who have close contact with immunocompromised persons.

[‡]Vaccination of pregnant women after the first trimester might be preferred to avoid coincidental association with spontaneous abortions, which are most common during the first trimester. However, no adverse fetal effects have been associated with influenza vaccination.

(Continued)

Copyright © 2010 by Saunders, an imprint of Elsevier Inc. All rights reserved.

Immunizations Strongly Recommended for Healthcare Personnel (HCP)—*cont'd*

Vaccine	Dose Schedule	Indications	Major Precautions and Contraindications	Special Considerations
Measles live-virus vaccine	One dose administered subcutaneously (SC); second dose ≥4 weeks later.	HCP who were born during or after 1957 without documentation of 1) receipt of 2 doses of live vaccine on or after their first birthday, 2) physician-diagnosed measles, or 3) laboratory evidence of immunity. Vaccine should also be considered for all HCP who have no proof of immunity, including those born before 1957.	Pregnancy; immunocompromised* state (including human immunodeficiency virus [HIV]-infected persons with severe immunosuppression); history of anaphylactic reactions after gelatin ingestion or receipt of neomycin; or recent receipt of antibody-containing blood products.	Measles, mumps, rubella (MMR) is the recommended vaccine, if recipients are also likely to be susceptible to rubella or mumps; persons vaccinated during 1963-1967 with 1) measles killed-virus vaccine alone, 2) killed-virus vaccine followed by live-virus vaccine, or 3) a vaccine of unknown type, should be revaccinated with two doses of live-virus measles vaccine.
Mumps live-virus vaccine	One dose SC; no booster.	HCP believed susceptible can be vaccinated; adults born before 1957 can be considered immune.	Pregnancy; immunocompromised state;* history of anaphylactic reaction after gelatin ingestion or receipt of neomycin.	MMR is the recommended vaccine.
Rubella live-virus vaccine	One dose SC; no booster.	HCP, both male and female, who lack documentation of receipt of live vaccine on or after their first birthday, or lack of laboratory evidence of immunity can be vaccinated. Adults born before 1957 can be considered immune, except women of childbearing age.	Pregnancy; immunocompromised†state; history of anaphylactic reaction after receipt of neomycin.	Women pregnant when vaccinated or who become pregnant within 4 weeks of vaccination should be counseled regarding theoretic risks to the fetus; however, the risk of rubella vaccine–associated malformations among these women is negligible. MMR is the recommended vaccine.
Varicella-zoster live-virus vaccine	Two 0.5 mL doses SC 4-8 weeks apart if aged ≥13 years.	HCP without reliable history of varicella or laboratory evidence of varicella immunity.	Pregnancy; immunocompromised†state; history of anaphylactic reaction after receipt of neomycin or gelatin; recent receipt of antibody-containing blood products; salicylate use should be avoided for 6 weeks after vaccination.	Because 71%-93% of U.S.-born persons without a history of varicella are immune, serologic testing before vaccination might be cost effective.

*Persons immunocompromised because of immune deficiencies, HIV infection, leukemia, lymphoma, generalized malignancy; or persons receiving immunosuppressive therapy with corticosteroids, alkylating drugs, antimetabolites; or persons receiving radiation.

Copyright © 2010 by Saunders, an imprint of Elsevier Inc. All rights reserved.

Work Restriction Guidelines for Healthcare Personnel with Infectious Diseases

Disease or Problem	Work Restriction	Duration
Conjunctivitis	Restrict from client contact and contact with client environment.	Until no discharge
Cytomegalovirus infection	No restriction.	
Diarrheal disease	Restrict from client contact, contact with client's environment, and food handling.	Until symptoms resolve
Enteroviral infection	Restrict from care of infants, neonates, and immunocompromised people and their environments.	Until symptoms resolve
Hepatitis A	Restrict from client contact, contact with client environment, and food-handling.	Until 7 days after onset of jaundice
Hepatitis B Personnel with acute or chronic hepatitis B surface antigenemia who do not perform exposure-prone procedures	No restriction*; refer to local regulations. Standard precautions should always be followed.	
Personnel with acute or chronic hepatitis B e-antigenemia who perform exposure-prone procedures	Do not perform exposure-prone invasive procedures until counsel from a review panel has been sought; panel should review and recommend procedures that personnel can perform, taking into account specific procedures as well as skill and technique. Standard precautions should always be observed. Refer to local regulations or recommendations.	Until hepatitis B e-antigen status is negative
Hepatitis C	No restrictions on professional activity.* HCV-positive healthcare personnel should follow aseptic technique and standard precautions.	
Herpes simplex (hands)	Restrict from client contact and contact with client's environment.	Until lesions heal
Herpes simplex (orofacial)	Evaluate need to restrict from care of clients who are at high risk.	
Human immunodeficiency virus infection; personnel who perform exposure-prone procedures	Do not perform exposure-prone invasive procedures until counsel from an expert review panel has been sought; panel should review and recommend procedures that personnel can perform, taking into account specific procedures as well as skill and technique. Standard precautions should always be observed. Refer to local regulations or recommendations.	
Measles (active)	Exclude from duty.	Until 7 days after the rash appears
Measles (postexposure of susceptible personnel)	Exclude from duty.	From fifth day after first exposure through twenty-first day after last exposure or 4 days after rash appears
Meningococcal infection	Exclude from duty.	Until 24 hours after start of effective therapy
Mumps (active)	Exclude from duty.	Until 9 days after onset of parotitis
Mumps (postexposure of susceptible personnel)	Exclude from duty.	From twelfth day after first exposure through twenty-sixth day after last exposure, or until 9 days after onset of parotitis
Pediculosis	Restrict from client contact.	Until treated and observed to be free of adult and immature lice
Pertussis (active)	Exclude from duty.	From beginning of catarrhal stage through third week after onset of paroxysms, or until 5 days after start of effective antibiotic therapy

(Continued)

Copyright © 2010 by Saunders, an imprint of Elsevier Inc. All rights reserved.

Work Restriction Guidelines for Healthcare Personnel with Infectious Diseases—cont'd

Disease or Problem	Work Restriction	Duration
Pertussis (postexposure-asymptomatic personnel)	No restriction; prophylaxis recommended.	
Pertussis (postexposure-symptomatic personnel)	Exclude from duty.	Until 5 days after start of effective antibiotic therapy
Rubella (active)	Exclude from duty.	Until 5 days after rash appears
Rubella (postexposure-susceptible personnel)	Exclude from duty.	From seventh day after first exposure through twenty-first day after last exposure
Staphylococcus aureus infection (active, draining skin lesions)	Restrict from contact with clients and client's environment or food handling.	Until lesions have resolved
Staphylococcus aureus infection (carrier state)	No restriction unless personnel are epidemiologically linked to transmission of the organism.	
Streptococcal group A infection	Restrict from client care, contact with patient's environment, and food handling.	Until 24 hours after adequate treatment started
Tuberculosis (active)	Exclude from duty.	Until proven noninfectious
Tuberculosis (PPD converter)	No restriction.	
Varicella (active)	Exclude from duty.	Until all lesions dry and crust
Varicella (postexposure-susceptible personnel)	Exclude from duty.	From tenth day after first exposure through twenty-first day (twenty-eighth day if varicella-zoster immune globulin [VZIG] administered) after last exposure
Zoster (localized, in healthy person)	Cover lesions, restrict from care of clients[†] at high risk.	Until all lesions dry and crust
Zoster (generalized or localized in immunosuppressed person)	Restrict from client contact.	Until all lesions dry and crust
Zoster (postexposure-susceptible personnel)	Restrict from client contact.	From tenth day after first exposure through twenty-first day (twenty-eighth day if VZIG administered) after last exposure; or, if varicella occurs, when lesions crust and dry
Viral respiratory illness, acute febrile	Consider excluding from the care of clients at high risk[‡] or contact with such clients' environments during community outbreak of respiratory syncytial virus and influenza.	Until symptoms resolve

Adapted from Bolyard EA: Hospital Infection Control Practices Advisory Committee. Guidelines for infection control in health care personnel, 1998, *Am J Infect Control* 26:289, 1998.
Adapted from recommendations of the Advisory Committee on Immunization Practices (ACIP).
*Unless epidemiologically linked to transmission of disease.
†Those susceptible to varicella and who are at increased risk of complications of varicella (e.g., neonates and immunocompromised persons of any age).
‡Patients at high risk as defined by ACIP for complications of influenza.

Copyright © 2010 by Saunders, an imprint of Elsevier Inc. All rights reserved.

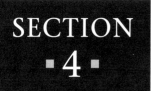

Medical Emergencies

American Society of Anesthesiologists (ASA) Physical Status Classification System to Determine Medical Risk

ASA I: Normal, healthy client without systemic disease.

ASA II: Client with a mild systemic disease or a significant risk factor (e.g., considerable anxiety, mild obesity, pregnancy, a smoker, well-controlled type 2 diabetes, controlled hypertension, well-controlled epilepsy, and/or well-controlled asthma). Person is able to walk up a flight of stairs or two level city blocks.

ASA III: Client with moderate or severe systemic disease that limits activity but is not incapacitating (e.g., massive obesity, symptomatic respiratory disease, stable angina, poorly controlled hypertension, exercise-induced asthma, prior myocardial infarction within 1 month or cerebrovascular accident with no residual signs and symptoms for more than 6 months before treatment).

ASA IV: Client with an incapacitating systemic disease that is a constant threat to life. Person is unable to walk up a flight of stairs or two level city blocks and is in distress at rest (e.g., unstable angina, liver failure, severe congestive heart failure, end-stage renal disease, myocardial infarction within 1 month or cerebrovascular accident within 6 months, uncontrolled epilepsy or uncontrolled diabetes).

ASA V: A moribund client not expected to survive 24 hours with or without an operation.

ASAE: Emergency operation. The *E* precedes the number to indicate the client's physical status (e.g., ASAE III).

Adapted from Malamed SF: *Medical emergencies in the dental office,* ed 6, St Louis, 2007, Mosby; Stefanac SJ, Nesbit SP: *Treatment planning in dentistry,* ed 2, St Louis, 2007, Mosby; and Little JW, Falace DA, Miller CS, et al: *Dental mangement of the medically compromised patient,* ed 7, St Louis, 2008, Mosby.

Summary of Techniques for Adult, Child, and Infant Cardiopulmonary Resuscitation

	Adult	**Child**	**Infant**
Hand Position	Two hands on the center of the chest	Two hands or one hand on the center of the chest	Two or three fingers on the center of the chest (just below the nipple line)
Compress	About 1½-2 inches	About 1-1½ inches	About ½-1 inch
Breathe	Until chest clearly rises (about 1 second per breath)	Until chest clearly rises (about 1 second per breath)	Until chest clearly rises (about 1 second per breath)
Cycle (one rescuer)	30 compressions, two breaths	30 compressions, two breaths	30 compressions, two breaths
Cycle (two rescuers)	30 compressions, two breaths	15 compressions, two breaths	15 compressions, two breaths
Rate	About 100 compressions per minute	About 100 compressions per minute	About 100 compressions per minute

Basic Emergency Drug Kit*

Drug/Route Administered	**Action**	**Indication**
Aromatic ammonia/inhaled	Chemical irritant	Syncope (fainting)
Epinephrine pen/subcutaneous	Cardiac stimulant and bronchodilator	Acute allergic reaction; acute bronchospasm (asthma)
Nitroglycerin/sublingual	Relaxes smooth muscle and dilates coronary arteries	Angina pectoris
Glucose/oral as sugar cubes, orange juice, or nondiet soft drink	Elevates blood sugar	Hypoglycemia
Bronchodilator/inhaled (albuterol, proventil, terbutaline)	Dilates bronchi	Bronchospasm; asthma
Antihistamine/oral (Benadryl)	Decreases the allergic response	Allergic reaction
Oxygen/inhaled	Increases oxygen to the brain	Respiratory distress

*Other medications may be included for use in advanced cardiac life support, but advanced training is needed to administer them.

Copyright © 2010 by Saunders, an imprint of Elsevier Inc. All rights reserved.

Information Given to the Emergency Medical Services Dispatcher

- Location of the emergency (with names of cross-streets, if possible)
- Number of telephone from which the call is made
- What happened (e.g., heart attack, seizure)
- Condition of the victim
- Aid being given to the victim
- Any other information requested
- Caller should hang up only when told to do so.

Rescue Breathing for the Adult Victim

- Give one breath every 5 to 6 seconds (10 to 12 breaths per minute).
- Give each breath in 1 second.
- Each breath must result in visible chest rise.
- Check the pulse again in about 2 minutes.

Adapted from American Heart Association: *BLS for healthcare providers student manual,* Dallas, 2006, American Heart Association.

Automated External Defibrillator Two-Rescuer Technique (Adult)

- First rescuer provides CPR.
- Second rescuer prepares to use the automated external defibrillator (AED).
- Second rescuer does the following while minimizing interruptions in chest compressions of no more than 10 seconds.
  1. Removes clothing covering the victim's chest to allow rescuers to provide chest compressions and to apply the AED electrode pads.
  2. Places the AED at the victim's side near the rescuer who will be operating it (i.e., the side of the victim opposite the rescuer performing chest compressions).
  3. Turns on the AED (POWER ON) and follows voice prompts.
  4. Attaches adult AED electrode pads.
  5. Removes the backing from the adhesive electrode pads.
  6. Attaches the adhesive electrode pads to the bare skin of the victim as per diagrams on electrodes.
  7. Attaches the electrode cable to the AED.
  8. Ensures that no one is touching the victim or resuscitation equipment while the AED is analyzing the heart rhythm (ANALYZE).
  9. Pushes ANALYZE button if needed.
  10. Ensures that no one is touching the victim or resuscitation equipment while following prompts to deliver a shock.
  11. Starts CPR immediately (beginning with chest compressions) after delivery of shock.
  12. If no shock is indicated, as per AED voice prompts, resumes CPR, beginning with chest compressions.

Signs of Complete Airway Obstruction

- Inability to speak
- Inability to breathe
- Inability to cough
- Universal sign for choking
- Panic

Copyright © 2010 by Saunders, an imprint of Elsevier Inc. All rights reserved.

Management of Specific Medical Emergencies

Condition	Signs and Symptoms	Management
Syncope (fainting)	Feeling of warmth, flushed skin, nausea, rapid heart rate, perspiration, pallor. Sudden, transient loss of consciousness.	Place in *Trendelenburg's position* (client's head lower than legs); loosen any binding clothes; maintain airway; administer oxygen; pass crushed ammonia capsule under victim's nose; place cool, damp cloth on forehead; reassure; monitor and record vital signs.
Shock	Skin pale and clammy, change in mental status and eventual unconsciousness if untreated, drop in blood pressure, increase in pulse and respiratory rate.	Position in Trendelenburg, maintain airway, monitor vital signs, administer oxygen, activate emergency medical services (EMS) and initiate Basic Life Support (BLS) and transport to nearest emergency room; start large-bore intravenous (if trained). (Maybe lactated Ringer's solution or blood, depending on the diagnosis.)
Hyperventilation	Rapid or excessively deep respirations, light-headedness, dizziness, tingling in extremities, tightness in the chest, rapid heartbeat, lump in throat, panic-stricken appearance.	Terminate procedure, use a quiet tone of voice to calm and reassure the client; encourage slow, deep breaths; have client breathe into a paper bag or cupped hands; *do not administer oxygen.*
Asthma	Coughing, shortness of breath, wheezing, pallor, anxiety, use of accessory muscles for breathing, cyanosis, increased pulse rate.	Assist client to a position that facilitates breathing (upright is usually best), have client self-medicate with inhaler, administer oxygen, monitor vital signs, if necessary activate EMS and initiate BLS.
Angina pectoris	Transient ischemia (lack of oxygenated blood) of the myocardium (heart muscle) manifested by crushing, burning, or squeezing chest pain, radiating to left shoulder, arms, neck, or mandible and lasting 2 to 15 minutes; shortness of breath; diaphoresis (sweating).	Terminate procedure, position client upright, monitor and record vital signs, administer oxygen, have client self-medicate with personal nitroglycerin supply (tablets, spray, or topical cream). If client does not have the medication, obtain nitroglycerin from the drug kit; if pain is not relived by rest and/or nitroglycerin (0.4 mg every five minutes for three doses), activate EMS and treat as a myocardial infarction.
Myocardial infarction (heart attack)	Mild to severe chest pain; pain in the left arm, jaw, and possibly teeth, not relieved by rest and nitroglycerin; cold, clammy skin; nausea; anxiety; shortness of breath; weakness; perspiration; burning feeling of indigestion.	Terminate procedure, activate EMS, place client supine, initiate BLS as needed, prepare nitroglycerin from the emergency kit, administer oxygen, monitor and record vital signs.
Cardiac arrest	Ashen, gray, cold clammy skin; no pulse; no heart sounds; no respirations; unconscious.	Activate EMS and initiate BLS.
Congestive heart failure	Shortness of breath, weakness, cough, swelling of lower extremities, pink frothy sputum, distention of jugular veins.	Terminate procedure, place chair back in upright position, administer oxygen, monitor vital signs, consult physician of record, activate EMS if necessary.
Stroke or cerebrovascular accident (CVA)	The supply of oxygen to the brain cells is disrupted by ischemia, infarction, or hemorrhage of the cerebral blood vessels; sudden weakness of one side, difficulty of speech, temporary loss of vision, dizziness, change in mental status, nausea, severe headache, and/or convulsions.	Terminate procedure, monitor vital signs, monitor airway, administer oxygen and initiate BLS as needed, activate EMS.
Hemorrhage	Arterial blood is red in color and "spurts." Venous blood is darker in color and "oozes."	Compression over hemorrhage: for bleeding from a dental extraction or surgical site, pack the area with gauze and have the client bite down until bleeding stops; for nosebleeds, apply pressure to bleeding side, or pack the bleeding nostril with gauze; for severe bleeding, watch for signs of shock and activate EMS.

(Continued)

Copyright © 2010 by Saunders, an imprint of Elsevier Inc. All rights reserved.

Management of Specific Medical Emergencies—*cont'd*

Condition	Signs and Symptoms	Management
Seizure		
Generalized tonic-clonic (grand mal) seizure	Aura (change in taste, smell, or sight preceding seizure), loss of consciousness, sudden cry, involuntary tonic-clonic muscle contractions, altered breathing, and/or involuntary defecation or urination.	Terminate procedure, lower dental chair and clear area of all sharp and dangerous objects, make no attempts to restrain the person; protect the head, assess and establish an airway, monitor vital signs, initiate BLS and activate EMS if needed—if stable, allow client to rest, arrange for medical follow-up, and arrange for assistance in leaving the dental facility.
Nonconvulsive (petit mal) seizure	Sudden momentary loss of awareness without loss of postural tone, a blank stare, and a duration of several to 90 seconds, muscle twitches.	Terminate procedure, observe closely, clear area of sharp objects, provide supportive care, may need physician evaluation.
Adrenal crisis (cortisol deficiency)	Confusion, weakness, lethargy, respiratory depression, hypercalcemia, shocklike symptoms—weak, rapid pulse and low blood pressure—abdominal pain, loss of consciousness.	Terminate procedure, activate EMS, place in Trendelenburg's position, monitor vital signs, administer oxygen, establish and maintain airway, initiate BLS as needed, transport to nearest emergency room.
Diabetic Emergency		
Hypoglycemia (hyperinsulinism)	Mood changes, hunger, headache, perspiration, nausea, confusion, irritation, dizziness and weakness, increased anxiety, possible unconsciousness.	Terminate procedure, administer oral sugar. If client conscious, ask when ate last and whether has taken insulin. Give concentrated form of oral sugar (e.g., sugar packet, cake icing, concentrated orange juice, apple juice, sugar-containing soda). If client is unconscious, activate EMS and place the sugar on the oral mucosa of the lower lip. Initiate BLS.
Hyperglycemia (ketoacidosis)	Polydipsia (excessive thirst); polyuria (excessive urination); polyphagia (excessive hunger); labored respirations; nausea; dry, flushed skin; low blood pressure; weak, rapid pulse; acetone breath ("fruity" smell), blurred vision, headache, unconsciousness.	Terminate procedure, activate EMS and provide BLS if necessary. If client is conscious, ask when ate last, whether has taken insulin, and whether client brought insulin to the appointment. Retrieve client's insulin. If able, client should self-administer the insulin; monitor and record vital signs.
Allergic Reaction		
Localized rash	Itching, skin redness, hives.	Call for assistance; prepare an antihistamine for administration; be prepared to administer BLS if needed.
Anaphylaxis	Urticaria (itchy wheals, also known as *hives*), angioedema (swelling of mucous membranes such as lips, tongue, larynx, pharynx), respiratory distress, wheezing, laryngeal edema, weak pulse, low blood pressure; may progress to unconsciousness and cardiovascular collapse.	Terminate procedure; immediately activate EMS; establish and maintain airway; place in supine position; monitor vital signs; administer oxygen; initiate BLS as needed; if qualified, administer epinephrine.
Reactions to local anesthesia	See Chapter 39 *Toxicity from local anesthesia:* light-headedness, blurred vision and slurred speech, confusion, drowsiness, anxiety, tinnitus, bradycardia, tachypnea. *Toxicity from vasopressor or vasoconstrictor:* anxiety, tachycardia, tachypnea, chest pain, dysrhythmias, cardiac arrest.	Assess airway, breathing, circulation; initiate BLS as needed, administer oxygen, activate EMS as needed.

Copyright © 2010 by Saunders, an imprint of Elsevier Inc. All rights reserved.

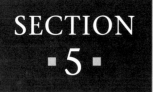

SECTION
▪ 5 ▪

Ergonomics

Grasp, Instrument Selection, Procedure, and Pressure

Grasp	Instrument	Procedure	Pressure
Modified pen	Mouth mirror	Oral inspection	Light
		Tongue and cheek retraction	Light to firm
		Transillumination	Light
		Reflective illumination	Light
	Periodontal probe	Periodontal assessment	Light
		Measure pathology or lesions	Light
	Explorer	Caries examination	Firm
		Calculus detection	Light
	Curets	Oral biofilm debridement	Light to firm
		Calculus removal	Firm
		Root debridement	Firm (lighten grasp as procedure is completed)
		Curettage	Light to firm
		Amalgam overhang removal	Firm
	Sickles	Calculus removal	Firm
		Amalgam overhang removal	Firm
	Hoes, files, etc.	Calculus removal	Firm
	Plastic instruments	Placing temporary fillings, periodontal pack, etc.	Light to firm
	Ultrasonic and sonic instruments	Calculus removal	Firm
		Oral biofilm and endotoxin removal	Light to firm
		Orthodontic cement and bonding removal	Firm
		Overhang removal	Firm
	Porte polisher	Selective polishing procedures for all surfaces except maxillary anterior teeth–facial surfaces	Firm
	Low-speed handpiece	Selective polishing procedures	Firm
		Amalgam polishing	Firm
		Sealant preparation	Firm
Palm	Curets, sickles, etc.	Instrument sharpening and maintenance	Firm
	Mouth mirror	Lip retraction with finger	Light
	Porte polisher	Selective polishing procedures on maxillary anterior teeth facials and maxillary posterior facial surfaces	Firm

Copyright © 2010 by Saunders, an imprint of Elsevier Inc. All rights reserved.

Fulcrum Finger Placement for Dominant Hand on the Mandibular and Maxillary Arch

Area in Dental Arch	Facial/Right Handed	Lingual/Right Handed	Facial/Left Handed	Lingual/Left Handed
Mandibular right molar area	Occlusal surface of mandibular right first molar or premolars	Occlusal or occlusolingual line angle of mandibular right premolars	Occlusofacial line angle of mandibular right first molar or premolars	Occlusofacial surface of mandibular right first molar or premolars
Mandibular right premolar area	Incisal edge of mandibular right lateral or central incisor	Incisal edge of mandibular central incisors	Incisofacial edge of mandibular right anterior teeth	Incisofacial edge of mandibular right lateral incisors or canine
Mandibular left molar area	Occlusofacial line angle of mandibular left first molar or premolars	Occlusofacial line angle of mandibular left first molar or second premolar	Occlusal surface of mandibular left first molar or premolar	Occlusal or occlusolingual line angle of mandibular left first molar or premolars
Mandibular left premolar area	Incisofacial edge of mandibular left canine or lateral incisor	Incisofacial edge of mandibular left canine or lateral incisor	Incisal edge of mandibular anterior teeth	Incisal edge of mandibular anterior teeth
Mandibular right canine (distal)	Incisal edge of mandibular incisors	Incisal edge of mandibular central incisors	Incisal edge of mandibular incisors	Incisal edge of mandibular central incisors
Mandibular left canine (mesial)	Occlusofacial line angle of mandibular left first premolar or canine	Occlusofacial line angle of mandibular left first premolar or canine	Occlusofacial line angle of mandibular left first or second premolar	Incisal edge of mandibular left canine
Mandibular left canine (distal)	Incisal edge of mandibular incisors	Incisofacial edge of mandibular central incisors	Incisal edge of mandibular incisors	Incisal edge of mandibular central incisors
Mandibular right canine (mesial)	Occlusofacial line angle of mandibular right premolars	Incisal edge of mandibular right canine	Occlusofacial line angle of mandibular right first premolar or canine	Occlusofacial line angle of mandibular right first premolar or canine
Maxillary right molar area	Occlusolingual line angle of maxillary right first molar or second premolar	Occlusolingual line angle of maxillary right molars	Occlusal surface of the tooth you are scaling or adjacent tooth	Occlusal surface of maxillary right first or second molar
Maxillary right premolar area	Incisolingual edge of maxillary right canine or premolars	Occlusolingual line angle of maxillary right first molar or premolars	Occlusal surface of the tooth you are scaling or adjacent tooth	Occlusal surface of maxillary right first premolar or second premolar
Maxillary left molar area	Occlusal surface of the tooth you are scaling or adjacent tooth	Occlusofacial line angle of maxillary left molars	Occlusolingual line angle of maxillary left first molar or second premolar	Occlusal surface of maxillary left molar area
Maxillary left premolar area	Occlusal surface of the tooth you are scaling or adjacent tooth	Occlusofacial line angle of maxillary left premolars	Incisolingual edge of maxillary canine or premolar	Occlusal surface of maxillary left premolar or molar area
Maxillary right canine (distal)	Incisofacial edge of maxillary incisors	Incisofacial edge of maxillary incisors	Incisolingual edge of maxillary right canine or lateral	Incisolingual edge of maxillary canine or lateral
Maxillary left canine (mesial)	Occlusofacial line angle of maxillary left premolars	Occlusofacial line angle of maxillary left first or second premolar	Occlusal surface of maxillary left first premolar or canine	Occlusal surface of maxillary left premolars

Copyright © 2010 by Saunders, an imprint of Elsevier Inc. All rights reserved.

Fulcrum Finger Placement for Dominant Hand on the Mandibular and Maxillary Arch—*cont'd*

Area in Dental Arch	Facial/Right Handed	Lingual/Right Handed	Facial/Left Handed	Lingual/Left Handed
Maxillary left canine (distal)	Incisolingual edge of maxillary left canine or lateral	Incisolingual edge of maxillary canine or lateral	Incisofacial edge of maxillary anterior teeth	Incisal edge of maxillary anterior teeth
Maxillary right canine (mesial)	Occlusal surface of maxillary right premolar or molar	Occlusolingual line angle of maxillary right premolars	Occlusofacial line angle of maxillary right premolars	Occlusolingual line angle of maxillary right premolars

Accessible Areas of the Client's Mouth

Right-Handed Clinician Clock Positions	Accessible Areas of the Client's Mouth	Left-Handed Clinician Clock Positions	Accessible Areas of the Client's Mouth
8 o'clock–9 o'clock	Mandibular right and left quadrants: all surfaces Maxillary right and left quadrants: all surfaces Exception: facial and lingual surfaces of maxillary and mandibular lingual teeth	3 o'clock–4 o'clock	Mandibular left and right quadrants: all surfaces Maxillary left and right quadrants: all surfaces Exception: facial and lingual surfaces of maxillary and mandibular anterior teeth
10 o'clock–2 o'clock	Mandibular right: mesial surfaces Mandibular anterior: all surfaces Mandibular left: posterior mesial surfaces	12 o'clock–2 o'clock	Mandibular right and left: mesial surfaces Mandibular anterior: all surfaces
12 o'clock–2 o'clock	Mandibular left: posterior mesial surfaces from the facial approach Maxillary right: posterior distal and lingual surfaces	10 o'clock–12 o'clock	Mandibular right: mesial posterior surfaces from the facial approach Maxillary left: distal and lingual posterior surfaces
2 o'clock–4 o'clock	Mandibular right: distal surfaces of last tooth in the quadrant	8 o'clock–10 o'clock	Mandibular left: distal surfaces of last tooth in the quadrant

Correct Clinician Positioning

Feet, Leg, and Thigh Position	Body Weight	Arm and Shoulder Position	Back Position	Head Position	Eyes
Feet flat on the floor	Centered on the seat of the clinician's stool	Shoulders are relaxed and in the neutral position (parallel to the floor)	Back is straight	Aligned with the spine (sit tall in the clinician's stool)	Directed downward
Thighs parallel with the floor	Supported by the legs and thighs	Upper arms are relaxed Elbows are in the neutral position (close to the body)	Lumbar curve is supported	Head is erect	Distance from eyes to client's oral cavity is approximately 14-16 inches

Copyright © 2010 by Saunders, an imprint of Elsevier Inc. All rights reserved.

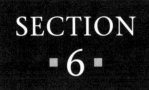

SECTION 6

Vital Signs

Vital Signs: Acceptable Ranges for Adults

Temperature
Range: 36° to 38° C (96.8° to 100.4° F)
Average oral or tympanic: 37° C (98.6° F)
Average rectal: 37.5° C (99.5° F)
Average axillary: 36.5° C (97.7° F)

Pulse
60 to 100 beats per minute
Average: 80 beats per minute

Respirations
12 to 20 breaths per minute

Blood Pressure
< 120/80 mm Hg
Pulse pressure: 30 to 50 mm Hg

Adapted from Potter PA, Perry AG: *Fundamentals of nursing,* ed 7, St Louis, 2009, Mosby.

Factors That Affect Body Temperature

Factors	Effects
Exercise	Increases body temperature
Hormonal influences	Decrease or increase body temperature
Before ovulation	Body temperature decreased below baseline
During ovulation	Body temperature increased to baseline or higher
Menopause	Periodic increase in body temperature
Time of day variations:	
Early morning	Temperature is lowest
Daytime	Body temperature rises
Evening	Body temperature peaks by 0.5°-1° F (0.3°-0.6° C)
Stress (physical and emotional)	Increases body temperature
Warm environment	Increases body temperature
Cold environment	Decreases body temperature
Infection	Increases body temperature
Tachypnea (rapid breathing)	Decreases oral temperature
Age	For persons >70 years of age, average oral body temperature is 96.8° F (36° C)
Hot liquids	Increase oral temperature for about 15 minutes
Cold liquids	Decrease oral temperature for about 15 minutes
Smoking	Increases oral temperature for about 30 minutes

Copyright © 2010 by Saunders, an imprint of Elsevier Inc. All rights reserved.

Acceptable Ranges of Heart (Pulse) Rate

Age	Heart Rate (Beats per Minute)
Infant	120-160
Toddler	90-140
Preschooler	80-110
School-age child	75-100
Adolescent	60-100
Adult	60-100

Adapted from Potter PA, Perry AG: *Fundamentals of nursing,* ed 7, St Louis, 2009, Mosby.

Factors That Influence Heart (Pulse) Rate

Factor	Increased Pulse Rate	Decreased Pulse Rate
Exercise	Short-term exercise	A conditioned athlete who participates in long-term exercise will have a lower heart rate at rest
Temperature	Fever and heat	Hypothermia
Emotions and stress	Acute pain and anxiety increase sympathetic stimulation, affecting heart rate	Unrelieved severe pain increases parasympathetic stimulation, affecting heart rate; relaxation
Medications	Positive chronotropic drugs, e.g., epinephrine	Negative chronotropic drugs, e.g., digitalis, beta and calcium blockers
Hemorrhage	Loss of blood increases sympathetic stimulation	
Postural changes	Standing or sitting	Lying down
Pulmonary conditions	Diseases causing poor oxygenation such as asthma, chronic obstructive pulmonary disease (COPD)	

From Potter PA, Perry AG: *Fundamentals of nursing,* ed 7, St Louis, 2009, Mosby.

Acceptable Ranges of Respiratory Rate According to Age

Age	Rate (Breaths per Minute)
Newborn	30-60
Infant (6 months)	30-50
Toddler (2 years)	25-32
Child	18-30
Adolescent	12-19
Adult	12-20

From Potter PA, Perry AG: *Fundamentals of nursing,* ed 7, St Louis, 2009, Mosby.

Average Optimal Blood Pressure According to Age

Age	Blood Pressure (mm Hg)
Newborn (3000 g [6.6 lb])	40 (mean)
1 month	85/54
6 years*	105/65
10-13 years*	110/65
14-17 years*	120/75
>18	<120/80

Data from Chobanian AV, Bakris GL, Black HR, et al: The seventh report of the Joint National Committee on Detection, Evaluation, and Treatment of High Blood Pressure, *JAMA* 289:2560, 2003.
*In children and adolescents, hypertension is defined as blood pressure that is, on repeated measurement, at the 95th percentile or higher, adjusted for age, height, and gender (NHBPEP, 1997).

Copyright © 2010 by Saunders, an imprint of Elsevier Inc. All rights reserved.

Factors That Influence Blood Pressure

Factors	Effects
Age	Blood pressure rises with age. Newborns have the lowest mean systolic blood pressure (75 mm Hg). As people age, elasticity in the arteries declines, producing an increase in blood pressure. Hypertension is common in the elderly (≥60 years).
Race	Prevalence of hypertension in African and Hispanic Americans is considerably higher than in the white population, and hypertension tends to appear earlier in life in these groups.
Weight	Blood pressure tends to be elevated in overweight and obese persons. Oversized blood pressure cuffs are necessary for accurate readings.
Gender	Hormonal variation causes females to have lower blood pressure after puberty than males; however, postmenopausal women tend to have higher blood pressure than men of similar age. Preeclampsia is abnormal hypertension experienced by some women during pregnancy. Postmenopausal women experience higher blood pressure.
Emotional stress	Stress stimulates the sympathetic nervous system, which in turn increases cardiac output and vasoconstriction. The outcome is elevated blood pressure.
Pain	Pain decreases blood pressure, and if severe can cause shock.
Oral contraceptives	These can increase blood pressure; however, the change is usually within normal limits.
Exercise	After exercise there is an increase in blood pressure for the first 30 minutes, followed by a decrease in blood pressure.
Eating	Older adults can have a 5– to 10–mm Hg fall in blood pressure 1 hour after eating.
Medications	Medications vary in their ability to increase and decrease blood pressure. Medications must be reviewed at each appointment to determine effects on blood pressure.
Diurnal variation	Blood pressure varies with metabolic rate. Pressure is lowest in the morning, then rises and peaks in the late afternoon or early evening.
Chronic disease	Diseases that affect cardiac output, blood volume, blood viscosity, or arterial elasticity will increase blood pressure.
Tobacco, alcohol, and caffeine use	Elevates blood pressure.
High fat and saturated fat intake	High blood cholesterol, especially high LDL cholesterol, and high triglycerides cause atherosclerosis, which in turn can cause an increase in blood pressure.
Dehydration	Accompanied by sudden changes in posture (lying to standing), can cause orthostatic or postural hypotension.
White-coat hypertension (isolated office hypertension)	Approximately 15%-20% of clients with stage 1 hypertension may have an elevated blood pressure in the presence of a healthcare worker, especially a physician.[*]
Body position	Blood pressure is lower when a person is lying down.

*Reference: Pickering TG, Hall JE, Appel LJ, et al: Recommendations for blood pressure measurement in humans and experimental animals, *Hypertension* 45:49, 2005.

Classification of Blood Pressure for Adults

Blood Pressure Classification	Systolic Blood Pressure[*] (mm Hg)	Diastolic Blood Pressure[*] (mm Hg)
Normal (routine dental treatment recommended)	<120	and <80
Prehypertension (routine dental treatment recommended)	120-139	or 80-89
Stage 1 hypertension (routine dental treatment recommended; assess risk factors, refer for consultation with physician of record)	140-159	or 90-99
Stage 2[†] hypertension (refer for consultation with physician of record)	≥160	or ≥100

National Institutes of Health (NIH): *The seventh report of the Joint National Committee on Detection, Evaluation, and Treatment of High Blood Pressure,* Bethesda, Md, 2004, NIH.
*Based on average of two or more properly measured, seated, blood pressure readings on each of two or more office visits.
†Note that if 160-179/100-109, routine dental care can be provided, but treatment should be delayed if care will be stressful or if client cannot handle stress. If local anesthesia is required, use 1:100,000 vasoconstrictor. If ≥180/≥110, delay treatment until blood pressure is controlled. If emergency dental care is needed, care should be provided in a hospital dental clinic where emergency life support personnel and equipment are located.

Copyright © 2010 by Saunders, an imprint of Elsevier Inc. All rights reserved.

Adult Blood Pressure Guidelines Used in the Dental Hygiene Process of Care

Blood Pressure (mm Hg)	ASA Physical Status Classification*	Dental and Dental Hygiene Therapy Considerations and Interventions Recommended
<140 systolic and <90 diastolic	I	No unusual precautions related to client management based on blood pressure readings Recheck in 6 months
140-159 systolic and/or 90-94 diastolic	II	No unusual precautions related to client management based on blood pressure readings needed unless blood pressure remains above normal after three consecutive appointments Recheck blood pressure before dental or dental hygiene therapy for three consecutive appointments; if all exceed these guidelines, seek medical consultation Stress-reduction protocol if indicated, such as administration of nitrous oxide–oxygen analgesia, should be considered
160-199 systolic and/or 95-114 diastolic	III	Recheck blood pressure in 5 minutes; if still elevated, seek medical consultation before dental or dental hygiene therapy No unusual precautions related to client management based on blood pressure readings after medical approval is obtained Stress reduction protocol if indicated, such as administration of nitrous oxide–oxygen analgesia
≥200 systolic and/or ≥115 diastolic	IV	Recheck blood pressure in 5 minutes; immediate medical consultation if still elevated No dental or dental hygiene therapy† until elevated blood pressure is corrected If blood pressure is not reduced using nitrous oxide–oxygen analgesia, only (noninvasive) emergency therapy with drugs (analgesics, antibiotics) is allowable to treat pain and infection Refer to hospital if immediate dental therapy is indicated

Adapted from Malamed SF: *Medical emergencies in the dental office,* ed 6, St Louis, 2007, Mosby.
*See Chapter 10 for an explanation of ASA Physical Status Classification.
†When the blood pressure is slightly above the cutoff for category IV and when anxiety is present, the use of inhalation sedation may diminish the blood pressure (via the elimination of stress) below the 200/115 level. The client should be advised that if the nitrous oxide and oxygen succeeds in decreasing the blood pressure below this level, the planned treatment can proceed. However, if the blood pressure remains elevated, the planned procedure must be postponed until the elevated blood pressure has been lowered to a more acceptable range.

Common Mistakes in Blood Pressure Assessment

Effect	Error	Effect	Error
False high reading	Bladder or cuff too narrow Cuff wrapped too loosely or unevenly Deflating cuff too slowly (false high diastolic reading) Arm below heart level Arm not supported Multiple examiners using different Korotkoff sounds Inflating too slowly or deflating too quickly (false high diastolic) Stethoscope that fits poorly or impairment of examiner's hearing causing sounds to be muffled (false high systolic) Repeating assessments too quickly (false high systolic)	False low reading	Failure to identify the auscultatory gap Bladder or cuff too wide Deflating cuff too quickly (false low systolic) Arm above heart level Stethoscope that fits poorly or impairment of examiner's hearing causing sounds to be muffled (false low systolic) Stethoscope pressed too firmly (false low diastolic) Inaccurate inflation level (false low systolic)

Copyright © 2010 by Saunders, an imprint of Elsevier Inc. All rights reserved.

Palpation Methods for Assessing the Oral Cavity

Type	Definition	Technique	Example
Digital palpation	Using index finger to move or press against tissue		Use to palpate the floor of the mouth and lingual border of the mandible
Bidigital palpation	Using fingers and thumb to move or compress tissue using a rolling motion		Use to palpate the lips, labial and buccal mucosa, and tongue
Manual palpation	Using all fingers of one hand to simultaneously move or compress tissues		Use to palpate the lymph nodes or thyroid gland
Bimanual palpation	Using index finger of one hand and fingers and thumb of other hand simultaneously to move or compress tissue, holding the fingers closely together to avoid missing areas		Use to palpate floor of the mouth, submandibular and sublingual glands, and lymph nodes
Bilateral palpation	Using a finger or fingers of both hands simultaneously to move or press tissue on contralateral (opposite) sides of the head and body		Use to palpate lymph nodes
Circular compression	Moving the fingertips in a deliberate, rotating fashion over tissues to be examined, exerting pressure		Use to palpate suspected lesion for more information

Copyright © 2010 by Saunders, an imprint of Elsevier Inc. All rights reserved.

Black's Classification of Dental Caries and Restorations

Classification	Description
Class I	Caries or restoration in the pits and fissures on the occlusal surfaces of molars and premolars, facial (buccal) or lingual pits and molars, and lingual pits of maxillary incisors
Class II	Caries or restoration on the proximal (mesial or distal) surfaces of the premolars and molars involving two or more surfaces
Class III	Caries or restoration on the proximal (mesial or distal) surfaces of incisors and canines
Class IV	Caries or restoration on the proximal (mesial or distal) surfaces of incisors and canines and also involving the incisal angle
Class V	Caries or restoration on the gingival third of the facial or lingual surfaces of any tooth
Class VI	Caries or restoration on the incisal edge of anterior teeth or the cusp tips of posterior teeth

Figures from Robinson DS, Bird DL: *Essentials of dental assisting,* ed 4, St Louis, 2007, Saunders.

Simple, Compound, and Complex Designations for Dental Caries and Restorations

Simple	Abbreviation	Compound	Abbreviation	Complex	Abbreviation
Buccal	B	Mesio-occlusal	MO	Mesioincisodistal	MID
Facial	F	Disto-occlusal	DO	Mesiolinguodistal	MLD
Gingival	G	Occlusobuccal	OB	Mesio-occlusobuccal	MOB
Incisal	I	Distolingual	DL	Mesio-occlusodistal	MOD
Lingual	Li	Disto-occlusal	DO	Mesio-occlusodistobuccolingual	MODBL
Labial	La				
Occlusal	O				

Copyright © 2010 by Saunders, an imprint of Elsevier Inc. All rights reserved.

Dentition Charting Symbols

Tooth Identification and Position

Term	Explanation	Ink Color	Procedure	Symbol
Missing teeth	Teeth not present due to extraction or congenitally missing	Blue	Place an X or vertical line through all views; label with CM if tooth is congenitally missing	
Unerupted or partially erupted teeth	Teeth that have not erupted	Blue	Circle all views of tooth; when partial eruption is present, label with PE above the buccal crown	
Impacted	Teeth that have not erupted because they are impacted	Red	Circle all views of the tooth and indicate by an arrow the direction the tooth is impacted	

Copyright © 2010 by Saunders, an imprint of Elsevier Inc. All rights reserved.

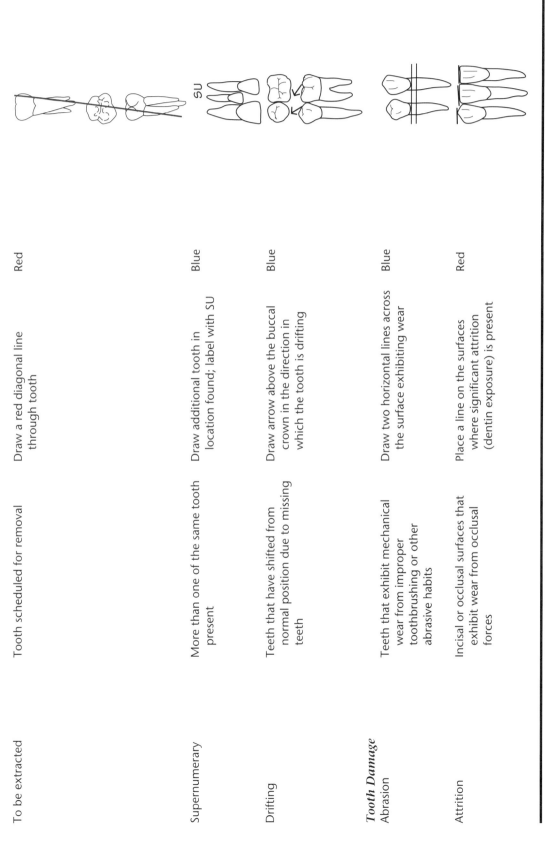

To be extracted	Tooth scheduled for removal	Draw a red diagonal line through tooth	Red
Supernumerary	More than one of the same tooth present	Draw additional tooth in location found; label with SU	Blue
Drifting	Teeth that have shifted from normal position due to missing teeth	Draw arrow above the buccal crown in the direction in which the tooth is drifting	Blue
Tooth Damage Abrasion	Teeth that exhibit mechanical wear from improper toothbrushing or other abrasive habits	Draw two horizontal lines across the surface exhibiting wear	Blue
Attrition	Incisal or occlusal surfaces that exhibit wear from occlusal forces	Place a line on the surfaces where significant attrition (dentin exposure) is present	Red

(Continued)

Copyright © 2010 by Saunders, an imprint of Elsevier Inc. All rights reserved.

Dentition Charting Symbols—cont'd

Term	Explanation	Procedure	Ink Color	Symbol
Caries	Surfaces exhibiting caries	Draw the outline as the carious lesion to be restored (i.e., MO, DO, MOD)	Red	
Incipient caries	Areas that have not cavitated and may be remineralized	Place a small dot on the affected area of the tooth	Red	
Decalcification	Surfaces that appear chalky white and are rough	Circle the area of decalcification and label with Decal or use a zigzag line over affected surface	Red	
Fracture	Areas of a tooth that have broken due to trauma or extensive caries	Draw a line on the fractured crown or root surface	Red	

Copyright © 2010 by Saunders, an imprint of Elsevier Inc. All rights reserved.

Restorative Therapy

Amalgam	Alloy of silver and mercury	Blue	Draw the shape of the restoration in all applicable charting views and color it in

Tooth-Colored Restorations

Composite resin	Tooth-colored restorative material commonly found on anterior teeth and is becoming more common on posterior teeth	Blue	Outline the exact size and shape of the restoration on all applicable charting views (do not fill in); label with CR
Ceramic/ceramic-metal crowns	Acrylic or porcelain facing bonded over white-gold alloy crown	Blue	Outline all charting views and label with PFM, GCPF, or GCAF or outline and fill in with diagonal lines using same labeling system

(Continued)

Copyright © 2010 by Saunders, an imprint of Elsevier Inc. All rights reserved.

Dentition Charting Symbols—*cont'd*

Term	Explanation	Procedure	Ink Color	Symbol
Veneer	Layer of acrylic or porcelain used on the facial surfaces of teeth	Outline and shade in surface where veneer is located; label with VE	Blue	
Metal Casting Full high noble and noble (gold)	Cast yellow-gold crown covering the entire surface or three-quarter crown covering less than three fourths of the surface	Outline showing the size, location, and shape of the crown; use diagonal lines within the outline	Blue	
Inlay	Cast yellow-gold restoration that does not extend over the cusps	Draw the shape of the restoration in all applicable charting views, and use diagonal lines to fill in shape or label with GI	Blue	
Onlay	Cast yellow-gold restoration that extends over the cusp tips	Draw the shape of the restoration and use diagonal lines to fill in shape or label with GO (gold onlay)	Blue	
Fixed crown and bridge (gold or porcelain)	Functional unit that serves to replace one or more missing teeth; consists of an abutment and pontic that are splinted together	Outline all aspects of the crown of each tooth involved indicating the type of restorative material used; draw one or two horizontal lines to connect the pontic to the crowns	Blue	

Copyright © 2010 by Saunders, an imprint of Elsevier Inc. All rights reserved.

(Continued)

Condition	Description	Charting	Color	Symbol
Temporary restorations and crowns	Placed as an intermediary during crown preparation, root canal therapy, or misplaced restoration	Outline the affected area indicating crown or restoration size, shape, and location; label with TEMP or TEMP AC (acrylic material)	Blue	TEMP.
Root canal	Pulp tissue is removed and canal is filled	Each canal restored is depicted by placing a vertical line through the affected root. If, based on periapical radiographs, there is reason to believe the root canal is faulty or periapical pathology exists, a red circle is drawn around the apex	Blue or red	
Stainless steel crown	Cast stainless steel crown covering entire surface	Outline crown of tooth and place SS on occlusal surface in red to complete and blue for already restored	Blue or red	
Implants	A surgically placed (osseointegrated) functional replacement for one or more missing teeth; composed of the anchor, abutment, and prosthetic tooth or appliance	Draw an X through the missing tooth and label with an I or IMPL; implant stamps are also available to use on the charting form; specific notations regarding the type of implant should be made. If implant is faulty, label in red ink	Blue or red	IMPL

Copyright © 2010 by Saunders, an imprint of Elsevier Inc. All rights reserved.

Dentition Charting Symbols—*cont'd*

Term	Explanation	Procedure	Ink Color	Symbol
Preventive Therapy				
Sealants	A clear or tinted resin coating that is bonded to the tooth in the pits and fissures	Outline the area showing size, location, and shape of the sealant; label using PF, PFS, or S above the occlusal surface. If a sealant is indicated for placement, outline the area in red and label using PF, PFS, or S above the occlusal surface; after sealant is placed, outline surface and PF in green or another color to identify completion	Red or green	PFS (or) PF
Amalgam polish	Polished amalgams retain less microbial plaque and resist tarnish and corrosion	Outline the existing restoration and label using AP above the restorations indicated for polishing; after polishing, outline AP in green or another color to identify that procedure was completed	Red or green	AP
Faulty Restorations				
Deficient or open margins	Restoration margins that are deficient or open will encourage microbial plaque retention and microleakage and should be replaced	Outline the existing restoration or crown and label appropriately; after replacement, outline in green or another color to identify that procedure was completed	Red or green	
Overhangs (Class I, II, or III)	An extension of restorative material beyond the curvature of the tooth; classified by the size of the extension; can be detected both clinically radiographically	Indicate the overhang on the surface on which it was detected by placing a < or > symbol on the lingual or buccal side of the occlusal view; to depict the size, add a + or ++ symbol for Classification II or III, respectively; after removal, outline the symbol in green or another color to identify that procedure was completed	Red or green	

Copyright © 2010 by Saunders, an imprint of Elsevier Inc. All rights reserved.

Recurrent or secondary caries	Signs of recurrent caries usually indicate the need to replace or expand the existing restoration	Draw the existing restoration in blue, and outline it in red as it would be restored	Blue or red

Prosthetic Appliances

Full denture	Removable appliance that replaces missing teeth	Chart the missing teeth with Xs or vertical lines through all surfaces; join with a horizontal line at the root apex or crowns; label to indicate upper or lower, CUD or CLD	Blue
Partial denture	Removable appliance that replaces missing teeth	Chart the missing teeth with Xs or vertical lines through all surfaces; join the Xs with a horizontal line at the root apex or crowns; label to indicate upper (PUD) or lower (PLD)	Blue

Adapted from Darby ML: *Mosby's comprehensive review of dental hygiene*, ed 6, St Louis, 2006, Mosby.

Copyright © 2010 by Saunders, an imprint of Elsevier Inc. All rights reserved.

Malrelationships of Individual Teeth or Groups of Teeth

Malrelationship	Description
Open bite	Abnormal vertical spaces between mandibular and maxillary teeth most frequently observed in the anterior teeth; however, may occur in posterior areas

Open bite

End-to-end (sometimes referred to as *edge-to-edge* in the anterior sextant)	The teeth occlude without the maxillary teeth overlapping the mandibular teeth. An end-to-end bite can occur anteriorly and posteriorly, unilaterally or bilaterally

Anterior   Posterior

Crossbite	Maxillary teeth are positioned lingually to the mandibular teeth; may occur unilaterally or bilaterally

Crossbite
Anterior   Posterior (bilateral)

Labioversion	A tooth positioned labial or facial to its normal position

Linguoversion	A tooth positioned lingual to its normal position

First three figures from Bath-Balogh M, Fehrenbach MJ: *Illustrated dental embryology, histology, and anatomy*, ed 2, St Louis, 2006, Saunders.

Copyright © 2010 by Saunders, an imprint of Elsevier Inc. All rights reserved.

Sequential Approach for Dentition Charting

- Complete a general appraisal of teeth, and note developmental anomalies and defects affecting tooth shape, number of teeth, tooth size, and presence of partial or complete dentures (e.g., generalized moderate fluorosis, amelogenesis imperfecta, peg laterals, number of teeth present, mandibular partial denture).
- Chart all missing or erupted supernumerary teeth before recording specific tooth-by-tooth information.
- Using radiographs, chart all unerupted or impacted teeth.
- Chart teeth indicated for extraction.
- Chart existing restorations (amalgam, tooth-colored, and temporary restorations; inlays, onlays, and gold foils; crowns, veneers, and bridges).

- Chart signs of tooth damage (dental caries, risk areas, attrition).
- Chart areas of plaque-retentive factors and defective restorations needing replacement (overhangs, deficient margins, unpolished amalgam restorations, fractured restorations, improper anatomic contour, occlusal surfaces indicated for pit-and-fissure sealants).
- When treatment has been completed on teeth indicated for restorative or supportive care, update chart using a different color ink to quickly identify teeth that were restored after original baseline charting.
- Update the dentition charting at each recare visit, and record any areas of change.

Adapted from Darby ML: *Mosby's comprehensive review of dental hygiene,* ed 6, St Louis, 2006, Mosby.

Types of Tooth Stains

Type	Source	Clinical Approach
Extrinsic Stains		
Green	Chromogenic bacteria and fungi (*Penicilium* and *Aspergillus* species) from poor oral hygiene; most often seen in children with enamel irregularities	Should not be scaled because of underlying demineralized enamel. Have client remove during toothbrush instruction or lightly polish; may use hydrogen peroxide to help with bleaching and removal.
Black stain	Iron in saliva; iron-containing oral solutions; *Actinomyces* species; industrial exposure to iron, manganese, and silver	Firmly scale because of calculus-like nature and selectively polish for complete removal.
Orange	Chromogenic bacteria (*Serratia marcescens* and *Flavobacterium lutescens*) from poor oral hygiene	Lightly scale and then polish selectively.
Brown stains	Tars from smoking, chewing, and	Lightly scale and then polish selectively.
Tobacco	dipping spit tobacco	Lightly scale and then polish selectively.
Food	Food and beverage pigment and tannins	
Topical medications	Stannous fluoride, chlorhexidine, or cetylpyridinium chloride mouth rinses	Lightly scale and then polish selectively.
Yellow	Oral biofilm	Have client remove during toothbrush instruction.
Blue-green stain	Mercury and lead dust	Lightly scale and then polish selectively.
Red-black stain	Chewing betel nut, betel leaf, and lime (pan); found in Western pacific and South Asian cultures	Firmly scale and then polish selectively.
Intrinsic Stains		
Dental fluorosis (white-spotted to brown-pitted enamel)	Excessive fluoride ingestion during enamel development	Cannot be removed by scaling or selective polishing.
Hypocalcification (white spots on enamel)	High fever during enamel formation	Cannot be removed by scaling or selective polishing.
Demineralization (white or brown spots on enamel, may be smooth or rough)	Acid erosion of enamel caused by oral biofilm	Cannot be removed by scaling or polishing. Recommend daily 0.05% sodium fluoride rinses for remineralization.
Tetracycline (grayish brown discoloration)	Ingestion of tetracycline during tooth development	Cannot be removed by scaling or selective polishing.

Copyright © 2010 by Saunders, an imprint of Elsevier Inc. All rights reserved.

CAMBRA Clinical Guidelines for Patients Age 6 Years and Older

Risk Level*	Frequency of Radiographs	Frequency of Caries Recall Examinations	Saliva Test (Saliva Flow and Bacterial Culture)	Antibacterials, Chlorhexidine, Xylitol†	Fluoride	pH Control	Calcium Phosphate Topical Supplements	Sealants (Resin-Based or Glass Ionomer)
Low risk	Bitewing radiographs every 24-36 months	Every 6-12 months to reevaluate caries risk	May be done as a baseline reference for new patients	Per saliva test if done	OTC fluoride-containing toothpaste twice daily, after breakfast and at bedtime Optional NaF varnish if excessive root exposure or sensitivity	Not required	Not required Optional for excessive root exposure or sensitivity	Optional or as per ICDAS sealant protocol
Moderate risk	Bitewing radiographs every 18-24 months	Every 4-6 months to reevaluate caries risk	May be done as a baseline reference for new patients or if there is suspicion of high bacterial challenge and to assess efficacy and patient cooperation	Per saliva test if done Xylitol (6-10 g/day) gum or candies; two tabs of gum or two candies four to five times daily	OTC fluoride-containing toothpaste twice daily plus 0.05% NaF rinse daily Initially, one or two applications of NaF varnish; one application at 4- to 6-month recall	Not required	Not required Optional for excessive root exposure or sensitivity	As per ICDAS sealant protocol
High risk‡	Bitewing radiographs every 6-18 months or until no cavitated lesions are evident	Every 3-4 months to reevaluate caries risk and apply fluoride varnish	Saliva flow test and bacterial culture initially and at every caries recall appointment to assess efficacy and patient cooperation	Chlorhexidine gluconate 0.12% 10-mL rinse for 1 minute daily for 1 week each month Xylitol (6-10 g/day) gum or candies; two tabs of gum or two candies four to five times daily	1.1% NaF toothpaste twice daily instead of regular fluoride toothpaste Optional 0.2% NaF rinse daily (one bottle) then OTC 0.05% NaF rinse two times daily Initially, one to three applications at 3- to 4-month recall	Not required	Optional: Apply calcium/phosphate paste several times daily	As per ICDAS sealant protocol

Copyright © 2010 by Saunders, an imprint of Elsevier Inc. All rights reserved.

| Extreme risk§ (high risk plus dry mouth or special needs) | Bitewing radiographs every 6 months or until no cavitated lesions are evident | Every 3 months to reevaluate caries risk and apply fluoride varnish | Saliva flow test and bacterial culture initially and at every caries recall appointment to assess efficacy and patient cooperation | Chlorhexidine 0.12% (preferably chlorhexidine in water base rinse) 10-mL rinse for 1 minute daily for 1 week each month Xylitol (6-10 g/day) gum or candies; two tabs of gum or two candies four to five times daily | 1.1% NaF toothpaste twice daily instead of regular fluoride toothpaste OTC 0.05% NaF rinse when mouth feels dry and after snacking, breakfast, and lunch Initially one to three applications of NaF varnish; one application at 3-month recall | Acid-neutralizing rinses as needed if mouth feels dry; after snacking, at bedtime, and after breakfast Baking soda gum as needed | Required: Apply calcium/phosphate paste twice daily | As per ICDAS sealant protocol |

From Jenson L, Brideny AW, Featherstone JDB, et al: Clinical protocols for caries management by risk assessment, *J Calif Dent Assoc* 35:716, 2007.

All restorative work to be done with the minimally invasive philosophy in mind. Existing smooth surface lesions that do not penetrate the dentoenamel junction and are not cavitated should be treated chemically, not surgically. For extreme-risk patients, use holding care with glass ionomer materials until caries progression is controlled. Patients with appliances (removable partial dentures, prosthodontics) require excellent oral hygiene together with intensive fluoride therapy, e.g., high-fluoride toothpaste and fluoride varnish every 3 months. Where indicated, antibacterial therapy should be administered in conjunction with restorative work.

ICDAS, International Caries Detection and Assessment System; *NaF,* sodium fluoride; *OTC,* over-the-counter.

*For all risk levels: Patients must maintain good oral hygiene and a diet low in frequency of fermentable carbohydrates.

†Xylitol is not good for pets (especially dogs).

‡Patients with one (or more) cavitated lesion(s) are high-risk patients.

§Patients with one (or more) cavitated lesion(s) and severe hyposalivation are extreme-risk patients.

Copyright © 2010 by Saunders, an imprint of Elsevier Inc. All rights reserved.

CAMBRA Clinical Guidelines for Patients Ages 0 to 5 Years

Risk Level*	Saliva Test†	Antibacterials	Fluoride	Frequency of Radiographs	Frequency of Periodic Oral Examination (POE)	Xylitol and/or Baking Soda‡	Sealant§	Existing Lesions
Low risk	Optional (baseline)	Not required or if saliva test was performed; treat main caregiver accordingly	Not required	After age 2: bitewing radiographs every 18-24 months	Every 6-12 months to reevaluate caries risk and give anticipatory guidance‖		Optional	
Moderate risk	Recommended	Not required or if saliva test was performed; treat main caregiver accordingly	OTC fluoride-containing toothpaste twice daily (a pea-sized amount) Sodium fluoride treatment gels and rinses	After age 2: bitewing radiographs every 12-18 months	Every 6 months to reevaluate caries risk and give anticipatory guidance	Xylitol gum or lozenges Two sticks of gum or two mints four to five times daily for the caregiver Xylitol food, spray, or drinks for the child	Sealants for deep pits and fissures after 2 years of age High-fluoride conventional glass iono-mer is recom-mended	Lesions that do not penetrate the DEJ and are not cavitated should be treated with fluoride toothpaste and fluoride varnish
High risk¶	Required	Chlorhexidine 0.12% 10-mL rinse for main caregiver of the infant or child for 1 week each month Bacterial test every caries recall Health pro-vider might brush infant's teeth with chlorhexidine	Fluoride var-nish at initial visit and caries recall examinations OTC fluoride-containing toothpaste and calcium phos-phate paste combination twice daily Sodium fluoride treatment gels and rinses	After age 2: two size No. 2 occlusal films and two bitewing radiographs every 6-12 months or until no cavitated lesions are evident	Every 3 months to reevaluate caries risk, apply fluoride varnish, and give anticipatory guidance	Xylitol gum or lozenges Two sticks of gum or two mints four to five times daily for the caregiver Xylitol food, spray, or drinks for the child	Sealants for deep pits and fissures after 2 years of age High-fluoride conven-tional glass ionomer is recommended	Lesions that do not penetrate the DEJ and are not cavitated should be treated with fluoride toothpaste and fluoride varnish ART might be recommended

Copyright © 2010 by Saunders, an imprint of Elsevier Inc. All rights reserved.

Extreme risk#	Required						
	Chlorhexidine 0.12% 10-mL rinse for 1 minute daily at bedtime for 2 weeks each month

Bacterial test at every caries recall

Health provider might brush infant's teeth with chlorhexidine | Fluoride varnish at initial visit, at each caries recall, and after prophylaxis

OTC fluoride-containing toothpaste and phosphate paste combination twice daily

Sodium fluoride treatment gels and rinses | After age 2: two size No. 2 occlusal films and two bitewing radiographs every 6 months or until no cavitated lesions are evident | Every 3 months to reevaluate caries risk, apply fluoride varnish, and give anticipatory guidance | Xylitol gum or lozenges

Two sticks of gum or two mints four to five times daily for the caregiver

Xylitol food, spray, or drinks for the child | Sealants for deep pits and fissures after 2 years of age

High fluoride conventional glass ionomer is recommended | Holding care with glass ionomer materials until caries progression is controlled (ART)

Fluoride varnish, and anticipatory guidance, self-management goals |

From Ramos-Gomez FJ, Crall J, Gansky SA, et al: Caries risk assessments appropriate for the age 1 visit (infants and toddlers). *J Calif Dent Assoc* 35:692, 2007.

ART, Atraumatic restorative treatment; *DEJ,* dentoenamel junction; *OTC,* over-the-counter.

*For all risk levels: Pediatric patients, through their caregivers, must maintain good oral hygiene and a diet low in frequency of fermentable carbohydrates. Patients with appliances (removable partial dentures, orthodontics) require excellent oral hygiene together with intensive fluoride therapy. Fluoride gel to be placed in removable appliances.

†Pediatric patients with daily medication such as inhalers or behavioral issues will have diminished salivary function.

‡Xylitol is not good for pets (especially dogs).

§ICDAS protocol presented by Jenson et al. This issue may be helpful on sealant decisions.

‖Anticipatory guidance: "Appropriate discussion and counseling should be an integral part of each visit for care." (AAPD)

¶Pediatric patients with one (or more) cavitated lesion(s) are high-risk patients.

#Pediatric patients with one (or more) cavitated lesion(s) and hyposalivary conditions or special needs are extreme-risk patients.

Parent/Caregiver Recommendations for Caries Prevention: Ages 0 to 5 Years

Daily Oral Hygiene
- Small amount of fluoride-containing toothpaste by cloth or brush twice daily
- Selective daily flossing

Diet
- Elimination of bottles with sugared fluids or juices
- Limited between-meal snacks, limited sodas; substitution of non-caries-causing snacks

Sugar-Free Gum
- For parent or caregiver of high-risk infant, use of xylitol-containing gum four to five times daily

Antibacterial Rinse
- For parent or caregiver, use of chlorhexidine gluconate (0.12%) once daily for 2 weeks every 2 to 3 months and use of fluoride rinse (0.05% NaF) daily in intervening weeks

Copyright © 2010 by Saunders, an imprint of Elsevier Inc. All rights reserved.

Characteristics of Periodontitis

Chronic Periodontitis
Onset at any age but is most prevalent in adults. Characterized by inflammation of the supporting structures of the teeth, loss of clinical attachment resulting from destruction of the periodontal ligament and loss of adjacent bone. Prevalence and severity increase with age. The following levels of chronic periodontal classifications have been identified.

Slight or early periodontitis
Progression of gingival inflammation into the alveolar bone crest and early bone loss resulting in slight attachment loss of 1 to 2 mm with periodontal probing depths of 3 to 4 mm.

Moderate periodontitis
A more advanced state of the previous condition, with increased destruction of periodontal structures, clinical attachment loss up to 4 mm, moderate-to-deep pockets (5 to 7 mm), moderate bone loss, tooth mobility, and furcation involvement not exceeding Class I in molars.

Severe or advanced periodontitis
Further progression of periodontitis with severe destruction of the periodontal structures, clinical attachment loss over 5 mm, increased bone loss, increased pocket depth (usually 7 mm or greater), increased tooth mobility, and furcation involvement greater than Class I in molars.

Aggressive Periodontitis
Occurs before age 35 and is associated with rapid rate of progression of tissue destruction, host defense defects, and composition of subgingival flora. The following subclassifications have been identified.

Prepubertal periodontitis
Onset occurs between eruption of the primary teeth and puberty; occurs in localized forms usually not associated with a systemic disease and generalized forms usually accompanied by alteration of neutrophil functioning; clinically manifests as attachment loss around primary and or permanent teeth.

Juvenile periodontitis
Localized and generalized forms. Generalized form (GJP) occurs late in the teenage years with a variable microbial cause that may include *Actinobacillus actinomycetemcomitans* (Aa) and *Porphyromonas gingivalis* (Pg) and affects most teeth.
Localized form (LJP) is associated with less acute clinical signs of inflammation than would be expected based on the severity of destruction. The localized form is associated with bone and attachment loss confined mostly to permanent first molars and/or incisors. Age of onset is at or around puberty; associated with *A. actinomycetemcomitans* (Aa) and neutrophil dysfunction.

Necrotizing Periodontal Diseases
Necrotizing ulcerative gingivitis (NUG)
A gingival infection with complex causes (e.g., plaque, temporary depression of polymorphonuclear leukocyte functioning, stress, poor diet) characterized by sudden onset of pain, necrosis of the tips of the gingival papillae (punched out appearance), and bleeding. Secondary features include fetid breath and a pseudomembrane covering. Fusiform bacteria, *Prevotella intermedia,* and spirochetes have been associated with gingival lesions.

Necrotizing ulcerative periodontitis (NUP)
Characterized by necrosis of gingival tissues, periodontal ligament and alveolar bone. Associated with immune disorders such as human immunodeficiency virus (HIV) infection and individuals on immunosuppressive therapies; characteristics include severe and rapid periodontal destruction. Extensive necrosis of the soft tissue occurs simultaneously with alveolar bone loss resulting in a lack of deep pocket formation.

Copyright © 2010 by Saunders, an imprint of Elsevier Inc. All rights reserved.

Clinical Gingival Characteristics in Health and Disease

Characteristic	Health	Disease
Color	Uniformly pale pink with or without generalized dark brown pigmentation	Bright red Dark red, blue-red Pink if fibrotic
Consistency	Firm, resilient	Soft, spongy, dents easily when pressed with probe Bleed readily on probing
Surface texture	Free gingiva—smooth Attached—stippled	Loss of stippling, shiny Fibrotic with stippling Nodular Hyperkeratotic
Contour	Gingival margin is 1-2 mm above CEJ in fully erupted teeth Marginal gingiva is knife-edge, flat; follows a curved line around the tooth and fits snugly around the tooth Papilla is pointed and pyramidal; fills interproximal spaces	Irregular margins from edema, fibrosis, clefting, and/or festooning May be rounded, rolled, or bulbous; therefore more coronal to CEJ May show recessions so that the anatomic root is exposed Bulbous, flattened, blunted, cratered
Size	Free marginal gingiva is near CEJ and adheres closely to the tooth	Enlarged from excess fluid in tissues or fibrotic from the formation of excess collagen fibers Free marginal gingiva may be highly retractable with air
Probing depth	0-4 mm; no apical migration of JE	More than 4 mm with or without apical migration of JE

CEJ, Cementoenamel junction; *JE,* junctional epithelium.

Clinical Characteristics in Gingivitis and Periodontitis

Characteristic	Gingivitis	Periodontitis
Gingival inflammation	Acute or chronic	Acute or chronic
Position of junctional epithelium	At the CEJ	Below the CEJ (attachment loss)
Position of gingival margin	Greater than 1-2 mm above the CEJ (gingival pocket)	Variable
Bleeding on probing	Present	May be present
Exudate	May be present	May be present
Furcation involvement	Absent	May be present
Tooth mobility	Absent	May be present
Bone loss	Absent	May be present

CEJ, Cementoenamel junction.

Copyright © 2010 by Saunders, an imprint of Elsevier Inc. All rights reserved.

Terminology Used to Describe Observations Associated with Clinical Assessment of Gingiva

Characteristic	Terminology	Description	Example
Gingival color	Location	Generalized or localized	Localized slight marginal redness lingual aspects of teeth 18, 19, 30, 31; all other areas coral pink, uniform in color
	Distribution	Diffuse, marginal, or papillary	
	Severity	Slight, moderate, severe	
	Quality	Red, bright red, pink, cyanotic	
Gingival contour	Location	Generalized or localized	Localized moderately cratered papilla teeth 6-11, 22-27; all other areas within normal limits
	Distribution	Diffuse, marginal, or papillary	
	Severity	Slight, moderate, severe	
	Quality	Bulbous, flattened, punched-out, cratered	
Consistency of gingiva	Location	Generalized or localized	Generalized moderate marginal sponginess more severe on facial aspect teeth 8, 9; all other areas firm
	Distribution	Diffuse, marginal, or papillary	
	Severity	Slight, moderate, severe	
	Quality	Firm (fibrotic), spongy (edematous)	
Surface texture of gingiva	Location	Generalized or localized	Localized smooth gingiva on facial aspect teeth 7, 8; all other areas with generalized stippling
	Distribution	Diffuse, marginal, or papillary	
	Quality	Smooth, shiny, eroded, stippling	

Classifications of Furcations

Class	Description
Class I	Beginning involvement. Concavity of furcation can be detected with an explorer or probe, but it cannot be entered. Cannot be detected radiographically.
Class II	The clinician can enter the furcation from one aspect with a probe or explorer but cannot penetrate through to the opposite side.
Class III	Through-and-through involvement, but the furcation is still covered by soft tissue. A definite radiolucency in the furcation area on a radiograph is visible.
Class IV	A through-and-through furcation involvement that is not covered by soft tissue. Clinically it is open and exposed.

Copyright © 2010 by Saunders, an imprint of Elsevier Inc. All rights reserved.

Guidelines for Writing Dental Hygiene Diagnoses

- Phrase the dental hygiene diagnosis as a client oral health problem, risk, or alteration in oral health state.
- Indicate what the problem is related to; problem and cause should be linked by the phrase *related to.*
- Indicate evidence for the problem and its cause by stating the defining characteristics as observed in the client; the defining characteristics should be linked to the diagnostic statement by the phrase *as indicated by.*
- Use language that avoids emotionalism or value judgment.
- Be sure that the dental hygiene diagnosis is not a medical or dental diagnosis.

Common Errors in Writing Dental Hygiene Diagnoses

Type of Error	Poor Dental Hygiene Diagnosis	Correction Required	Corrected Dental Hygiene Diagnosis
Emotionalism expressed in the diagnosis	Inadequate self-care related to laziness	Eliminate words that express emotionalism.	Unmet need for responsibility for oral health related to lack of adherence to self-care regimen, as evidenced by heavy biofilm accumulation and client's self-report.
Dental diagnosis instead of a dental hygiene diagnosis	Moderate, localized aggressive periodontitis	Avoid using dental diagnostic terms.	Unmet need in skin and mucous membrane integrity due to heavy plaque and cigarette smoking, as indicated by continued loss of clinical attachment since the last 3-month continued-care appointment. Refer to dentist for dental diagnosis.
Citing cause as the diagnosis	Deficit related to nonadherence	Use human need framework.	Unmet need for responsibility for oral health related to a lack of manual dexterity and self-care, as evidenced by a plaque index score of 3 and an inability to grasp a toothbrush.
Identifying signs and symptoms as the client problem	Generalized gingival bleeding and attachment levels of 5-8 mm	Use signs and symptoms to define and validate the actual problem.	Unmet need for skin and mucous membrane integrity related to inadequate oral self-care and smoking, as manifested by generalized, clinical attachment loss of 5-8 mm and signs of nicotine stomatitis.
Writing the diagnosis in terms of what the dental hygienist will do	Needs education on the disease process	Write the diagnosis in terms of the client rather than what the dental hygienist needs to do.	Unmet need in conceptualization and problem solving related to a lack of knowledge about disease process, as evidenced by client's misconceptions about caries cause and prevention.

Copyright © 2010 by Saunders, an imprint of Elsevier Inc. All rights reserved.

Guidelines for Writing Client-Centered Goals

Prepare each goal, or set of goals, from only one dental hygiene diagnosis.

Ensure that goals, if met, will resolve the problem reflected in the dental hygiene diagnosis.

Collaborate with dentist to ensure that the dental hygiene and dental care plans are mutually supportive.

Involve client in goal setting.

Validate that client values and is ready to achieve the delineated goals.

Write observable and measurable goals that include target times when each will be met by the client.

Use active verbs such as the following to denote client behavior expected in the goal:

affirm	detect	plan
attend	discuss	purchase
choose	eliminate	remove
communicate	exhibit	replace
complete	explain	report
decrease	finish	stop
define	guide	use
demonstrate	increase	verbalize
describe	perform	

Common Phrases to Maximize Client Involvement

- Here is a hand mirror. Let's examine your mouth together.
- What was your primary reason for seeking dental hygiene care?
- Is this set of treatment priorities acceptable to you?
- Is this care plan acceptable to you?
- What would you like to achieve as a result of dental hygiene care?
- How will you feel if this goal is attained?
- Are you satisfied with the plan of care we just discussed?
- How important is your oral health?
- Where would you like me (the dental hygienist) to start first?
- When and where is it easiest for you to clean your mouth (or your dependent's mouth)?
- Can you think of a better way that we can accomplish this goal?
- Let's compare how your gingiva looks today with how it looked 2 weeks ago.
- What are you willing to do to keep your mouth healthy?

Client Reasons for Refusal of Care, Dental Hygiene Actions, and Documentation of Informed Refusal

Client Reasons	Clinician Actions	Documentation
Cost of service	Acknowledge client's concerns	Include brief explanation of recommended care
Fear of pain	Clarify proposed plan of care	Identify specific treatment procedure being declined
Lack of understanding	Discuss consequences of not receiving recommended care	List risks and consequences to client's health without treatment
Low value placed on dental care	Recommend alternative treatment options when appropriate	Indicate date of informed refusal
Lack of dental insurance coverage		Include signatures of client, dentist, and a witness

Copyright © 2010 by Saunders, an imprint of Elsevier Inc. All rights reserved.

Insurance Codes for Nonsurgical Periodontal Therapy

Code	Procedure	Description
D0120	Periodic oral evaluation	An evaluation performed on a patient of record to determine any changes in the patient's dental and medical health status since a previous comprehensive or periodic evaluation. This includes an oral cancer evaluation and periodontal screening where indicated, and may require interpretation of information acquired through additional diagnostic procedures. Report additional diagnostic procedures separately.
D0140	Limited oral evaluation: problem focused	An evaluation limited to a specific oral health problem or complaint. This may require interpretation of information acquired through additional diagnostic procedures. Report additional diagnostic procedures separately. Definitive procedures may be required on the same date as the evaluation. Typically, patients receiving this type of evaluation have been referred for a specific problem and/or have dental emergencies, trauma, acute infection, etc.
D0150	Comprehensive oral evaluation	Used by a general dentist and/or a specialist when evaluating a patient comprehensively. This applies to new patients; established patients who have had a significant change in health conditions or other unusual circumstances, by report; or established patients who have been absent from active treatment for 3 or more years, It is a thorough evaluation and recording of the extraoral and intraoral hard and soft tissues. It may require interpretation of information acquired through additional diagnostic procedures. Additional diagnostic procedures should be reported separately. This includes an evaluation for oral cancer where indicated, the evaluation and recording of the patient's dental and medical history, and a general health assessment. It may include the evaluation and recording of dental caries, missing or unerupted teeth, restorations, existing prostheses, occlusal relationships, periodontal conditions (including periodontal screening and/or charting), hard- and soft-tissue anomalies, etc.
D0160	Detailed and extensive oral evaluation: problem focused, by report	A detailed and extensive problem-focused evaluation entails extensive diagnostic and cognitive modalities based on the findings of a comprehensive oral evaluation. Integration of more extensive diagnostic modalities to develop a treatment plan for a specific problem is required. The condition requiring this type of evaluation should be described and documented. Examples of conditions requiring this type of evaluation may include dentofacial anomalies, complicated perioprosthetic conditions, complex temporomandibular dysfunction, facial pain of unknown origin, conditions requiring multidisciplinary consultation, etc.
D0180	Comprehensive periodontal evaluation	This procedure is indicated for patients showing signs or symptoms of periodontal disease and for patients with risk factors such as smoking or diabetes. It includes evaluation of periodontal conditions, probing and charting, evaluation and recording of the patient's dental and medical history, and general health assessment. It may include the evaluation and recording of dental caries, missing or unerupted teeth, restorations, and occlusal relationships and oral cancer evaluation.
D0277	Vertical bitewings: seven or eight films	
D0415	Collection of microorganisms for culture and sensitivity testing	
D0415	Bacteriologic studies for determination of pathologic agents	May include, but is not limited to, tests for susceptibility to periodontal disease.
D0421	Genetic test for susceptibility to oral diseases	Sample collection for the purpose of certified laboratory analysis to detect specific genetic variations associated with increased susceptibility for oral diseases such as severe periodontal disease.
D1110	Prophylaxis: adult	Removal of plaque, calculus, and stains from the tooth structures in the permanent and transitional dentition. It is intended to control local irritational factors.
D1120	Prophylaxis: child	Removal of plaque, calculus, and stains from the tooth structures in the primary and transitional dentition. It is intended to control local irritational factors.

(Continued)

Copyright © 2010 by Saunders, an imprint of Elsevier Inc. All rights reserved.

Insurance Codes for Nonsurgical Periodontal Therapy—*cont'd*

Code	Procedure	Description
D1310	Nutritional counseling for control of dental disease	Counseling on food selection and dietary habits as a part of treatment and control of periodontal disease and caries.
D1320	Tobacco counseling for the control and prevention of oral disease	Tobacco prevention and cessation services reduce client risk of developing tobacco-related oral diseases and conditions and improve prognosis for certain dental therapies.
D1330	Oral hygiene instructions	This may include instructions for home care. Examples include toothbrushing technique, flossing, and use of special oral hygiene aids.
D4341	Periodontal scaling and root planing, four or more teeth per quadrant	This procedure involves instrumentation of the crown and root surfaces of the teeth to remove plaque and calculus from these surfaces. It is indicated for patients with periodontal disease and is therapeutic, not prophylactic, in nature. Root planing is the definitive procedure designed for the removal of cementum and dentin that is rough and/or permeated by calculus or contaminated with toxins or microorganisms. Some soft-tissue removal occurs. This procedure may be used as a definitive treatment in some stages of periodontal disease and/or as a part of presurgical procedures in others.
D4342	Periodontal scaling and root planing, one to three teeth per quadrant	This procedure involves instrumentation of the crown and root surfaces of the teeth to remove plaque and calculus from these surfaces. It is indicated for patients with periodontal disease and is therapeutic, not prophylactic, in nature. Root planing is the definitive procedure designed for the removal of cementum and dentin that is rough, and/or permeated by calculus or contaminated with toxins or microorganisms. Some soft-tissue removal occurs. This procedure may be used as a definitive treatment in some stages of periodontal disease and/or as a part of presurgical procedures in others.
D4355	Full-mouth debridement to enable comprehensive periodontal evaluation and diagnosis	The gross removal of plaque and calculus that interfere with the ability of the dentist to perform a comprehensive oral examination. This is a preliminary procedure and does not preclude the need for additional procedures.
D4381	Localized delivery of antimicrobial agents via a controlled release vehicle into diseased crevicular tissue, per tooth, by report	U.S. Food and Drug Administration (FDA)–approved subgingival delivery devices containing antimicrobial medication(s) are inserted into periodontal pockets to suppress the pathogenic microbiota. These devices slowly release the pharmacologic agents so they can remain at the intended site of action in a therapeutic concentration for a sufficient length of time.
D4910	Periodontal maintenance	This procedure is instituted after periodontal therapy and continues at varying intervals, determined by the clinical evaluation of the dentist, for the life of the dentition or any implant replacements. It includes removal of the bacterial plaque and calculus from supragingival and subgingival regions, site-specific scaling and root planing where indicated, and polishing of teeth. If new or recurring periodontal disease appears, additional diagnostic and treatment procedures must be considered.
D9910	Application of desensitizing medicament	Includes in-office treatment for root sensitivity. Typically reported on a "per visit" basis for application of topical fluoride. This code is not to be used for bases, liners, or adhesives used under restorations.
D9911	Application of desensitizing resin for cervical and/or root surface, per tooth	Typically reported on a "per tooth" basis for application of adhesive resins. This code is not to be used for bases, liners, or adhesives used under restorations.

From American Dental Association (ADA): *Current dental terminology 2007-2008,* Chicago, 2008, ADA.

Copyright © 2010 by Saunders, an imprint of Elsevier Inc. All rights reserved.

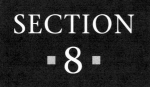
Toothbrushing Methods and Indications for Use

Method	Technique	Indications
Bass (sulcular)	Filaments are directed apically at a 45-degree angle to the long axis of the tooth; gentle force is applied to insert bristles into sulcus; use gentle but firm vibratory strokes without removing filament ends from sulcus.	Sulcular cleansing Periodontal health Periodontal disease Periodontal maintenance
Stillman	Filaments are directed apically and angled similar to Bass method; filaments are placed partly on cervical portion of teeth and partly on adjacent gingiva; short back-and-forth vibratory strokes are employed, and the brush head is moved occlusally with light pressure.	Progressive gingival recession; gingival stimulation
Charter	Filaments are directed toward the crown of the tooth; filaments are placed at the gingival margin and angled 45 degrees to the long axis of the tooth; short back-and-forth vibratory strokes are used for activation. (Distinguished from the Bass and Stillman methods in that the bristles are directed away from the gingiva towards the occlusal or incisal edge.)	Orthodontics Temporary cleaning of surgical sites Fixed prosthetic appliances
Roll stroke	Filaments are directed apically and rolled occlusally in a vertical motion.	Used in conjunction with Bass, Stillman, and Charter methods
Modified Bass, Stillman, and Charter methods	Add a roll stroke; roll tufts occlusally in a vertical motion after cervical area is cleaned by prescribed method.	Cleaning of entire facial and lingual surfaces
Fones	Filaments are activated in a circular motion.	Young children with primary teeth; otherwise not recommended

Illustrations from Newman MG, Takei HH, Klokkevold PR, Carranza FA: *Carranza's clinical periodontology,* ed 10, St Louis, 2006, Saunders.
Photographs from Daniel SJ, Harfst SA, Wilder RS: *Mosby's dental hygiene,* ed 2, St Louis, 2008, Mosby.

Copyright © 2010 by Saunders, an imprint of Elsevier Inc. All rights reserved.

Fluoride Supplements Dosage Schedule (milligrams of fluoride per day)*

Client Age	Level of Fluoride in Primary Water Supply		
	<0.3 ppm Fl	0.3-0.6 ppm Fl	>0.6 ppm Fl†
Birth to 6 months	None	None	None
6 months to 3 years	0.25 mg	None†	None†
3 years to 6 years	0.50 mg	0.25 mg	None
6 years to at least 16 years	1.00 mg	0.50 mg	None

Data from American Dental Association Chicago, Illinois; American Academy of Pediatric Dentistry, Chicago, Illinois; and American Academy of Pediatrics, Elk Grove Village, Illinois.

Fl, fluoride; *ppm,* parts per million.

*2.2 mg of sodium fluoride provides 1 mg of fluoride ions.

†Infants receiving their total diet from breast-feeding need a 0.25-mg supplement.

Nutrition- and Exercise-Related Formulas and Calculations

Formula or Calculation	Definition	Use	Disadvantage
Body Mass Index (BMI) Weight in lb × 703 ÷ Height in inches²	Measurement of weight in relation to height	Useful in determining if client is underweight or overweight	Does not measure lean tissue in relation to fat (i.e., bodybuilders may have a higher BMI owing to a larger amount of lean tissue but are not overweight or obese).
Ideal Body Weight (IBW) For men, 106 lb for the first 5′ of height and 6 lb for each inch above 5′; for women, 100 lb for the first 5′ and 5 lb for each inch after 5′	Determines ideal body for height of individual	Useful in determining if client is underweight or overweight	Does not measure lean tissue in relation to fat. A client may be considered underweight but may still be "overfat."
Basal Energy Expenditure (BEE) For men, 66.5 + (13.8 × Weight in kg) + (5 × Height in cm) − (6.8 × Age) For women, 655.1 + (9.6 × Weight in kg) + (1.9 × Height in cm) − (4.7 × Age)	Determines the calories needed to maintain the client's body at current weight	Useful as a part of determining total daily energy expenditure	Does not account for the desire to lose or gain weight and must be adjusted accordingly in that case. A measurement of only the calories needed to keep a human body alive.
Total Daily Energy Expenditure (TDE) BEE × Activity factor* (× Injury factor†)	Determines the calories required per day to maintain the client's current weight while taking into account activity levels and, if necessary, calories expended as a result of illness or injury	Useful when used with weight loss, weight gain, or weight maintenance plans	Most clients will overestimate their energy expenditure. Injury factors are used at the discretion of the clinician and may be overestimated or underestimated.

*Activity factors include 1.2, confined to bed; 1.3, ambulatory; 1.5 to 1.75, normally active; and 2.0, extremely active.

†Injury factors include 1.2, minor surgery; 1.35, skeletal trauma; 1.44, elective surgery; 1.6 to 1.9, major sepsis; 1.88, trauma plus steroids; and 2.1 to 2.5, severe thermal burns.

Copyright © 2010 by Saunders, an imprint of Elsevier Inc. All rights reserved.

Healthy Snack Ideas for Children and Adults

Breads, Crackers, Grains
Unsweetened cereal
Plain crackers
Toast (whole wheat)
Unbuttered popcorn
Tortillas
Dried rice and corn cakes
Baked tortilla chips
Pizza

Vegetables
Raw and cut-up carrots, celery, broccoli, cauliflower,
   cucumbers, tomatoes
Low-sodium vegetable juice, 6- to 8-ounce serving

Fruits
Apples, peaches, pears, plums, oranges, tangerines
Bananas (with peanut butter)
Cut-up watermelon, cantaloupe, or other melon
Berries
Unsweetened fruit juice, 4- to 6-oz serving
Canned fruit in natural juice

Meat and Protein
Sliced chicken or turkey or deli meat
Tuna on crackers
Bean and legumes
Hummus on crackers
Nuts (not recommended for young children because
   of choking hazard)

Dairy
Milk
Yogurt
Cheese
Cottage cheese
Sugar-free pudding

Other
Sugar-free ice pops
Sugar-free candy and chewing gum
Sugar-free gelatin

Adapted from U.S. Department of Health and Human Services, National Institutes of Health, National Institute of Dental and Craniofacial Research: *Snack smart for healthy teeth.* Available at: www.nidcr.nih.gov/HealthInformation/DiseasesAndConditions/ChildrensOralHealth/ SnackSmart. Accessed October 22, 2007.

Vitamins and Minerals Required for Calcified Structures

Vitamin or Mineral	Recommended Dietary Allowance (RDA) (for Adults)	Food Sources
Vitamin A (fat soluble)	900 μg (men); 700 μg (women)	Only found in animal foods: meats, milk, cheese, etc. Beta carotene found in orange fruits and vegetables (carrots, squash, pumpkin, sweet potato, apricots) and green leafy vegetables such as spinach
Vitamin D (fat soluble)	Adequate intake (AI) is 5 μg in the absence of sunlight; no set RDA	Sunshine, fortified milk
Vitamin E (fat soluble)	15 μg	Sweet potato, shrimp, sunflower seeds, canola oil, corn oil
Vitamin K (fat soluble)	AI is 120 μg (men); 90 μg (women)	Produced in the large intestine; cabbage, spinach, cauliflower, milk, eggs, garbanzo beans, beef liver
Vitamin C (water soluble)	90 mg (men)/75 mg (women)	Citrus fruits such as oranges, grapefruit; vegetables such as potatoes, green pepper, broccoli, and Brussels sprouts
Calcium	AI is 1000 mg; no set RDA	Dairy products such as milk, cheese, fortified soy milk; tofu, sardines, almonds. Vegetables such as broccoli, turnip greens, cauliflower, kale, bok choy
Phosphorus	700 mg	Dairy products such as milk, cottage cheese; meat and fish products such as salmon, sirloin steak
Magnesium	420 mg (men); 320 mg (women)	Vegetables such as black-eyed peas, spinach, baked potato. Other sources include oysters, dried figs, sunflower seeds
Fluoride	4 mg (men); 3 mg (women)	Fluoridated water, fluoridated dental products, teas, marine fish
Copper	900 μg	Shellfish, liver, nuts, seeds, legumes, whole-grain products
Manganese	No RDA Estimates of safe and adequate daily dietary intake = 2.3 mg (men); 1.8 mg (women)	Nuts, legumes, whole-grain cereals, leafy vegetables
Molybdenum	45 μg	Legumes, whole-grain products, nuts
Selenium	70 μg (men)/55 μg (women)	Animal products such as meats and shellfish. Vegetables and grains grown in selenium-rich soil (common in the United States)

Copyright © 2010 by Saunders, an imprint of Elsevier Inc. All rights reserved.

Anatomy of MyPyramid

One size doesn't fit all

USDA's new MyPyramid symbolizes a personalized approach to healthy eating and physical activity. The symbol has been designed to be simple. It has been developed to remind consumers to make healthy food choices and to be active every day. The different parts of the symbol are described below.

Activity

Activity is represented by the steps and the person climbing them, as a reminder of the importance of daily physical activity.

Moderation

Moderation is represented by the narrowing of each food group from bottom to top. The wider base stands for foods with little or no solid fats or added sugars. These should be selected more often. The narrower top area stands for foods containing more added sugars and solid fats. The more active you are, the more of these foods can fit into your diet.

Personalization

Personalization is shown by the person on the steps, the slogan, and the URL. Find the kinds and amounts of food to eat each day at MyPyramid.gov.

Proportionality

Proportionality is shown by the different widths of the food group bands. The widths suggest how much food a person should choose from each group. The widths are just a general guide, not exact proportions. Check the Web site for how much is right for you.

Variety

Variety is symbolized by the 6 color bands representing the 5 food groups of the Pyramid and oils. This illustrates that foods from all groups are needed each day for good health.

Gradual Improvement

Gradual improvement is encouraged by the slogan. It suggests that individuals can benefit from taking small steps to improve their diet and lifestyle each day.

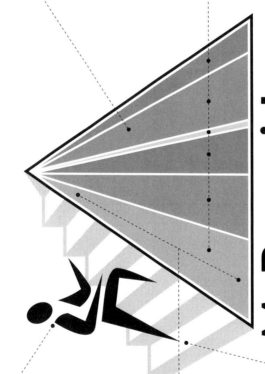

MyPyramid.gov
STEPS TO A HEALTHIER YOU

GRAINS   VEGETABLES   FRUITS   OILS   MILK   MEAT & BEANS

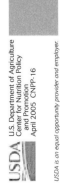

U.S. Department of Agriculture
Center for Nutrition Policy
and Promotion
April 2005 CNPP-16

USDA is an equal opportunity provider and employer.

Copyright © 2010 by Saunders, an imprint of Elsevier Inc. All rights reserved.

Body Mass Index Table

BMI	Normal						Overweight					Obese										Extreme Obesity															
	19	20	21	22	23	24	25	26	27	28	29	30	31	32	33	34	35	36	37	38	39	40	41	42	43	44	45	46	47	48	49	50	51	52	53	54
Height (inches)																					Body Weight (pounds)															
58	91	96	100	105	110	115	119	124	129	134	138	143	148	153	158	162	167	172	177	181	186	191	196	201	205	210	215	220	224	229	234	239	244	248	253	258
59	94	99	104	109	114	119	124	128	133	138	143	148	153	158	163	168	173	178	183	188	193	198	203	208	212	217	222	227	232	237	242	247	252	257	262	267
60	97	102	107	112	118	123	128	133	138	143	148	153	158	163	168	174	179	184	189	194	199	204	209	215	220	225	230	235	240	245	250	255	261	266	271	276
61	100	106	111	116	122	127	132	137	143	148	153	158	164	169	174	180	185	190	195	201	206	211	217	222	227	232	238	243	248	254	259	264	269	275	280	285
62	104	109	115	120	126	131	136	142	147	153	158	164	169	175	180	186	191	196	202	207	213	218	224	229	235	240	246	251	256	262	267	273	278	284	289	295
63	107	113	118	124	130	135	141	146	152	158	163	169	175	180	186	191	197	203	208	214	220	225	231	237	242	248	254	259	265	270	278	282	287	293	299	304
64	110	116	122	128	134	140	145	151	157	163	169	174	180	186	192	197	204	209	215	221	227	232	238	244	250	256	262	267	273	279	285	291	296	302	308	314
65	114	120	126	132	138	144	150	156	162	168	174	180	186	192	198	204	210	216	222	228	234	240	246	252	258	264	270	276	282	288	294	300	306	312	318	324
66	118	124	130	136	142	148	155	161	167	173	179	186	192	198	204	210	216	223	229	235	241	247	253	260	266	272	278	284	291	297	303	309	315	322	328	334
67	121	127	134	140	146	153	159	166	172	178	185	191	198	204	211	217	223	230	236	242	249	255	261	268	274	280	287	293	299	306	312	319	325	331	338	344
68	125	131	138	144	151	158	164	171	177	184	190	197	203	210	216	223	230	236	243	249	256	262	269	276	282	289	295	302	308	315	322	328	335	341	348	354
69	128	135	142	149	155	162	169	176	182	189	196	203	209	216	223	230	236	243	250	257	263	270	277	284	291	297	304	311	318	324	331	338	345	351	358	365
70	132	139	146	153	160	167	174	181	188	195	202	209	216	222	229	236	243	250	257	264	271	278	285	292	299	306	313	320	327	334	341	348	355	362	369	376
71	136	143	150	157	165	172	179	186	193	200	208	215	222	229	236	243	250	257	265	272	279	286	293	301	308	315	322	329	338	343	351	358	365	372	379	386
72	140	147	154	162	169	177	184	191	199	206	213	221	228	235	242	250	258	265	272	279	287	294	302	309	316	324	331	338	346	353	361	368	375	383	390	397
73	144	151	159	166	174	182	189	197	204	212	219	227	235	242	250	257	265	272	280	288	295	302	310	318	325	333	340	348	355	363	371	378	386	393	401	408
74	148	155	163	171	179	186	194	202	210	218	225	233	241	249	256	264	272	280	287	295	303	311	319	326	334	342	350	358	365	373	381	389	396	404	412	420
75	152	160	168	176	184	192	200	208	216	224	232	240	248	256	264	272	279	287	295	303	311	319	327	335	343	351	359	367	375	383	391	399	407	415	423	431
76	156	164	172	180	189	197	205	213	221	230	238	246	254	263	271	279	287	295	304	312	320	328	336	344	353	361	369	377	385	394	402	410	418	426	435	443

Source: Adapted from *Clinical Guidelines on the Identification, Evaluation, and Treatment of Overweight and Obesity in Adults: The Evidence Report.*

Copyright © 2010 by Saunders, an imprint of Elsevier Inc. All rights reserved.

Over-the-Counter Pharmacotherapies for Tobacco Cessation[*]

Pharmacotherapy	Contraindications	Dose	Duration	Side Effects	Cost per Day[‡]
Nicotine gum	Recent myocardial infarction Life-threatening arrhythmias Severe or worsening angina Pregnancy[†] Lactation Stomach ulcer Active temporo-mandibular joint disease Dentures, fixed dental bridges, loose teeth	1-20 cigs/day: 2 mg gum (up to 24 pieces/day) 20+ cigs/day: 4 mg gum (up to 24 pieces/day)	Up to 12 weeks	Mouth soreness Aphthous ulcers Jaw muscle ache Improper use: Dyspepsia Hiccups Gastrointestinal disturbance	2 mg: $3.28-$6.58 (9 pieces) 4 mg: $4.31-$6.58 (9 pieces)
Nicotine lozenge	Recent myocardial infarction Life-threatening arrhythmias Severe or worsening angina Pregnancy[†] Lactation Stomach ulcer	Initial dose based on time to first cigarette: within 30 minutes of waking, begin with 4-mg lozenge; after 30 minutes of waking, begin with 2-mg lozenge; at least 9/day, limit 20/day	Up to 12 weeks	Sore mouth and jaw Improper use: Nausea Hiccups Flatulence	2 mg: $3.66-$5.26 (9 pieces) 4 mg: $3.66-$5.26 (9 pieces)
Nicotine patch[§]	Recent myocardial infarction Life-threatening arrhythmias Severe or worsening angina Pregnancy[†] Lactation Stomach ulcer Psoriasis, eczema	21 mg/24 hours 14 mg/24 hours 7 mg/24 hours 15 mg/16 hours	4 weeks then 2 weeks then 2 weeks	Local skin reaction Insomnia In first hour, mild itching, burning, tingling After patch removal the skin may appear red for the next 24 hours If skin stays red more than 4 days or swells, or if a rash appears, contact healthcare provider; do not put on a new patch Improper use: Nightmares (dose is too high) Insomnia and/or headache (dose is too low)	$1.90-$3.89 (1 patch)

Adapted from Fiore MC, Bailey WC, Cohen SJ, et al: *Treating tobacco use and dependence: quick reference guide for clinicians,* Rockville, Md, 2000, U.S. Department of Health and Human Services, Public Health Service.

[*]The information contained within this table is not comprehensive. Please see package insert for additional information.

[†]Controversy surrounds pregnant women's use of the patch. However, some feel that nicotine replacement poses less risk to the mother and fetus than smoking because it is not inhaled and mainstream smoke effects are eliminated.

[‡]Average wholesale price from Wolters Kluwer Health: Medi-Span Electronic Drug File, Indianapolis, September 2008.

[§] Generic brands of the patch recently became available and may be less expensive.

Copyright © 2010 by Saunders, an imprint of Elsevier Inc. All rights reserved.

Prescription Pharmacotherapies for Tobacco Cessation*

Pharmacotherapy	Contraindications	Dose	Duration	Side Effects	Cost per Day[‡]
Bupropion SR[†]	History of seizure, eating disorder, head injury, bipolar disorder, anxiety disorder Use of Wellbutrin, monoamine oxidase inhibitor, sedatives, stimulants, excess alcohol, alcohol or sedative withdrawal	150 mg every morning for 3 days then 150 mg twice daily (begin treatment 1-2 weeks before quit date)	7-12 weeks maintenance up to 6 months	Insomnia Dry mouth	$3.62-$7.40 (2 tablets)
Chantix[†] (varenicline)	Less than 18 years of age; pregnancy; breast-feeding; kidney problems may prescribe a lower dose	Days 1-3 white tablet (0.5 mg), one tablet each day Days 4-7 white tablet (0.5 mg) twice a day—one in the morning and one in the evening Day 8 to end of treatment blue tablet (1 mg) twice a day—one in the morning and one in the evening	12 weeks	Nausea Changes in dreaming Constipation Gas Vomiting	$4.49-$4.75 (2 tablets)
Nicotine inhaler[†]	Recent myocardial infarction Life-threatening arrhythmias Severe or worsening angina Pregnancy[§] Lactation Stomach ulcer	6-16 cartridges/day	Up to 6 months	Local irritation of mouth and throat Dyspepsia, rhinitis, hiccups, headaches, unpleasant taste, cough	$5.29 (6 cartridges)
Nicotine nasal spray[†]	Recent myocardial infarction Life-threatening arrhythmias Severe or worsening angina Pregnancy[§] Lactation Stomach ulcer	8-40 doses/day	3-6 months	What to expect in the first week: Sneezing Coughing Watery eyes Runny nose Hot peppery feeling in back of throat or nose Side effects lessen over a few days	$3.72 (8 doses)

Adapted from Fiore MC, Bailey WC, Cohen SJ, et al: *Treating tobacco use and dependence: quick reference guide for clinicians,* Rockville, Md, 2000, U.S. Department of Health and Human Services, Public Health Service.
*The information contained within this table is not comprehensive. Please see package insert for additional information.
[†]First-line pharmacotherapies (approved for use for smoking cessation by the U.S. Food and Drug Administration).
[‡]Average wholesale price from Wolters Kluwer Health: Medi-Span Electronic Drug File, Indianapolis, September 2008.
[§]Controversy surrounds pregnant women's use of the patch. However, some feel that nicotine replacement poses less risk to the mother and fetus than smoking because it is not inhaled and mainstream smoke effects are eliminated.

Copyright © 2010 by Saunders, an imprint of Elsevier Inc. All rights reserved.

Calculation of Total Daily Calorie Intake for an Oral Surgery Client

A 35-year-old woman weighs 118 pounds and is 5 feet 6 inches tall. Her exercise includes walking 4 miles every evening. She has undergone oral and maxillofacial reconstructive surgery to correct her malocclusion.
- Conversion of pounds to kilograms: divide pounds by 2.2
- Conversion of inches to centimeters: multiply inches by 2.54

- *BEE:* $655.1 + 9.6(54) + 1.9(168) - 4.7(35) = 1327$ calories per day
- *TDE:* $1327 \times 1.5 \times 1.4 = 2787$ calories per day postsurgery to promote healing without a resultant weight loss
A registered dietitian should be the individual who adjusts specific nutrient values in the client's diet.

BEE, Basal energy expenditure; *TDE,* total daily energy expenditure.
The activity factor or injury factor may be adjusted to better describe the amount of activity or injury.

Strategies to Decrease Incidence of Early Childhood Caries

- Determine if the water supply that serves the client's home is fluoridated. If there is no fluoride in the water, or an inadequate amount, discuss supplement options with the parent. Fluoride is also found in over-the-counter mouth rinses, some bottled waters, and some foods and beverages (see Chapters 31 and 33).
- Put babies to bed without a bottle or with a bottle containing only water; do not let babies fall asleep with a bottle containing formula, milk, fruit juice, or other carbohydrate-dense liquid in the mouth. This is especially important because of decreased saliva flow during sleep and an opportunity for disease-causing bacteria to grow.
- Encourage children to drink from a cup as they approach their first birthday; wean children from bottle at 12 to 14 months of age.
- Instead of pacifying a baby with a bottle, rely on strategies such as cuddling, patting, talking, singing, reading, or playing.
- Give babies a clean pacifier. Do not give them pacifiers that have been dipped in sugar, honey, syrup, or other sugary substances or that have been "cleaned" in the mother or father's mouth.
- Never "clean off" a pacifier in another person's mouth. This practice can infect a baby's mouth with bacterial pathogens that cause dental caries and periodontal disease (vertical transmission of disease from parent or caregiver to infant).
- Never share eating utensils with an infant. Infectious *Streptococcus mutans,* the initiators of the caries disease process, can be transferred from the parent's mouth to the baby's mouth. Caries can develop as early as 11 months of age. The danger of infecting an infant's teeth is increased when the mother already has dental caries herself (vertical transmission of disease).
- Cleaning a child's teeth after ingestion of sugar-containing medication can prevent caries formation. Many over-the-counter medications and prescription drugs such as oral antibiotic liquid formulations contain up to 50% sucrose.
- Consult with a dentist and pediatrician about the need for fluoride supplementation and/or home-use fluoride gels if the fluoride history reveals a fluoride deficiency (see Chapter 10, section on dental history, and Chapter 31).
- Even before teeth begin to erupt, thoroughly clean the infant's gums after each feeding with a water-soaked infant washcloth or gauze pad to stimulate the gum tissue and remove food. When the baby's teeth begin to erupt, brush them gently with a small, soft-bristled toothbrush.
- Do not use fluoridated toothpaste until age 2 to 3 years (unless at a moderate to high risk of caries); fluoride is also found in some over-the-counter mouth rinses, community water supplies, some bottled waters, and some foods.
- Using a small amount (size of a pea or a smear) of fluoridated toothpaste inhibits decay and minimizes the chance of developing fluorosis when used after 2 to 3 years of age.
- When child is 2 or 3 years old, begin to teach child proper brushing techniques. But remember, parents or caregivers need to follow up with brushing and gentle flossing until age 7 or 8, when the child has the dexterity to do it alone.
- Thumbsucking should be discouraged after age 4; most children stop by age 2.
- Children should be supervised when using fluoridated toothpaste and oral rinses. If not monitored, they may swallow over four times the recommended daily amount of fluoride.
- Keep dentifrices and oral rinses away from children to avoid accidental ingestion.
- Schedule regular oral health appointments starting around child's first birthday. The oral health professional will check for cavities in the primary teeth and watch for developmental problems, as well as help to create a positive experience that may alleviate fear at future visits.
- Fluoride varnish can be used on very young children who are at moderate to high risk of early childhood caries.
- The use of 0.12% chlorhexidine gel or rinse is an intervention for early childhood caries because it inhibits growth of *S. mutans.*
- Xylitol-containing gum and mints (1.55 g therapeutic dose at least four to five times daily throughout the day) is used as a healthy treat to inhibit growth of *S. mutans.*
- Sealant applications are used to protect the chewing surfaces of children's teeth.
- Encourage the child to discuss any fears about oral health visits; do not mention the word *hurt* or *pain.* Saying "it won't hurt" instills the possibility of pain in the child's thought process.
- Determine if the water supply that serves the home is fluoridated. If a water filter is used, determine if it takes fluoride out of the water. If there is not fluoride in the water, discuss supplement options with the dental hygienist.

Copyright © 2010 by Saunders, an imprint of Elsevier Inc. All rights reserved.

Clinical Signs of Moderate Anxiety

Reception Area
Questions receptionist regarding injections or use of
     sedation
Nervous conversations with others in reception area
History of emergency dental care only
History of canceled appointments for nonemergency
     treatment
Cold, sweaty palms

In Dental Chair
Unnaturally stiff posture
Nervous play with tissue or handkerchief
White-knuckle syndrome
Perspiration on forehead and hands
Overwillingness to cooperate with clinician
Quick answers

Communication Strategies for Managing Dental Anxiety

Practice the tell-show-do technique.
Provide full disclosure of "unseen fears."
- Radiation
- Infection control
- Mercury exposure
- Nitrous oxide exposure

Provide full disclosure of financial matters.
- Costs of procedures per procedure
- Prioritizing as finances dictate
- Payment options
- Consider payment plans and financing options

Minimize waiting time in reception and treatment rooms.
- Occupy client by asking for form completion
- Choose treatment room music carefully
- Consider offering refreshments

Offer respectful care that gives client some control.
- Inquire into comfort: stop and alleviate pain or
  discomfort
- Offer contracted pauses
- Encourage client to use stop signal (e.g., raising
  hand or other device) when experiencing discomfort
  or when in need of a break

Stress-Reduction Protocols

Normal, Healthy, Anxious Client (ASA I)
- Recognize the client's level of anxiety.
- Premedicate the evening before the dental
  appointment, as needed.*
- Premedicate immediately before the dental
  appointment, as needed.*
- Schedule the appointment in the morning.
- Minimize the client's waiting time.
- Consider psychosedation during therapy.
- Administer adequate pain control during therapy.
- Length of appointment variable.
- Follow up with postoperative pain and anxiety control.
- Telephone the highly anxious or fearful client later the
  same day that treatment was delivered.

Medical Risk Client (ASA II, III, IV)
- Recognize the client's degree of medical risk.
- Complete medical consultation before care, as needed.
- Schedule the client's appointment in the morning.
- Monitor and record preoperative and postoperative
  vital signs.
- Consider psychosedation during therapy.
- Administer adequate pain control during therapy.
- Length of appointment variable; do not exceed the
  client's limits of tolerance.
- Follow up with postoperative pain and anxiety control.
- Telephone the higher medical risk client later on the
  same day that treatment was delivered.
- Arrange the appointment for the highly anxious or
  fearful, moderate- to high-risk client during the first few
  days of the week (Monday through Wednesday in most
  countries; Saturday or Sunday through Monday in
  many Middle Eastern countries) when the office is open
  for emergency care and the treating doctor is available.

*Antianxiety medication is prescribed by a dentist or physician.

Copyright © 2010 by Saunders, an imprint of Elsevier Inc. All rights reserved.

Recommended Maximum Doses of Epinephrine

Epinephrine Concentration (mcg/ Cartridge)	CARTRIDGES (ROUNDED OFF)	
	Normal, Healthy Patient (ASA I)*	Patient with Clinically Significant Cardiovascular Disease (ASA III or IV)†
1:50,000 (36)	5.5	1
1:100,000 (18)	11‡	2
1:200,000 (9)	22‡	4

From Malamed SF: *Handbook of local anesthesia,* ed 5, St Louis, 2004, Mosby.
ASA, American Society of Anesthesiologists.
*Maximum epinephrine dose of 0.2 mg or 200 mcg per appointment.
†Maximum recommended dose of 0.04 or 40 mcg per appointment.
‡Actual maximum volume of administration is limited by the dose of local anesthetic drug.

Calculation of Maximum Doses and Number of Cartridges (Single Drug)

Patient: 22 Years Old, Healthy, Female, 110 lb

Local anesthetic: lidocaine HCl + epinephrine 1:100,000
Lidocaine 2% = 36 mg/cartridge
Lidocaine: 2 mg/lb = 220 mg (MRD-a)
              3 mg/lb = 330 mg (MRD-m)
No. of cartridges: Malamed: 220/36 = approx. 6
              Manufacturer: 330/36 = approx. 9

Patient: 40 Years Old, Healthy, Male, 200 lb

Local anesthetic: prilocaine HCl + epinephrine 1:200,000
Prilocaine 4% = 72 mg/cartridge
Prilocaine: 2.7 mg/lb = 540 mg (MRD-a and MRD-m)
              Absolute maximum = 400 mg
No. of cartridges: Malamed and manufacturer: 400/72 = 5.5

Patient: 6 Years Old, Healthy, Male, 40 lb

Local anesthetic: mepivacaine HCl, no vasoconstrictor
Mepivacaine 3% = 54 mg/cartridge
Mepivacaine: 2 mg/lb = 80 mg (MRD-a)
              3 mg/lb = 120 mg (MRD-m)
              Absolute maximum = 400 mg
No. of cartridges: Malamed: 80/54 = approx. 1.5
              Manufacturer: 120/54 = 2

From Malamed SF: *Handbook of local anesthesia,* ed 5, St Louis, 2004, Mosby.
HCl, Hydrochloride; *MRD-a,* Malamed's maximum recommended dose; *MRD-m,* manufacturer's maximum recommended dose.

Local Anesthetic Agents and Duration of Pulpal and Soft-Tissue Anesthesia

Agent	DURATION (APPROXIMATE MINUTES)*	
	Pulpal	Soft Tissue
Short Duration		
Lidocaine HCl 2%	5-10	60-120
Prilocaine HCl 4% (by infiltration)	5-10	90-120
Mepivacaine HCl 3%	20-40	120-180
Intermediate Duration		
Lidocaine HCl 2%, epinephrine 1:50,000	60	180-240
Lidocaine HCl 2%, epinephrine 1:100,000	60	180-240
Prilocaine HCl 4% (block)	60	120-240
Articaine HCl 4%, epinephrine 1:100,000	75	180-300
Prilocaine HCl 4%, epinephrine 1:200,000	60-90	120-240
Long Duration		
Bupivacaine HCl 0.5%, epinephrine 1:200,000	>90	240-540

Adapted from Malamed SF: *Handbook of local anesthesia,* ed 5, St Louis, 2004, Mosby.
HCl, Hydrochloride.
*Short-duration agents provide pulpal anesthesia for 30 minutes or less; intermediate-duration agents for approximately 60 minutes; long-term duration agents for longer than 90 minutes. The classification of duration is approximate. Variations may be noted.

Copyright © 2010 by Saunders, an imprint of Elsevier Inc. All rights reserved.

Maximum Recommended Doses (MRDs) of Local Anesthetics Available in North America

LOCAL ANESTHETIC	MANUFACTURER'S MRD (MRD-m)			MALAMED'S MRD (MRD-a)		
	mg/kg	mg/lb	MRD (mg)	mg/kg	mg/lb	MRD (mg)
Articaine						
With vasoconstrictor	7	3.2	500	7	3.2	500
Bupivacaine						
With vasoconstrictor	1.3	0.6	90	1.3	0.6	90
Lidocaine						
No vasoconstrictor	4.4	2	300	4.4	2	300
With vasoconstrictor	6.6	3	500	4.4	2	300
Mepivacaine						
No vasoconstrictor	6.6	3	400	4.4	2	300
With vasoconstrictor	6.6	3	400	4.4	2	300
Prilocaine						
No vasoconstrictor	6	2.7	400	6	2.7	400
With vasoconstrictor	6	2.7	400	6	2.7	400

CALCULATION OF MILLIGRAMS OF LOCAL ANESTHETIC PER DENTAL CARTRIDGE (1.8-mL CARTRIDGE)

Local Anesthetic	Percent Concentration	mg/mL	×1.8 mL = mg/Cartridge
Articaine	4	40	72*
Bupivacaine	0.5	5	9
Lidocaine	2	20	36
Mepivacaine	2	20	36
	3	30	54
Prilocaine	4	40	72

From Malamed SF: *Handbook of local anesthesia*, ed 5, St Louis, 2004, Mosby.
*Cartridges of articaine hydrochloride in the United States read, "Minimum content of each cartridge is 1.7 mL."

Health Conditions That Require Special Consideration When Local Anesthetics Are Administered

Health Condition	Reason for Modification	Recommended Action
Hyperthyroidism	Possible exaggerated response to vasoconstrictors	Avoid or limit use (uncontrolled) of vasoconstrictors; use 3% mepivacaine or 4% prilocaine.
Atypical plasma cholinesterase	Toxic overdose to esters	Use amide anesthetic agents.
Methemoglobinemia	Potential for cyanosis-like state, respiratory distress, and lethargy in response to prilocaine and articaine	Use other anesthetic agents.
Malignant hyperthermia	Life-threatening syndrome caused by administration of certain drugs in combination with amide agents	Use amides or esters in normal doses; seek medical consultation.
Significant liver dysfunction	Difficulty metabolizing amide agents, potential for overdose	Seek medical consultation; use amide agents judiciously.
Significant renal dysfunction	Difficulty excreting local anesthetic agents, potential for overdose	Seek medical consultation; use anesthetic agents judiciously.
Pregnancy	Potential for complications with pregnancy	Avoid elective treatment during first trimester; use local anesthetics judiciously.

Copyright © 2010 by Saunders, an imprint of Elsevier Inc. All rights reserved.

Medications That Affect the Selection of Local Anesthetic Agents or Vasoconstrictors

Medication	Type of Contraindications	Drugs to Avoid	Potential Problem(s)	Action or Alternative Drug
CVS depressants, CNS depressants	Relative	Large doses of local anesthetics	Increased depression of CVS or CNS	Minimize dose of local anesthetic
Tricyclic antidepressants	Relative	Large doses of vasoconstrictors	Potentiate the action of epinephrine and increase blood pressure	Epinephrine concentrations of 1:200,000 or 1:100,000 used judiciously or mepivacaine 3% or prilocaine 4%
Phenothiazines	Relative	Large doses of vasoconstrictors	Potentiate the action of epinephrine and increase blood pressure	Epinephrine concentrations of 1:200,000 or 1:100,000 used judiciously or mepivacaine 3% or prilocaine 4%
Beta-receptor blockers	Relative	Large doses of vasoconstrictors	Potentiate the action of epinephrine and increase blood pressure	Epinephrine concentrations of 1:200,000 or 1:100,000 used judiciously or mepivacaine 3% or prilocaine 4%
Adrenergic neuron blockers	Relative	Large doses of vasoconstrictors	Potentiate the action of epinephrine and increase blood pressure	Epinephrine concentrations of 1:200,000 or 1:100,000 used judiciously or mepivacaine 3% or prilocaine 4%
Sulfonamides	Relative	Esters	Esters inhibit action of sulfonamides	Amides

CNS, Central nervous system; *CVS,* cardiovascular system.

Copyright © 2010 by Saunders, an imprint of Elsevier Inc. All rights reserved.

Clinical Manifestations and Management of a Local Anesthetic Overdose Reaction

Signs and symptoms	Management
Minimal to Moderate Blood Levels (Mild Overdose Reaction)	
Confusion	Terminate procedure.
Talkativeness	Reassure client.
Apprehension	Position client comfortably.
Excitedness	Administer oxygen.
Lightheadedness	Provide basic life support as
Dizziness	indicated.
Ringing in ears (tinnitus)	Monitor vital signs.
Headache	Summon medical assistance if
Slurred speech	needed.
Generalized stutter	Allow client to recover, and
Muscular twitching and tremor of face and extremities	discharge.
Blurred vision, unable to focus	
Numbness of perioral tissues	
Flushed or chilled feeling	
Drowsiness, disorientation	
Elevated blood pressure	
Elevated heart rate	
Elevated respiratory rate	
Loss of consciousness	
Moderate to High Blood Levels (Severe Overdose Reaction)	
Tonic-clonic seizure, followed by:	Terminate procedure.
Central nervous system depression	Position client supine, legs elevated.
Depressed blood pressure, heart rate, and respiratory rate	Summon medical assistance.
	Manage seizure: protect client from injury.
Unconsciousness	Provide basic life support as indicated.
	Administer oxygen.
	Monitor vital signs.
	Administer an anticonvulsant (prolonged seizure).
	Transport client to hospital after stabilization.

Some data from Malamed SF: *Medical emergencies in the dental office*, ed 6, St Louis, 2007, Mosby.

Clinical Manifestations and Management of a Client with an Epinephrine Overdose Reaction

Signs and Symptoms	Management
Fear, anxiety	Terminate procedure.
Tenseness	Position client upright.
Restlessness	Reassure client.
Throbbing headache	Provide basic life support as
Tremor	indicated.
Perspiration	Monitor vital signs.
Weakness	Summon medical assistance
Dizziness	if needed.
Pallor	Administer oxygen if
Respiratory difficulty	needed.
Palpitations	Allow client to recover, and
Sharp elevation in blood pressure, primarily systolic	discharge.
Elevated heart rate	
Cardiac dysrhythmias	

Some data from Malamed SF: *Medical emergencies in the dental office*, ed 6, St Louis, 2007, Mosby.

Copyright © 2010 by Saunders, an imprint of Elsevier Inc. All rights reserved.

Clinical Manifestations and Management of an Allergic Reaction

Type of Allergic Response	Signs and Symptoms	Management
Delayed		
Skin	Erythema	Administer antihistamine.
	Urticaria (hives)	Obtain medical consultation.
	Pruritus (itching)	
	Angioedema (localized swelling of extremities, lips, tongue, pharynx, larynx)	
Respiration	Bronchospasm	Terminate procedure.
	Distress	Position client semierect.
	Dyspnea	Reassure client.
	Wheezing	Provide basic life support as indicated.
	Perspiration	Summon medical assistance if needed.
	Flushing	Administer epinephrine.
	Cyanosis	Monitor vital signs.
	Tachycardia	Administer antihistamine.
	Anxiety	Allow client to recover, and discharge.
Laryngeal edema	Swelling of vocal apparatus and subsequent obstruction of airway	Terminate procedure.
	Respiratory distress	Position client supine.
	Exaggerated chest movements	Summon medical assistance.
	High-pitched sound to no sound	Administer epinephrine.
	Cyanosis	Maintain airway.
	Loss of consciousness	Administer oxygen.
		Additional drug management: antihistamine, corticosteroid.
		Cricothyrotomy if needed.
		Transfer client to hospital.
Immediate Anaphylaxis		
Skin	Pruritus (itching)	Terminate procedure.
	Flushing	Position client supine, legs elevated.
	Urticaria (face and upper chest)	Provide basic life support as indicated.
	Feeling of hair standing on end	Summon medical assistance.
	Conjunctivitis, vasomotor rhinitis	Administer epinephrine.
		Administer oxygen.
		Monitor vital signs.
		Additional drug management: antihistamine, corticosteroid.
		Transport client to hospital.
Gastrointestinal or genitourinary	Abdominal cramps	Same as management of anaphylaxis related to skin.
	Nausea, vomiting	
	Diarrhea	
Respiratory	Substernal tightness or chest pain	Same as management of anaphylaxis related to skin.
	Cough, wheezing	
	Dyspnea	
	Cyanosis of mucous membranes, nail beds	
	Laryngeal edema	
Cardiovascular	Pallor	Same as management of anaphylaxis related to skin.
	Lightheadedness	
	Palpitations, tachycardia	
	Hypotension	
	Cardiac dysrhythmias	
	Unconsciousness	
	Cardiac arrest	

Copyright © 2010 by Saunders, an imprint of Elsevier Inc. All rights reserved.

Calculating the Percentage of Gas Being Delivered

$$\text{Percentage of } N_2O = \frac{L/\min N_2O}{L/\min O_2 + L/\min N_2O}$$

$$\text{Percentage of } O_2 = \frac{L/\min O_2}{L/\min O_2 + L/\min N_2O}$$

Signs and Symptoms in Response to Nitrous Oxide and Oxygen Conscious Sedation

Concentration N₂O	Response
10%-20%	Body warmth
	Tingling of hands and feet
20%-30%	Circumoral numbness
	Numbness of thighs
20%-40%	Numbness of tongue
	Numbness of hands and feet
	Droning sounds present
	Hearing distinct but distant
	Dissociation begins and reaches peak
	Mild sleepiness
	Analgesia (maximum at 30%)
	Euphoria
	Feeling of heaviness or lightness of body
30%-50%	Sweating
	Nausea
	Amnesia
	Increased sleepiness
40%-60%	Dreaming, laughing, giddiness
	Further increased sleepiness, tending toward unconsciousness
	Increased nausea and vomiting
50% and over	Unconsciousness and light general anesthesia

From Bennett CR: *Conscious sedation in dental practice,* ed 2, St Louis, 1978, Mosby.

Copyright © 2010 by Saunders, an imprint of Elsevier Inc. All rights reserved.

Clients with Special Needs

CARDIOVASCULAR DISEASE

Commonly Prescribed Cardiovascular Medication

Brand Name	Generic Name	Indications for Use	Oral Implications
Glycosides			
Lanoxin	Digoxin	Congestive heart failure (CHF), atrial fibrillation	Excessive salivation, sensitive gag reflex
Diuretics			
Dyazide	Triamterene	CHF, hypertension	Decreased salivary flow
Maxzide	Hydrochlorothiazide		
Lasix	Furosemide		
Beta-Blockers			
Tenormin	Atenolol	Hypertension, angina	Xerostomia
Inderal	Propranolol		
Lopressor	Metoprolol		
Calcium Channel Blockers			
Cardizem	Diltiazem	Hypertension, angina	Decreased salivary flow, gingival enlargement
Procardia	Nifedipine		
Calan	Verapamil		
Catapres	Clonidine		
ACE (Angiotensin-Converting Enzyme) Inhibitors			
Capoten	Captopril	Hypertension	Xerostomia, taste impairment, oral ulceration
Vasotec	Enalapril		
Zestril	Lisinopril		
Vasodilators			
Nitroglycerin	Nitroglycerin	Angina	Burning under tongue

Copyright © 2010 by Saunders, an imprint of Elsevier Inc. All rights reserved.

Quick Reference—Dental Hygiene Care Implications for Individuals with Cardiovascular Disease

Disease	Implications for Dental Hygiene Care	Dental Hygiene Actions
Rheumatic heart disease	Special attention to oral self-care practices; self-inflicted bacteremias may occur when oral disease is present.	Careful manipulation of soft tissues during instrumentation; ADA-accepted antibacterial mouth rinse to reduce transient bacteremia.
Infective endocarditis	Client susceptible to reinfection with transient bacteremia. Prophylactic antibiotic premedication is indicated for invasive dental hygiene procedures.	Careful manipulation of soft tissue; antibacterial mouth rinse to reduce transient bacteremia.
Valvular heart defects	Infective endocarditis may occur after dental hygiene procedures that cause transient bacteremias. Clients receiving anticoagulant medication may have a prolonged bleeding time.	If anticoagulant medication is being used and scaling procedures are planned, dosage of anticoagulant medication should be discussed with client's cardiologist.
Mitral valve prolapse	Special attention to oral self-care practices because self-inflicted bacteremias may occur when oral disease is present.	Careful manipulation of soft tissues during instrumentation to reduce transient bacteremia.
Cardiac dysrhythmias and arrhythmias	Electrical interference can cause unshielded pacemaker to malfunction.	Use of electrical dental equipment is contraindicated.
Hypertension	Stress and anxiety about treatment may increase blood pressure.	Use stress reduction strategies; if blood pressure is uncontrolled, dental hygiene care is contraindicated.
Coronary (ischemic) heart disease	Stress and anxiety about treatment may precipitate angina.	Have nitroglycerin available during treatment. Implement stress reduction strategies; create atmosphere conducive to relaxation.
Congestive heart failure Congenital heart disease	None if person is under appropriate medical care.	Keep client in upright position to decrease lung fluid.

Basic Steps in a Cardiac Emergency Situation

Make certain client is comfortable; loosen restricting garments, elevate head slightly, provide reassurance.

Angina Pectoris
- Immediately administer nitroglycerin sublingually and 100% oxygen with a face mask or nasal cannula to prevent disease transmission.*
- Monitor vital signs.

Myocardial Infarction
- Transfer client to an emergency facility as soon as possible.
- Apply automated external defibrillator and/or administer cardiopulmonary resuscitation if necessary.
- Stay with the client until physician or emergency medical technician takes over.

*Note: An overdose of nitroglycerin can cause headache.

Copyright © 2010 by Saunders, an imprint of Elsevier Inc. All rights reserved.

DIABETES MELLITUS

Warning Signs of Diabetes

Type 1 diabetes mellitus is characterized by sudden appearance of the following:
- Constant urination
- Excessive thirst
- Extreme hunger
- Dramatic weight loss
- Irritability
- Weakness and fatigue, nausea and vomiting

Type 2 diabetes mellitus is characterized by slow onset; includes any of the type 1 symptoms and/or the following:
- Recurring or hard-to-heal skin, gum, or bladder infections
- Fatigue
- Blurred vision
- Tingling or numbness in hands or feet
- Itching

Adapted from American Diabetes Association: *Diabetes symptoms.* Available at: http://www.diabetes.org/diabetes-symptoms.jsp. Accessed October 8, 2008.

Hypoglycemia Compared with Hyperglycemia

Signs and Symptoms	Hypoglycemia (40-50 mg/dL)	Hyperglycemia (400-600 mg/dL)
Onset	Rapid (minutes)	Slow (days/weeks)
Thirst	Absent	Increased
Nausea and vomiting	Absent	Frequent
Vision	Double	Dim
Respirations	Normal	Difficult, hyperventilation
Skin	Moist, pale	Hot, dry, flushed
Tremors	Frequent	Absent
Blood pressure	Normal	Hypotension

Signs and Symptoms of Hypoglycemia

Lack of Glucose to the Brain (Neuroglycopenia)
- Confusion
- Blurred vision
- Paresthesia (tingling, burning, prickling sensation in arms and legs)
- Fatigue
- Stupor
- Convulsions
- Unconsciousness (coma)
- Irritability
- Impaired concentration
- Headache
- Somnolence (sleepiness or drowsiness)
- Psychiatric disorders (stupor)
- Transient sensory or motor defects (weakness, slurred speech)

Nervous System Compensations (Adrenergic Discharge)
- Anxiety
- Sweating
- Pallor
- Tachycardia
- Palpitations
- Hunger
- Restlessness
- Excitability
- Trembling
- Headache
- Nausea
- Dizziness

Features of Severe Diabetic Ketoacidosis

Features	Possible Causes
Symptoms	
Thirst	Dehydration
Polyuria	Hyperglycemia, osmotic dieresis
Fatigue	Dehydration, protein loss
Weight loss	Dehydration, protein loss, catabolism*
Anorexia	*
Nausea, vomiting	Ketones,* gastric stasis, ileus
Abdominal pain	Gastric stasis,* ileus, electrolyte deficiency*
Muscle cramps	Potassium deficiency*
Signs	
Hyperventilation	Acidemia
Dehydration	Osmotic diuresis, vomiting
Tachycardia	Dehydration
Hypotension	Dehydration, acidemia
Warm, dry skin	Acidemia (peripheral vasodilation)
Hypothermia	Acidemia-induced peripheral vasodilation (when infection is present)
Impaired consciousness or coma	Hyperosmolality
Ketotic breath	Hyperketonemia (acetone)

*Indicates speculated or unknown cause.

Copyright © 2010 by Saunders, an imprint of Elsevier Inc. All rights reserved.

Oral Complications of Diabetes Mellitus

Clinical Signs and Symptoms	Pathophysiology
Salivary and Oral Changes	
Xerostomia	Increased fluid loss
Bilateral, asymptomatic parotid gland swelling with increased salivary viscosity	Increased fatty acid deposition
	Increased salivary glucose levels
	Compensatory hypertrophy due to a decrease in saliva production
Increased dental caries, especially in cervical region	Secondary to xerostomia and salivary glucose levels
Unexplained odontalgia and percussion sensitivity (acute pulpitis)	Pulpal arteritis from microangiopathies
Lingual erosion of anterior teeth*	Complications of anorexia nervosa and bulimia
Periodontal Changes	
Periodontal disease†	Induction and accumulation of AGEs
Tooth mobility	
Rapidly progressive pocket formation	Degenerative vascular changes
Gingival bleeding	Microangiopathies
	Local factors
Subgingival polyps	Cause unknown
Infection and Wound Healing	
Slow wound healing (including periapical lesions after endodontics) and increased susceptibility to infection	Hyperglycemia reduces phagocytic activity
	Ketoacidosis may delay chemotaxis of granulocytes
	Vascular changes lead to decreased blood flow
	Abnormal collagen production
Oral ulcers refractory to therapy, especially in association with a prosthesis	Microangiopathies
	Neuropathies
Irritation fibromas	Altered wound healing
Increased incidence and prolonged healing of dry socket	Degenerative vascular changes
	Postextraction infection
Tongue Changes	
Glossodynia	Neuropathic complications
	Xerostomia
	Candidiasis
Median rhomboid glossitis (glossal central papillary atrophy)	*Candida albicans*
Other Changes	
Opportunistic infections: *Candida albicans* and mucormycosis	Repeated use of antibiotics
	Compromised immune system
Acetone or diabetic breath (seen when the person is close to a diabetic coma)	Ketoacidotic state
Increased incidence of lichen planus (as high as 30%)	Compromised immune system

Adapted from Lalla RV, D'Ambrosio JA: Dental management considerations for the patient with diabetes mellitus, *J Am Dent Assoc* 132:1425, 2001.
AGE, Advanced glycation end product.
*Although not a complication of diabetes per se, this pattern is seen when the person wants to maintain the weight-loss aspect of diabetes while ignoring or tolerating the hyperglycemic side effects. Client may not be taking proper insulin doses and may not be truthful when asked about this.
†Periodontal disease is seen in up to 40% of diabetic patients. Adequate periodontal therapy may result in decreased insulin requirements.

Copyright © 2010 by Saunders, an imprint of Elsevier Inc. All rights reserved.

CANCER

Common Signs of Oral Cancer

- Swelling, lump, growth, or area of induration or hardness anywhere in or about the mouth or neck, which is usually painless
- Erythroplakia patch (velvety, deep red)
- Leukoplakia patch (white or red-and-white patch)
- Any sore (ulcer, irritation) that does not heal after 2 weeks
- Repeated bleeding from the mouth or throat
- Difficulty in swallowing or persistent hoarseness

Management of Oral Manifestations of Cancer Therapies

Manifestation	Prevention	Palliative Measures and Management	Dental Hygiene Care Guidelines
Mucositis or stomatitis (related to direct effect of radiation therapy and cytotoxic chemotherapy).	Caused by toxicity of the cancer therapy. Early onset and severity can be minimized by consistent hydration and excellent bacterial plaque control. Gentle tooth and gingival brushing with extra-soft toothbrush. Discontinue toothpastes with strong, irritating flavoring agents and replace with baking soda and water paste. Discontinue alcohol-based rinses, full-strength peroxide, and irritating foods.	Increased hydration with water, saliva substitutes, ice chips, or sugar-free Popsicles. Cool-mist humidifiers may be helpful, especially in dry environments. Baking soda and water solutions (1 tsp baking soda, ½ tsp salt, and 16 oz water) may be used as rinses or placed in disposable irrigation bag (let solution flow through mouth to gently rinse). Topical anesthetics.	Do not schedule dental hygiene procedures while client is experiencing oral ulcerations and pain.
Salivary gland dysfunction or xerostomia (related to direct radiation damage to salivary gland tissue and possible indirect effect of chemotherapeutic agents. Salivary gland dysfunction is permanent after radiation therapy, whereas function usually returns after chemotherapy.	Eliminate use of products with alcohol and irritating agents. Diminish caffeine intake. Discontinue tobacco use. Humidify air with cool-mist humidifier. Consult with oncologist for salivary gland stimulant prescription.	Suggest over-the-counter saliva substitutes. Stimulate functional salivary gland tissue by chewing xylitol gum or wax bolus. Consult physician for salivary gland stimulant prescription. Lubricate lips with balm or cream (not pure petrolatum). Increase hydration with water, ice chips, or high-moisture foods. Thin foods with liquids. Recommend cool-mist humidifier, especially while client is sleeping. Suggest baking soda and water rinsing for ropy saliva (see details under mucositis).	To prevent rampant caries, encourage improved oral hygiene measures, diet low in sucrose, and fluoride supplementation (e.g., daily use of 1.1% neutral-pH sodium fluoride gels for 5 to 10 minutes in customized fluoride trays for home use).

Copyright © 2010 by Saunders, an imprint of Elsevier Inc. All rights reserved.

Management of Oral Manifestations of Cancer Therapies—*cont'd*

Manifestation	Prevention	Palliative Measures and Management	Dental Hygiene Care Guidelines
Infection: fungal, viral, and bacterial (related to chemotherapy-induced immunosuppression). Oral infections may not cause typical signs and symptoms. Candidiasis is common during radiation therapy.	Frequent and consistent oral hydration with water, ices, and/or saliva substitutes. Increase bacterial plaque control. Oral infections may be unrelenting when the client is severely immunosuppressed during chemotherapy.	Oral microbiologic culturing and assessment. Alert oncologist at first signs of oral infection. Encourage use of antifungals that are sugar-free.	Do not proceed with dental hygiene procedures while a client has an acute oral infection. Schedule dental hygiene procedures when the client's absolute neutrophil count is >1000/mm^3. If the client has a central venous catheter, the American Heart Association antibiotic prophylactic protocol should be followed for invasive dental hygiene procedures, including dental prophylaxis.
Bleeding (related to chemotherapy-induced myelosuppression).	Bleeding is not preventable, but bacterial plaque can exacerbate the complication if not consistently removed.	Refer to oncologist for management.	Dental hygiene procedures should be delayed until the client has a platelet count over 50,000/mm^3 or has a blood transfusion.
Rampant dental caries or demineralization (related to therapy-induced salivary gland dysfunction).	Bacterial plaque control. Frequent oral hydration with water, ices, or saliva substitutes. Daily 5- to 10-minute application of 1.1% sodium fluoride gel in custom gel carriers (soft vinyl trays adapted to extend beyond the cervical line of the teeth) or topical fluoride. In-office application of fluoride varnish to exposed cementum. Dietary guidelines to discourage frequent snacking on cariogenic foods, sugared beverages, or acidic beverages (diet sodas with citric or phosphoric acid). If there is evidence of dental decay despite daily fluoride application, place client on 2-week chlorhexidine regimen and in-office fluoride varnish application.	Same as prevention measures.	Encourage participation of client in planning oral hygiene homecare, and ensure strict adherence by frequent monitoring. Establish a 2- to 3-month continued-care interval until client demonstrates ability to care for teeth and acute side effects of therapy have resolved.

(Continued)

Copyright © 2010 by Saunders, an imprint of Elsevier Inc. All rights reserved.

Management of Oral Manifestations of Cancer Therapies—*cont'd*

Manifestation	Prevention	Palliative Measures and Management	Dental Hygiene Care Guidelines
Trismus or temporomandibular disorder (related to direct effect of radiation on muscles of mastication and/or temporomandibular joint [TMJ]).	Daily exercise for muscles of mastication: instruct client to open and close mouth 20 times without causing pain to the TMJ. This exercise should be repeated three times a day.	Same as prevention. Also instruct client to encourage further opening of the mouth by placing increasing numbers of tongue blades between posterior teeth for several minutes a day.	Dental hygiene procedures may need to be altered for clients with trismus to avoid exacerbating the associated pain (e.g., shortened appointments or sedation).
Soft-tissue necrosis and osteoradionecrosis (related to direct effect of radiation on tissue and bone; tissue becomes hypovascular, hypoxic, and hypocellular; damage to the bone and soft tissue is permanent).	All teeth within the field of radiation that have a poor lifelong prognosis should be extracted 14 to 21 days before the initiation of radiation therapy. Avoid all surgical insult to irradiated bone throughout the client's lifetime.	Referral to an oral surgeon for possible hyperbaric oxygen therapy and surgical management of the necrotic tissue and bone.	Frequent and regular dental hygiene continued-care interval to ensure prevention of periodontal disease and adherence to oral hygiene homecare protocol.

Copyright © 2010 by Saunders, an imprint of Elsevier Inc. All rights reserved.

HUMAN IMMUNODEFICIENCY VIRUS

AIDS-Defining Conditions and Diagnostic Criteria

Condition	Signs and Symptoms
Candidiasis	Of the bronchi, trachea, lungs, or esophagus
Cervical cancer	Invasive
Coccidioidomycosis	Disseminated or extrapulmonary
Cryptococcosis	Extrapulmonary
Cryptosporidiosis	Chronic intestinal (>1 month duration)
Cytomegalovirus disease	Other than liver, spleen, or nodes
Cytomegalovirus retinitis	With loss of vision
Encephalopathy	HIV-related
Herpes simplex	Chronic ulcer(s) (>1 month duration), or bronchitis, pneumonitis, or esophagitis
Histoplasmosis	Disseminated or extrapulmonary
Isosporiasis	Chronic intestinal (>1 month duration)
Kaposi's sarcoma	Intraoral or extraoral
Lymphoma	Burkitt's lymphoma
	Immunoblastic
	Primary, in the brain
Mycobacterium avium complex or *Mycobacterium kansasii*	Disseminated or extrapulmonary
Mycobacterium tuberculosis	Any site (pulmonary or extrapulmonary)
Pneumocystis carinii	Pneumonia
Pneumonia	Recurrent
Progressive multifocal leukoencephalopathy	—
Salmonella septicemia	Recurrent
Toxoplasmosis	Of brain
Wasting syndrome	HIV-related

Adapted from Centers for Disease Control and Prevention: *1993 revised classification system for HIV infection and expanded surveillance case for AIDS among adolescents and adults, December 18, 1992.* Available at: http://www.cdc.gov/mmwr/preview/mmwrhtml/00018871.htm. Accessed October 9, 2008.

Copyright © 2010 by Saunders, an imprint of Elsevier Inc. All rights reserved.

Recommended HIV Postexposure Prophylaxis (PEP) for Percutaneous Injuries

	INFECTION STATUS OF SOURCE				
Exposure Type	HIV-Positive Class 1*	HIV-Positive Class 2*	Source of Unknown HIV Status†	Unknown Source‡	HIV-Negative
Less severe§	Recommend basic two-drug PEP	Recommend expanded three-drug PEP	Generally, no PEP warranted; however, consider basic two-drug PEP‖ for source with HIV risk factors¶	Generally, no PEP warranted; however, consider basic two-drug PEP‖ in settings where exposure to HIV-infected persons is likely	No PEP warranted
More severe#	Recommend expanded three-drug PEP	Recommend expanded three-drug PEP	Generally, no PEP warranted; however, consider basic two-drug PEP‖ for source with HIV risk factors¶	Generally, no PEP warranted; however, consider basic two-drug PEP‖ in settings where exposure to HIV-infected persons is likely	No PEP warranted

*HIV-Positive, Class 1—asymptomatic HIV infection or known low viral load (e.g., <1500 RNA copies/mL). HIV-Positive, Class 2—symptomatic HIV infection, AIDS, acute seroconversion, or known high viral load. If drug resistance is a concern, obtain expert consultation. Initiation of postexposure prophylaxis (PEP) should not be delayed pending expert consultation, and, because expert consultation alone cannot substitute for face-to-face counseling, resources should be available to provide immediate evaluation and follow-up care for all exposures.

†Source of unknown HIV status (e.g., deceased source person with no samples available for HIV testing).

‡Unknown source (e.g., a needle from a sharps disposal container).

§Less severe (e.g., solid needle and superficial injury).

‖The designation "consider PEP" indicates that PEP is optional and should be based on an individualized decision between the exposed person and the treating clinician.

¶If PEP is offered and taken and the source is later determined to be HIV-negative, PEP should be discontinued.

#More severe (e.g., large-bore hollow needle, deep puncture, visible blood on device, or needle used in patient's artery or vein).

Copyright © 2010 by Saunders, an imprint of Elsevier Inc. All rights reserved.

SEIZURES

Management of Generalized Tonic-Clonic (Grand Mal) Seizures

1. Terminate procedure.
   - Remove instruments and dental appliances from client's mouth.
2. Position the client supine with legs elevated.
   - Turn client onto his or her side to minimize aspiration of secretions.
   - Place nothing in mouth or between teeth.
   - Loosen tight clothing.
3. Summon medical assistance.
4. Assess and perform, when necessary, Basic Life Support.
   - Perform head tilt–chin lift to maintain airway.
   - Protect client from injury.
5. After seizure, reassure client and allow him or her to recover.
   - Assess oral cavity for injury to teeth and tissues.
6. Discharge client to hospital, physician, or home with a responsible adult.

Adapted from Malamed SF: *Medical emergencies in the dental office,* ed 6, St Louis, 2008, Mosby.

Copyright © 2010 by Saunders, an imprint of Elsevier Inc. All rights reserved.

AUTOIMMUNE DISEASES

Autoimmune Diseases

Disease	Oral Manifestation(s)	Systemic Signs and Symptoms	Dental Hygiene Interventions	Pharmacologic Treatment
Cicatricial pemphigoid	Vesicles or bullae that rupture, leaving large areas of superficial, ulcerated, and denuded mucosa; lesions are painful and may persist for weeks or months if untreated	Involvement of other mucosal sites: conjunctiva, nose, esophagus, larynx, and vagina	Client education: practice of meticulous oral hygiene may decrease severity of lesions; demonstration on use of flexible mouthguard as a medicine carrier	Topical corticosteroids Systemic corticosteroids Immunosuppressive agents (cyclophosphamide)
Pemphigus	Superficial "ragged" erosions and ulcerations, haphazard distribution; most common areas are palate, labial mucosa, buccal mucosa, ventral surface of the tongue, and gingivae	Skin lesions: flaccid vesicles ("without tone") and bullae that rupture quickly, producing erythematous, denuded surface Positive Nikolsky sign Lesions persist and involve more surface area (without treatment)	Referral to physician and/or dermatologist is necessary Client education: side effects of long-term systemic corticosteroids on oral cavity and systemic health	Systemic corticosteroids Other immunosuppressive agents
Erythema multiforme (EM)	Erythematous patches that undergo epithelial necrosis; become large, shallow erosions and ulcerations with irregular borders; lesions emerge quickly; very painful; diffuse distribution; hemorrhagic, crusted lips common; gingivae and hard palate lesions rare	Diffuse sloughing and ulceration of entire skin and mucosal surfaces (in its severe form) Prodromal period: fever, malaise, headache, cough, and sore throat Skin lesions (50% of cases): variety of lesions present ("many forms"); early lesions flat, round, "dusky-red"; appear on extremities; may evolve into bullae with necrotic centers; "target lesions" may develop (highly characteristic of disease)	Referral to physician and/or dermatologist as necessary Client education: side effects of systemic or topical corticosteroid therapy	Topical corticosteroid syrups or elixirs Topical anesthetic agents (for painful oral lesions) Intravenous rehydration (in severe forms of disease) Systemic corticosteroids
Immune-mediated (type I) diabetes mellitus	In poorly controlled diabetes: cheilosis, xerostomia, glossodynia Enlarged salivary glands Increased glucose in saliva Fungal infections (candidiasis) Common: gingivitis, periodontitis, dental caries	Sudden onset: Constant urination Excessive thirst Extreme hunger Dramatic weight loss Irritability Obvious weakness and fatigue Nausea and vomiting	Immediate referral to physician necessary Client education: caries and diet; importance of recall frequency; periodontal disease and diabetes connection; blood sugar monitoring and regular insulin dosing; meticulous oral homecare	Fluoride therapy Salivary replacement therapy Amorphous calcium phosphate therapy Use of xylitol products Antimicrobial subgingival irrigation of periodontal pockets Antifungal therapy (if necessary)
Hashimoto's thyroiditis	Thickened lips Enlarged tongue	Lethargy, weakness, fatigue; dry coarse skin; swelling of face and extremities; huskiness of voice; constipation; slow heart rate (bradycardia); reduced body temperature (hypothermia)	Client education: referral to physician if suspected; stress importance of thyroid replacement therapy	Thyroid replacement therapy

Copyright © 2010 by Saunders, an imprint of Elsevier Inc. All rights reserved.

Disease	Oral Manifestations	Clinical/Systemic Manifestations	Dental Management	Medications
Rheumatoid arthritis	Temporomandibular joint (TMJ) involvement (75% of cases)	Swelling, stiffness, and pain (usually in joints of extremities); joint deformity; disability	Client education: risk of TMJ involvement; regular panoramic radiographs to assess mandibular condylar wear and TMJ; Premedication when indicated before dental services	Nonsteroidal anti-inflammatory drugs; Corticosteroids; Disease-modifying antirheumatic drugs (e.g., Plaquenil); Minocycline biologic agents (e.g., Enbrel); Immunosuppressants (e.g., methotrexate, azathioprine)
Sarcoidosis	Chronic, violaceous (of violet color) indurated lesions on lips; enlarged salivary glands; xerostomia; mucoceles may occur (oral manifestations are uncommon); Occasionally: submucosal mass, isolated papule, or area of granularity; may be normal in color, brownish-red, violaceous, or hyperkeratotic; bony involvement may mimic periodontal disease	Dyspnea, dry dry cough, chest pain, fever, malaise, fatigue, arthralgia, and weight loss; 20% have no symptoms; Granulomatous inflammation of skin (25%); Erythema nodosum (scattered, nonspecific, tender, erythematous nodules) may occur on lower legs; Xerophthalmia	Referral to physician if necessary; Client education: xerostomia's effect on teeth and tissues; increased risk of dental caries; salivary substitute; fluoride regimen (at home); Use of xylitol products; Amorphous calcium phosphate therapy	Case dependent
Systemic sclerosis (scleroderma)	Radiographically: widened periodontal ligament spaces; Microstomia; Limited opening of the mouth; Loss of attached gingival mucosa and generalized recession; Difficulty swallowing; Firm, hypomobile tongue	Raynaud's phenomenon; Skin develops a diffuse, hard texture; Fibrosis of organs (may lead to organ failure): lungs, heart, kidneys, gastrointestinal tract	Client education: augmentation of oral hygiene regimen in cases of limited manual dexterity	Immunosuppressive agents
Sjögren's syndrome	Erythematous oral mucosa; Xerostomia; Difficulty swallowing; Altered taste; Difficulty wearing dentures; Fissured tongue; atrophy of papillae	General malaise, fatigue; Dry skin; Xerophthalmia; Rheumatoid arthritis; Diffuse, firm enlargement of major salivary glands (usually bilateral), may be nonpainful, tender, or intermittent; Retrograde bacterial sialadenitis	Referral to physician or ophthalmologist if necessary; Client education: daily fluoride application at home to prevent xerostomia-induced dental caries; Daily fluoride regimen; Amorphous calcium phosphate therapy; Use of artificial tears and saliva; Antifungal therapy for secondary candidiasis; Xylitol gum and candy to stimulate salivary flow and therapeutic doses to interfere with *Streptococcus mutans*	Sialagogues (pilocarpine); Evoxac (cevimeline hydrochloride)

(Continued)

Copyright © 2010 by Saunders, an imprint of Elsevier Inc. All rights reserved.

Autoimmune Diseases—cont'd

Disease	Oral Manifestation(s)	Systemic Signs and Symptoms	Dental Hygiene Interventions	Pharmacologic Treatment
Lichen planus	White, interlacing lines over erythematous areas (Wickham's striae) Sites of involvement: bilateral posterior buccal mucosa, but may be found on lateral and dorsal of tongue, the gingivae, and the palate	Skin lesions are purple, pruritic, polygonal papules; located on flexor surfaces of extremities; itch and are painful; may exhibit Wickham's striae on surface of papules Other sites affected: glans penis, vulvar mucosa, and the nails	Referral to physician if necessary Client education: meticulous oral hygiene may lessen severity of gingival involvement	No treatment for reticular type Antifungal therapy needed if secondary candidal infection present Erosive lesions: topical corticosteroids (e.g., fluocinonide gel); follow-up for 3 months required (small chance of malignant transformation)
Systemic lupus erythematosus (SLE)	Oral lesions (5%-25% of patients) Location of lesions: palate, buccal mucosa, gingivae May appear lichenoid, may look nonspecific or granulomatous Ulceration, pain, erythema, hyperkeratosis	Fever, weight loss, arthritis, malaise Characteristic "butterfly rash" over malar area and nose (40%-50%) Kidneys affected (40%-50%); may lead to kidney failure Cardiac involvement common: warty vegetations on heart valves	Referral to physician if necessary Client education: meticulous oral hygiene; analgesic rinses when necessary; avoid excessive sun exposure	Systemic corticosteroids Other immunosuppressive agents
Chronic cutaneous lupus erythematosus (CCLE)	Painful lesions are practically identical to lesions of erosive lichen planus	Skin lesions: discoid lupus erythematosus (scaly, erythematous patches frequently on sun-exposed skin; head and neck areas)	Referral to dermatologist or physician if necessary Client education: avoid exposure to acidic or salty foods if painful intraoral lesions are present; avoid excessive sun exposure	Systemic corticosteroids Antimalarial drugs may be effective
Subacute cutaneous lupus erythematosus (SCLE)	Features intermediate between SLE and CCLE	Arthritis or musculoskeletal problems Photosensitivity Features intermediate between SLE and CCLE Skin lesions most prominent feature	Referral to dermatologist or physician if necessary Client education: avoid excessive sun exposure	Systemic corticosteroids Antimalarial drugs may be effective

Copyright © 2010 by Saunders, an imprint of Elsevier Inc. All rights reserved.

RESPIRATORY DISEASES

Signs and Symptoms of an Acute Asthmatic Attack

- Wheezing
- Cough
- Nasal flaring
- Dyspnea
- Feeling of pressure or tightness in the chest
- Need to stand, sit upright, or lean forward
- Increased anxiety and apprehension
- Perspiration
- Respiratory rate of more than 30 rpm
- Increased pulse rate of more than 120 bpm
- Rise in blood pressure (particularly in severe attacks)
- Confusion
- Agitation
- Cyanosis

Techniques to Be Avoided in Individuals with Certain Respiratory Diseases

Disease	Techniques Contraindicated or Used with Precautions	Rationale
Asthma	Use of air polisher	Aerosols created by air polisher may precipitate asthma attack
	Use of power-driven polisher	Polisher may exacerbate existing breathing problems
	Use of ultrasonic scaler	Pathogens found in bacterial plaque and periodontal pockets may be aspirated into the lungs
COPD: chronic bronchitis and emphysema	Avoid use of rubber dam	Rubber dam may cause more breathing difficulties
	Use of power-driven polisher	Polisher may exacerbate existing breathing problems
	Use of ultrasonic scaler	Pathogens found in bacterial plaque and periodontal pockets may be aspirated into lungs
	Nitrous oxide–oxygen analgesia	May produce cessation of respiration (apnea)
Tuberculosis	Use of air polisher	Airborne pathogens of communicable diseases may be transmitted by aerosols emitted by air polisher
	Use of ultrasonic scaler	Airborne pathogens of communicable diseases may be transmitted by aerosols emitted by ultrasonic instrumentation

COPD, Chronic obstructive pulmonary disease.

Copyright © 2010 by Saunders, an imprint of Elsevier Inc. All rights reserved.

COGNITIVE AND DEVELOPMENTAL DISABILITIES

Some Oral Manifestations Observed in Clients with Intellectual and Developmental Disabilities

- Self-biting
- Bruxism
- Thick, flaccid lips
- Microdontia
- Malocclusion
- Delayed tooth eruption
- Dental attrition and sensitivity
- Temporomandibular joint disorder
- Periodontal disease
- Heavy oral biofilm accumulation

Some Oral Manifestations Observed in Persons with Down Syndrome

- Underdeveloped maxilla
- Narrow palate with broadened alveolar ridges
- Congenitally missing teeth
- Malocclusion
- Enamel hypoplasia
- High rate of tooth loss caused by periodontal disease
- Shortened roots
- Enlarged tonsils and adenoids
- Mouth open with protruding tongue
- Fissured tongue
- Enlarged vallate papillae on tongue
- Microdontia
- Tetracycline tooth staining
- Periodontal diseases
- Heavy oral biofilm accumulation
- Low caries risk

Copyright © 2010 by Saunders, an imprint of Elsevier Inc. All rights reserved.

Medical and Dental Hygiene Considerations for Clients with Down Syndrome*

Concern	Clinical Expression	When Seen	Dental Hygiene Care Implications and Management Issues
Congenital heart disease (CHD)	Septal defects Tetralogy of Fallot Valvular defects Pulmonary artery hypertension	Newborn or first 6 weeks	Increased susceptibility to infection Prevention of infective endocarditis via antibiotic premedication Assess symptoms of secondary concerns before dental hygiene care
Hypotonia	Reduced muscle tone Increased range of joint movement Motor function problems	Throughout life Improvement with maturity	Important to address client's comfort while in dental chair Limited neck movement and pain Motor function problems making oral care difficult May exhibit spastic movements Considerations with client positioning Alterations in oral hygiene aids
Delayed growth	Typically at or near the third percentile of general population	Throughout life	Evaluate mental age Nutrition assessment and counseling During assessment may see delays in tooth development and facial growth
Intellectual and developmental delays	Some global delay, degree varies Specific processing problems Specific expressive language delay	First year, monitor Throughout life	Assess client's mental age to appropriately plan oral care instruction Use caregiver to communicate with client as needed
Hearing deficits	Otitis media Small ear canals Conductive impairment	Assess by 6 months Review annually	May need to speak clearly and use visual aids Thorough health history to identify hearing problems Involve the caregiver to determine what mode of communication would work best with the client
Eye disease	Refractive errors Strabismus Cataracts Tear duct abnormalities Amblyopia Nystagmus	Eye examination in early months Regular follow-up	Tactile communication important Assist client to prevent injury Thorough health history to identify ocular problems Involve caregiver to determine severity of problem When giving oral care instruction, be in clear view Adjust instruction to client need (e.g., do not expect client to see small anatomy on a radiograph) Avoid glare of dental light in the eyes
Cervical spine problem	Atlantoaxial instability Skeletal cervical anomalies Possible spinal cord compression	X-ray examination by 3 years of age	May require shorter appointments for comfort Aid client in walking to treatment area as needed Place client in comfortable position for treatment

(Continued)

Copyright © 2010 by Saunders, an imprint of Elsevier Inc. All rights reserved.

Medical and Dental Hygiene Considerations for Clients with Down Syndrome*—*cont'd*

Concern	Clinical Expression	When Seen	Dental Hygiene Care Implications and Management Issues
Thyroid disease	Hypothyroidism (rarely hyperthyroidism) Decreased growth, activity	Some congenital, most second decade or older Check by age 1, repeat	Be cognizant of room temperature for client comfort (may be cold and require a blanket) Assess pharmacologic history Create a low-stress environment Stress good oral hygiene to prevent infection Gingiva may appear spongy; tongue may be swollen
Obesity	Excessive weight gain	Especially 2-3 years old, 12-13 years old, and in adult life	May require large blood pressure cuff Nutritional counseling If client is in a group home, may consider doing an in-service May have an exaggerated inflammatory response
Seizure disorder	Primarily generalized tonic-clonic (grand mal) Also, myoclonic, hypsarrhythmia	Any time	Assess pharmacologic history Minimize stress Avoid flashing dental light into client's eyes Avoid stress-inducing situations Dental sealants and fluoride beneficial If gingival enlargement is present, more frequent continued care may be needed
Emotional problems	Inappropriate behavior, depression	Mid to late childhood, adulthood	Praise client to build self-esteem and cooperation Treat client with respect Assess client's frame of mind (via caregiver or healthcare decision maker) before appointment; validate at appointment Assess pharmacologic history
Premature senescence	Behavioral changes; functional losses	Fifth decade and older	Evaluate mental age Treat client with respect and concern Assess client's frame of mind with the caregiver before the appointment Assess pharmacologic history

*Also variable occurrence of congenital gastrointestinal anomalies such as Hirschsprung's disease (an extreme dilation of the colon), imperforate anus, duodenal obstruction, and tracheoesophageal fistula, as well as other conditions such as celiac disease, leukemia, Alzheimer's disease, attention deficit hyperactivity disorder, autistic spectrum disorders, hepatitis B carrier state, keratoconus (conical protrusion of the center of the cornea), dry skin, hip dysplasia, diabetes, and mitral valve prolapse.

Copyright © 2010 by Saunders, an imprint of Elsevier Inc. All rights reserved.

SUBSTANCE ABUSE

Oral Manifestations of Alcohol Abuse

- Xerostomia
- Poor oral hygiene
- Gingival bleeding on probing
- Coated tongue
- Glossitis due to nutritional deficiency
- Attrition related to bruxism
- Erosion related to vomiting
- Broken teeth due to accidents related to intoxication
- Buccal cervical caries

Red Flags for Suspicion of Substance Abuse

- Unreliable; frequently misses appointments
- Careless in appearance and hygiene
- Lapses in memory and/or concentration
- Alcohol on breath
- Speech is slurred; appearance of intoxication
- Needle marks on arm
- Rapid mood swings (within minutes)
- Frequently requests written excuses from work
- Frequently requests specific medication for pain
- Calls the dental office and complains of severe pain and requests that a prescription for pain medication be given without making an appointment with the dentist
- High tolerance to sedatives and analgesics
- Pupils are abnormally dilated or constricted

Assessment Findings Associated with Substance Abuse

Abused Substance	Eye Signs	Oral Findings	Treatment Considerations
Amphetamines	Dilated pupils Slow or no reaction of pupil to light	Xerostomia, increased caries, bruxism (extreme tooth wear in ecstasy users) leading to trismus.	Drugs can increase bleeding and interfere with coagulation. Chronic abusers should have blood tests before surgery or periodontal treatment.
Alcohol	Red, puffy	Tooth erosion from sugar in alcohol or regurgitation. Sialosis, xerostomia, glossitis. Stomatitis due to nutritional deficiencies and anemia. Orofacial injuries from accidents or violence. Severe infections due to immunosuppression.	Increased dosage of drugs for anesthesia and sedation. Increase in bleeding after surgery. Increased healing time due to immunosuppression.
Cocaine	Dilated pupils Slow or no reaction of pupil to light	Placement of cocaine in maxillary premolar area to test the purity of a drug sample can cause localized gingival and alveolar bone necrosis. Increased caries from carbohydrates added to cocaine as filler.	Possible spontaneous gingival bleeding from thrombocytopenia. Interaction between cocaine and anesthetics containing epinephrine.

(continued)

Copyright © 2010 by Saunders, an imprint of Elsevier Inc. All rights reserved.

Assessment Findings Associated with Substance Abuse—*cont'd*

Abused Substance	Eye Signs	Oral Findings	Treatment Considerations
Opiates and opioids (heroin, morphine, methadone)	Constricted pupils Nonreactive to light	Methadone is sugary syrup taken orally, which may increase caries.	Increased possibility of hepatitis, HIV infection from drug injection. Poor pain tolerance. Increased possibility of bacterial endocarditis in scaling procedures. Increased bleeding from thrombocytopenia. Interactions between opioids and dentally prescribed medications.
Barbiturates and benzodiazepines	Constricted pupils	Xerostomia, lesions on oral mucosa in the area of drug use.	Tolerance to sedative drugs.
Cannabis (marijuana)	Reddened sclera, swollen eyelids, tears	Leukoplakia and increased incidence of lingual carcinoma; gingival enlargement.	Interaction between cannabis and anesthetics containing epinephrine.
LSD, PCP	Dilated pupils Swollen eyelids	Orofacial injuries experienced while "tripping." Bruxism resulting in trismus.	Flashback that may cause panic attacks can occur owing to a stressful dental environment. Respiratory depression if opioids are prescribed.
Methamphetamine	Bloodshot eyes	Caries on buccal surfaces and interproximal surface of anterior teeth, bruxism, clenching, xerostomia	Be cautious if administering local anesthetic agents, sedatives, or nitrous oxide conscious sedation, or prescribing drugs; numerous drug interactions
Inhalants		"Glue-sniffer's rash," erythema around the labial borders, oral frostbite.	Anesthetic toxicity is increased, sensitization to epinephrine can occur; increased risk of seizures.
Anabolic steroids		High carbohydrate diet may cause increased caries.	Cardiac dysfunction can result from anesthetics containing epinephrine, increase in bleeding.

HIV, Human immunodeficiency virus; *LSD,* lysergic acid diethylamide; *PCP,* phencyclidine.

Copyright © 2010 by Saunders, an imprint of Elsevier Inc. All rights reserved.

EATING DISORDERS

Oral Health Education for the Client with an Eating Disorder

Oral health education programs should include discussion of the following:
- Cause of the observed oral signs and symptoms of eating disorder behaviors
- Effect of eating disorder behaviors on the oral environment and dental structures
- Oral health–systemic health connections
- Current oral status
- Potential progression of oral problems
- Harm reduction strategies (e.g., mouth guard use during vomiting; rinsing mouth with neutralizing rinse after vomiting)
- Effect of dietary habits on dental and oral health
- Frequency of eating
- Types of foods and drinks consumed
- Individualized oral hygiene education

Oral health promotion should include the following:
- Specific management and control of oral and dental manifestations of the disorder
- Amelioration of existing problems
- Prevention of progression of other characteristics
- Management of oral discomfort associated with dentinal hypersensitivity
- Recommendation for daily, at-home use of a neutral sodium fluoride rinse or gel
- Recommendation of sodium bicarbonate or magnesium hydroxide rinses, or saliva substitute, as necessary
- Construction of an oral mouth guard for protection during vomiting episodes
- Interprofessional collaboration for client-centered care

Possible Causes for Oral Findings Commonly Associated with Clients Who Have Eating Disorders

Perimolysis and Erosion
- Gastric or physical disturbances with associated vomiting (e.g., previous pregnancies, chemotherapy, hiatal hernia, duodenal or peptic ulcers, cancer-related therapy)
- High citric acid fruit or fruit juice intake
- Antabuse therapy (and associated vomiting) for alcoholism
- Habitual eating or sucking on vitamin C tablets or sweet-and-sour candies
- Medications containing hydrochloric acid
- Exposure to industrial acids

Parotid Enlargement
- Salivary neoplasms
- Inflammatory diseases (e.g., mumps, infectious mononucleosis, tuberculosis, sarcoidosis, histoplasmosis)
- Metabolic disturbances (e.g., malnutrition, alcoholic cirrhosis, diabetes mellitus)
- Autoimmune diseases such as Sjögren's syndrome
- Parotid duct obstruction
- Acquired immunodeficiency syndrome (AIDS)

Xerostomia
- Medications (e.g., antihypertensives, antidepressants, antipsychotics, antihistamines)
- Systemic diseases (e.g., diabetes, Sjögren's syndrome)
- Side effect of radiation therapy for cancer of the head and neck area
- Dehydration from recent flulike illnesses or high fever

Commissure Lesions
- Loss of vertical dimension or overclosure
- Vitamin B deficiency
- Yeast infection

Copyright © 2010 by Saunders, an imprint of Elsevier Inc. All rights reserved.

OLDER ADULTS

Alterations in Dental Hygiene Care of the Older Adult

Condition	Potential Risk Relating to Dental Hygiene Care	Prevention of Medical Complications	Dental Hygiene Care Plan Modification	Oral Complications

Angina pectoris	Stress and anxiety related to oral healthcare visit may precipitate angina attack in the oral healthcare setting
	
	Myocardial infarction may occur when older adult is in the oral healthcare setting
	
	Sudden death caused by disruption of cardiac rhythm or cardiac arrest without acute myocardial infarction may occur in the oral healthcare setting
		1. Detect older adult with history of angina pectoris.
		2. Refer older adult thought to have untreated or unstable angina based on health history for medical evaluation and treatment.
		3. Older adult under medical treatment for angina; during oral healthcare visit, every attempt should be made to reduce stress:
		  a. Concern and warm approach from oral healthcare professionals.
		  b. Make older adult feel free to talk about fears.
		  c. Morning appointments; however, some evidence supports early afternoon appointments as possibly better.
		  d. Short appointments.
		  e. Premedication—diazepam (Valium), 5-10 mg; one tablet preoperatively and/or night before; consider prophylactic nitroglycerin.
		  f. Nitrous oxide–oxygen analgesia or low-flow oxygen via nasal canula may be beneficial.
		  g. Effective local anesthetic—maximum dose of epinephrine 0.036 mg or levonordefrin 0.20 mg can and should be used; aspirate; inject slowly (do not use vasoconstrictors in patients with a serious arrhythmia).
		  h. Avoid epinephrine-impregnated retraction cords.
		  i. Avoid anticholinergic drugs.
		  j. Daily aspirin or other antiplatelet aggregation drugs do not usually cause clinically significant bleeding.
		4. Reinforce importance of risk factors that can be influenced by older adults.
		5. Terminate appointment if patient becomes fatigued or develops change in pulse rate or volume.
		6. If older adult develops chest pain during hygiene care, stop procedure and give nitroglycerin tablet sublingually.
		  a. If pain is relieved, let older adult rest and then continue with appointment or terminate appointment and reschedule for another day.
		  b. If pain continues longer than 5 minutes, monitor vital signs and give up to two nitroglycerin tablets one at a time during the next 10 minutes; if after three nitroglycerin tablets within a 15-minute time period pain persists and older adult's condition is stable, transport to hospital emergency room and call physician; if patient is unstable,
			Usually none; however, on rare occasions older adults may have lower jaw pain of cardiac origin (referral pain); history of what initiates the pain and how it is relieved should provide clue to its cardiac origin

		Older adults with stable form of angina, any routine oral healthcare Older adults with unstable form of angina, only care needed to deal with oral pain and/or infection		

Copyright © 2010 by Saunders, an imprint of Elsevier Inc. All rights reserved.

Congestive heart failure	Sudden death resulting from cardiac arrest or arrhythmia
	Myocardial infarction
	Cerebrovascular accident
	Infection
	Infective endocarditis (see Chapter 10)
	Shortness of breath
	Drug side effects
	a. Orthostatic hypertension (diuretics, vasodilators)
	b. Arrhythmias (digoxin, overdosage)
	c. Nausea, vomiting (digoxin, vasodilators)
	d. Palpitations (vasodilators)
		call for medical aid and be prepared to render cardiopulmonary resuscitation.
		1. Detect and refer to physician.
		2. No routine dental care until under good medical management.
		3. In older adults under good medical management with no complications, any indicated dental care can be performed. Cause of heart failure and any other complications must be considered in the dental hygiene care plan.
		  a. Hypertension
		  b. Prosthetic cardiac valve, prosthetic cardiac material used for cardiac valve repair, cardiac valvulopathy
		  c. Congenital heart disease
		  d. Myocardial infarction
		  e. Renal failure
		  f. Thyrotoxicosis
		  g. Chronic obstructive lung disease
		4. For older adults in the less-severe stages, Class I and II, use maximum dose of 0.036 mg epinephrine or 0.20 mg levonordefrin; avoid vasoconstrictors in Class III and IV older adults.
		5. Older adults should be in the semisupine or upright position during care to decrease collection of fluid in lung.
		6. Terminate appointment if older adult becomes fatigued.
		7. Drug considerations:
		  a. Digitalis—older adult more prone to nausea and vomiting
		  b. Anticoagulants—dosage should be reduced so that prothrombin time is two times normal value or less (takes 3 to 4 days)
		  c. Antidysrhythmic drugs (see cardiac arrhythmias)
		  d. Antihypertensive agents (hypertension)
		  e. Avoidance of outpatient general anesthesia
			In older adults under good medical management with no complications, any indicated dental care can be performed.	Infection
				Bleeding
				Petechiae
				Ecchymoses
				Drug-related
				a. Xerostomia
				b. Lichenoid mucosal lesions

Hypertensive disease	Stress and anxiety related to oral healthcare visit may cause increase in blood pressure; in older adult with already elevated blood pressure as a result of hypertensive disease, myocardial infarction or cerebrovascular accident may be precipitated
	Older adults being treated with antihypertensive agents may become nauseated or hypotensive or may develop postural hypotension
		1. Detect and refer older adults with marked elevation of blood pressure and those with moderate prolonged elevation of blood pressure for medical evaluation and treatment. For older adults with blood pressure higher than 180/110, delay elective care and refer to a physician.
		2. Older adults being treated with antihypertensive agents.
		  a. Reduce stress and anxiety of oral healthcare visit by premedication, short appointments, morning appointments, and concerned attitude from oral healthcare professionals; let older adult talk about fears and concerns related to oral healthcare visit; nitrous oxide–oxygen analgesia can be used, but hypoxia must be avoided.
		  b. If older adult becomes stressed, terminate appointment.
		  c. Avoid orthostatic hypotension by changing chair positions slowly and supporting client when he or she gets out of chair.
			In older adults under good medical management with no complications, such as renal failure, any indicated treatment may be provided.
			In older adults with complications, refer for evaluation.
				Xerostomia secondary to diuretic agents and other antihypertensive medications
				Mercurial diuretics may cause oral ulceration or stomatitis
				Lichenoid reactions may be seen with thiazides, methyldopa, propranolol, and labetalol

(Continued)

Copyright © 2010 by Saunders, an imprint of Elsevier Inc. All rights reserved.

Alterations in Dental Hygiene Care of the Older Adult—*cont'd*

Condition	Potential Risk Relating to Dental Hygiene Care	Prevention of Medical Complications	Dental Hygiene Care Plan Modification	Oral Complications
	Excessive use of vasopressors may cause significant elevation of blood pressure Sedative medications used in older adults taking certain antihypertensive agents may bring about hypotensive episodes	d. Avoid stimulating gag reflex. e. Select sedative medication and dosage cautiously. 3. Drug considerations: a. Use of local anesthetics with small concentration of vasopressor (epinephrine 0.036 mg; levonordefrin 0.20 mg); aspirate before injection and inject slowly. b. Use caution when using vasoconstrictors in older adults taking a nonselective beta blocker. c. Do not use gingival packing material that contains epinephrine. d. Reduce dose of barbiturates and other sedatives whose actions may be enhanced by many antihypertensive agents. e. Avoid use of general anesthesia in the office.		Lupuslike reaction, rarely seen with hydralazine
Myocardial infarction	Cardiac arrest Myocardial infarction Angina pectoris Congestive heart failure Bleeding tendency secondary to anticoagulant Electrical interference with unshielded pacemaker	1. No routine oral healthcare until at least 6 months after infarction because of increased risk of new infarction and arrhythmias. 2. Consultation with older adult's physician before starting routine oral healthcare to confirm older adult's current status. 3. Morning appointments. 4. Short appointments. 5. Termination of appointment if older adult becomes fatigued or short of breath or develops change in pulse rate or rhythm; inform physician. If older adult develops chest pain during appointment, manage as described for a client with unstable angina. 6. Use of local anesthetic with maximum epinephrine 0.036 mg and levonordefrin 0.20 mg; aspirate before injecting; inject slowly; avoid use of vasopressors to control local loss of blood; also avoid use of vasopressors in gingival packing material; do not use epinephrine in local anesthetics with severe arrhythmias. 7. Premedication before appointment and/or the night before to reduce stress associated with oral healthcare visit—diazepam 5-10 mg.	Older adults 6 months or more after infarction with no complication, any routine oral healthcare can be performed If complications such as congestive heart failure are present, oral healthcare should be limited to immediate needs only	

Copyright © 2010 by Saunders, an imprint of Elsevier Inc. All rights reserved.

(Continued)

8. Anticoagulant medication—if surgery or scaling procedures are planned for older adults taking warfarin, physician should be contacted to confirm that PT ratio (prothrombin time) will be two times normal or less, or international normalized ration (INR) less than 3.0; patients taking aspirin or other antiplatelet aggregation drug may have increased bleeding, but it is not usually clinically significant.
9. Digitalis—older adult more prone to nausea and vomiting; avoid stimulating gag reflex.
10. Antisialagogues—atropine and scopolamine may cause tachycardia; check with older adult's physician before using.
11. Antiarrhythmic agents—quinidine, procainamide—nausea and vomiting may occur; hypotension may occur; oral ulceration may indicate agranulocytosis.
12. Antihypertensive agents (refer to section in table).
13. Avoid use of instruments such as ultrasonic scaler with older adults who have unshielded pacemaker.

Asthma — Precipitation of acute asthmatic attack

1. Identify asthmatic older adult by health history.
2. Determine character of asthma:
   a. Type (allergic or nonallergic)
   b. Precipitating factors
   c. Age at onset
   d. Frequency and severity of attacks
   e. How usually managed
   f. Medications being taken
   g. Necessity for past emergency care
3. Avoidance of known precipitating factors.
4. Consultation with physician for severe, active asthma.
5. Older adult should bring medication inhaler to each appointment and use before appointment.
6. Drug considerations—avoid:
   a. Aspirin
   b. Nonsteroidal anti-inflammatory drugs (NSAIDs)
   c. Narcotics and barbiturates
   d. Macrolide antibiotics (erythromycin) if older adult is taking theophylline
7. May want to avoid sulfite-containing local anesthetic solution.
8. Chronic corticosteroid use may necessitate supplementation.
9. Premedicate anxious older adult (nitrous oxide–oxygen analgesia or diazepam).
10. Provide stress-free environment.

None required

Oral candidiasis reported with use of inhaler without spacer but is rare

Copyright © 2010 by Saunders, an imprint of Elsevier Inc. All rights reserved.

Alterations in Dental Hygiene Care of the Older Adult—cont'd

Condition	Potential Risk Relating to Dental Hygiene Care	Prevention of Medical Complications	Dental Hygiene Care Plan Modification	Oral Complications

Tuberculosis	Tuberculosis may be contracted by dental hygienist from actively infectious older adult
	
	Older adults can be infected by oral health-care professionals
		Many older adults with infectious diseases cannot be identified by history or examination; therefore all older adults should be approached using universal precautions.
		1. In older adults with active sputum-positive tuberculosis:
		  a. Consultation with physician before dental hygiene care
		  b. Care limited to emergency care only
		  c. Care in hospital setting with proper isolation, sterilization, mask, gloves, gown, ventilation
		  d. When older adult produces consistently negative sputum and remains in chemotherapy, is provided same care as normal patient
		2. In older adults with past history of tuberculosis:
		  a. Approach with caution; obtain good history of disease and its treatment (treatment of at least 6 to 18 months' duration); appropriate review of systems is mandatory
		  b. Should give history of periodic chest x-ray films and examination to rule out reactivation
		  c. Consult with physician and postpone care if:
		    (1) Questionable history of proper care
		    (2) Lack of appropriate medical supervision since recovery
		    (3) Signs or symptoms of relapse
		  d. If present status "free of active disease," care provided is same as for normal older adult
		3. In older adults with recent conversion to positive skin test (PPD):
		  a. Should have been evaluated by physician to rule out active disease
		  b. May be receiving isoniazid (INH) for 1 year prophylactically
		  c. Care provided same as for normal patient when physician authorizes care
		4. In older adults with signs or symptoms of tuberculosis:
		  a. Refer to physician and postpone treatment
		  b. If treatment necessary, care provided as in category 1
			None required	Oral ulceration (rare), tongue most common
				Tuberculosis involvement of cervical and submandibular lymph nodes (scrofula)

Joint disease: osteoarthritis	Joint pain, stiffness, and loss of mobility
	Increased bleeding from aspirin or NSAIDs
		1. Short appointments.
		2. Ensure physical comfort:
		  a. Position changes
		  b. Comfortable chair position
		  c. Physical supports
			Dictated by severity of disability; if severe, extensive care not indicated; encourage and facilitate oral	Temporomandibular joint involvement

Copyright © 2010 by Saunders, an imprint of Elsevier Inc. All rights reserved.

(Continued)

Condition	Complications	Management	Considerations	Oral Manifestations
		3. Aspirin or NSAIDs may result in increased bleeding but it usually is not clinically significant. 4. If client has joint prosthesis, antibiotics not necessary unless "high risk" (rheumatoid arthritis, diabetic, immunosuppressed or previous infection).	health–promoting behaviors	

Joint disease: rheumatoid arthritis	Joint pain and immobility
	Increased bleeding secondary to aspirin and NSAIDs
	Bone marrow suppression from immunosuppressives resulting in anemia, agranulocytosis, thrombocytopenia, and/or increased vulnerability to infection
		1. Short appointments.
		2. Physical comfort:
		  a. Position changes
		  b. Comfortable chair position
		  c. Physical supports
		3. Management of drug complications:
		  a. Aspirin or NSAIDs may result in increased bleeding but it is not usually clinically significant.
		  b. Gold salts, penicillamine, sulfasalazine, corticosteriods, immunosuppressives, or biologic agents; obtain complete blood count with differential and bleeding time.
		4. If joint prosthesis within 2 years of placement, prophylactic antibiotics recommended.
			Dictated by severity of disability and temporomandibular joint involvement; if severe, extensive care not indicated; temporomandibular joint surgery may be helpful; encourage oral health–promoting behaviors	Temporomandibular joint involvement; anterior open bite possible
				Stomatitis secondary to gold salts, penicillamine, and immunosuppressives

Joint prosthesis		1. Deep infection around joint prosthesis secondary to bacteremia caused by acute infection elsewhere in body; there is no evidence that transient bacteremias caused by invasive dental procedures can infect these prostheses after 2 years since placement. 2. Several authors have suggested that patients with active rheumatoid arthritis, severe type 1 diabetes mellitus, congenital or acquired immunodeficiency, hemophilia, loose prostheses, or history of infection of prostheses may be at risk, but there again are few data to support this concept (see Chapter 10).	Obtain good health history Few data support use of antibiotic prophylaxis In contrast, most orthopedic surgeons still recommend prophylaxis Obtain medical consultation regarding need for prophylaxis If orthopedic consultant does not recommend prophylaxis, proceed without it If orthopedic consultant recommends prophylaxis, consult with dentist and patient to determine best course of action	None

Copyright © 2010 by Saunders, an imprint of Elsevier Inc. All rights reserved.

Alterations in Dental Hygiene Care of the Older Adult—*cont'd*

Condition	Potential Risk Relating to Dental Hygiene Care	Prevention of Medical Complications	Dental Hygiene Care Plan Modification	Oral Complications

Stroke	Dental hygiene care could precipitate stroke
	Bleeding secondary to drug therapy
		1. Identify stroke-prone older adult from health history (hypertension, smoking, transient ischemic attacks).
		2. Reduce older adult's risk factors for stroke.
		3. For past history of stroke:
		  a. For current transient ischemic attacks (TIAs)—no elective care
		  b. Drug considerations—aspirin and dipyridamole (Persantine), obtain pretreatment bleeding time (less than 20 minutes); warfarin (Coumadin), obtain prothrombin time, which should be <20 seconds on the day of the scheduled procedure
		  c. Short morning appointments
		  d. Monitor blood pressure
		  e. Use minimum amount of vasoconstrictor in local anesthetic
		  f. No epinephrine in retraction cord
			Dependent on physical impairment
			All restorations should be readily cleansable; avoid porcelain occlusals
			Modified oral hygiene aids may be needed
				None

Diabetes	In uncontrolled diabetes:
	  a. Infection
	  b. Poor wound healing
	In older adult treated with insulin, insulin reaction
	In older diabetic clients, early onset of complications relating to cardiovascular system, eyes, kidneys, and nervous system (angina, myocardial infarction, cerebrovascular accident, renal failure, peripheral neuropathy, blindness, hypertension, congestive heart failure)
		1. Detect by:
		  a. Health history
		  b. Clinical findings
		  c. Screening blood glucose level
		2. Refer for medical diagnosis and treatment.
		3. Monitor and control hyperglycemia.
		4. Older adult receiving insulin—prevent insulin reaction.
		  a. Advise older adult to eat normal meals before appointments.
		  b. Schedule appointments in morning or midmorning.
		  c. Advise older adult to inform you of any symptoms of insulin reaction when they first occur.
		  d. Have sugar in some form to give in case of insulin reaction.
		5. Older adults with diabetes being treated with insulin who develop oral infection may require increase in insulin dosage; consult with physician in addition to performing aggressive local and systemic management of infection (including antibiotic sensitivity testing).
		6. Drug considerations:
		  a. Insulin reaction
		  b. Hypoglycemic agents, on rare occasions aplastic anemia, and so on
		  c. In clients with severe diabetes, avoid general anesthesia
			In well-controlled diabetes, no alteration of dental hygiene care plan is indicated unless complications of diabetes present, such as:
			Hypertension
			Congestive heart failure
			Myocardial infarction
			Angina
			Renal failure
				Accelerated periodontal disease
				Periodontal abscesses
				Xerostomia
				Poor healing
				Infection
				Oral ulcerations
				Mucormycosis
				Numbness, burning, or pain in oral tissues

Copyright © 2010 by Saunders, an imprint of Elsevier Inc. All rights reserved.

| Cirrhosis | Bleeding tendencies; unpredictable drug metabolism | 1. Identify alcoholic older adult:
  a. Health history
  b. Clinical examination
  c. Repeated detection of odor on breath
  d. Information from friends or relatives
2. Consult with physician to verify current status.
3. Attempt to direct older adult into treatment.
4. Laboratory screening:
  a. Complete blood count with differential
  b. Aspartate aminotransferase (AST), alanine aminotransferase (ALT)
  c. Bleeding time
  d. Thrombin time
  e. Prothrombin time
5. Minimize drugs metabolized by liver.
6. If screening test results abnormal, consult physician. | Because oral neglect is commonly seen in alcoholics, older adults should demonstrate interest in and ability to care for dentition before any significant dental hygiene care is performed | Neglect
Bleeding
Ecchymoses
Petechiae
Glossitis
Angular cheilosis
Impaired healing
Parotid enlargement
Candidiasis
Oral cancer
Alcohol breath odor
Bruxism
Dental attrition
Xerostomia |

Adapted from Little JW, Falace DA: *Dental management of the medically compromised patient*, ed 7, St Louis, 2008, Mosby. See Chapter 10 for prophylactic antibiotic premedication guidelines.

Copyright © 2010 by Saunders, an imprint of Elsevier Inc. All rights reserved.

FIXED AND REMOVABLE DENTURES

Types of Oral Soft-Tissue Lesions in Denture-Wearing Clients Indicating an Unmet Need for Skin and Mucous Membrane Integrity of the Head and Neck		
Oral Manifestation	**Due to**	**As Evidenced by**
Reactive Lesions		

Acute ulcers	Ill-fitting dentures
	Chemical agent irritation:
	   Denture adhesive
	   Denture cleanser
	   Self-medication
		Yellow-white exudates
		Red halo
		Varying pain and tenderness

Chronic ulcers	Same as above	Yellow membrane Elevated margin Little or no pain
Focal (frictional) hyperkeratosis	Chronic rubbing or friction of dentures	White patch Asymptomatic
Denture-induced fibrous hyperplasia (epulis fissurata, denture hyperplasia)	Ill-fitting denture	Folds of fibrous connective tissue Varying color Asymptomatic Typical on vestibular mucosa at denture flange contact
Infectious Lesions		

Denture stomatitis (denture sore mouth)	Chronic *Candida albicans* infection
	Poor oral hygiene care
	Continuous wear of dentures
	Ill-fitting dentures
	Systemic factors: anemia, diabetes, immunosuppression, menopause
	Systemic antibiotics
	Chemical agent irritation:
	   Denture adhesive
	   Denture cleanser
	   Self-medication
	Denture base allergy
		Generalized redness of mucosa
		Velvetlike appearance
		Pain and burning sensations
		Typical under maxillary denture

Angular cheilitis	Chronic *C. albicans* infection Pooling of saliva in commissural folds Riboflavin deficiency	Fissured at angles of mouth Eroded Encrusted Moderate pain
Mixed Lesions		
Papillary hyperplasia	Chronic *C. albicans* infection Chronic low-grade denture trauma	Multiple round to ovoid nodules: "cobblestone" appearance Generalized red mucosa background Rarely ulcerated Typical under maxillary denture

Copyright © 2010 by Saunders, an imprint of Elsevier Inc. All rights reserved.

Nutritional Guidelines for Maintenance of Oral Health in Edentulous and Partially Edentulous Clients

Nutritional Goal	Rationale
Eat a variety of foods.	Essential for repair and maintenance of structurally and functionally competent body parts; increases likelihood of getting necessary nutrients.
Select foods high in complex carbohydrates: fruits, vegetables, whole-grain bread, and cereals.	Blood glucose levels rise less if complex carbohydrates are consumed rather than simple sugars. Also, fiber in these foods promotes normal bowel function and may reduce serum cholesterol.
Protein-rich foods including lean meat, poultry, fish, dried peas, and beans are required daily.	Maintains strength and integrity of tissues, especially when exposed to physiologic stress.
Obtain calcium from dairy products; some nondairy foods also contain substantial amounts of calcium.	Calcium intake is critical to maintain bone mass. Alveolar bone is an early site of calcium withdrawal if dietary calcium intake is low.
Consume fruit juices containing vitamin C and citrus fruit daily.	Essential for repair and healing of wounds and for absorption of other vitamins and minerals.
Limit intake of processed foods high in saturated and hydrogenated fats and sodium.	Evidence links high fat intake to heart disease, certain cancers, and obesity. High sodium intake may cause hypertension.
Limit intake of bakery products high in fat and simple sugars.	Bakery products are often high in calories and/or low in nutrients.
Drink eight glasses of water daily.	Essential nutrient for all body functions.

Adapted from Zarb GA, Bolender CL, Carlson GE: *Boucher's prosthodontic treatment for edentulous patients,* ed 11, St Louis, 1997, Mosby.

Inexpensive, Safe, and Effective Cleaning Solution for Oral Appliances Devoid of Metal

- 1 tablespoon (15 mL) sodium hypochlorite (household bleach)
- 1 teaspoon (4 mL) detergent (e.g., Calgon)
- 4 ounces (114 mL) water

After soaking, the oral appliance must be rinsed thoroughly with water before reinsertion into the oral cavity.

Copyright © 2010 by Saunders, an imprint of Elsevier Inc. All rights reserved.

DENTAL IMPLANTS

Indications and Contraindications for Using Dental Implants

Indications
- Good general physical and mental health to facilitate client acceptance of the dental implant
- A commitment to a daily oral biofilm–control regimen to avoid peri-implantitis
- Manual dexterity to ensure that oral biofilm–control procedures can be performed effectively on a daily basis
- A sufficient quantity and quality of alveolar bone to retain the dental implant
- Continuous cooperation and communication between client and oral healthcare team

Contraindications
- Blood dyscrasias (prevent proper healing and clotting)
- Certain cardiovascular diseases
- Chronic renal diseases
- Corticosteroid use
- Debilitating or uncontrollable disease or compromised healing conditions, such as that resulting from radiation therapy
- Diabetic clients susceptible to gingival and periodontal disease
- Hypersensitivity of tissues to specific implant materials
- Inability of client to maintain optimal daily hygiene care
- Inadequate client motivation
- Local gingival infection
- Metabolic diseases
- Noncorrectable heavy bruxing problem
- Pregnant client
- Psychiatric disorders
- Rheumatoid disease
- Systemic infection
- Unattainable prosthetic reconstruction
- Unrealistic client expectations

Assessment Questions to Determine Whether Client Is a Good Candidate for Dental Implants

- When you eat, do your dentures cause you pain?
- Do your dentures fit adequately?
- Are your teeth mobile or displaced?
- Do you have any concerns about your dentures?
- Will you commit time daily to take care of your dental implants?
- Will you keep your appointments?
- Will you be able to wait 6 months for the final dental implant system?
- Are you willing to stop using tobacco?

Benefits and Risks of Dental Implants

Benefits
- Improved ability to masticate and speak adequately
- Enhanced self-confidence and esteem due to improved esthetics and function
- Decreased amount of bone resorption
- Decreased tissue ulceration and unnecessary pressure
- Elimination of direct force on the gingival tissue and alveolar crest
- Increased retention of the prosthetic appliance
- Preservation of the remaining bone structure

Risks
- Failure to osseointegrate
- Improper client selection
- Improper control of immediate stress or load force
- Improper oral hygiene care
- Inadequate allowance of healing time and interface development
- Inadequate control of manufacture quality
- Inadequate implant or prosthetic design
- Periimplantitis
- Surgical complications

Continuing-Care Schedule for Clients with Dental Implants

Care	Care Schedule
Once implant is placed	Oral hygiene education and instruction
Radiographic evaluation of bone and periodontal structures	Every 3 months for first year and annually thereafter, unless necessary earlier
Continued-care appointment	Every 3 months for first year; thereafter evaluate for 4-month continued-care appointments
Removal and cleaning of implant superstructure	Annually, during continued-care appointment
Any signs of infection	Return to general dentist in 10-14 days, or refer to specialist

Be sure to commit client to the next continued-care appointment before appointment ends.

Copyright © 2010 by Saunders, an imprint of Elsevier Inc. All rights reserved.

ORTHODONTIC APPLIANCES

Oral Hygiene Recommendations for Clients with Fixed Appliances

- Brush three times a day with fluoride dentifrice (0.22% sodium fluoride).
- Aim toothbrush bristles at the gingival margin to stimulate and debride the gingival margin area.
- Brush around brackets, placing the bristles above and aiming them down toward the brackets, then placing the bristles below and aiming them up toward the brackets.
- Consider using specialized orthodontic brushes.
- Consider using power toothbrushes.
- Use floss threader or super floss to clean subgingivally on proximal surfaces.
- Use Proxabrush or Stim-U-Dent to get under the archwire and between teeth if the space is wide enough.
- Use the oral irrigator on low power at least once a day. Aim it perpendicularly to contact just above the papilla.
- Use disclosing tablets to check for plaque removal.
- Rinse with 0.05% sodium fluoride rinse for 1 minute after brushing or "rinse, spit, go to bed."
- Use chlorhexidine 0.1% to 0.2% as a 1-minute rinse twice daily for short periods (i.e., a few weeks); however, there should be at least 30 to 60 minutes between this and fluoride treatment for effective use of each.

Foods to Avoid and to Include When Wearing Fixed Orthodontic Appliances

Foods to Avoid
- Chewing gum, sugarless or otherwise
- Sticky foods (e.g., peanut butter, sticky candy such as caramels, Sugar Daddies, Tootsie Rolls)
- Hard foods (e.g., nuts, corn on the cob, popcorn, hard candy, bagels, apples, whole carrots, hard pretzels, hard chips, jerky)
- Ice

Foods to Include
- Foods low in sugar
- Fresh fruits and vegetables cut in pieces
- Applesauce
- Yogurt
- Pasta
- Representatives from all areas of the food pyramid cut in pieces if needed (see Chapter 33)

Copyright © 2010 by Saunders, an imprint of Elsevier Inc. All rights reserved.

ABUSE AND NEGLECT

Indicators of Abuse and Neglect in Clients

Type of Abuse	Indicators
Physical abuse	Unexplained bruises in various stages of healing
	Multiple bruises on face, lips, arms, legs
	Bruising on nonbony protrusions*
	Shaped or patterned injuries or bruises such as belt or belt buckle marks, iron burns, hand slap or finger markings, rope burns
	Cigarettes burns
	Scalding injuries (glovelike immersion burns)
	Broken nose
	Black eyes
	Inappropriate seasonal dress (long sleeves in the summer to cover bruises)
	Cuts or lacerations especially on the face or neck
	Oral trauma including:
	Torn frenum
	Avulsed teeth
	Discolored teeth (due to pulpal necrosis), indicator of past traumatic injury
	Fractured teeth
	Gingival abrasions
	Burns from scalding liquids or hot utensils
	Oral lacerations due to forced feeding
	Trauma to the corners of the mouth (may indicate the use of gags)
	Gingival contusions
	Petechiae or bruising (may indicate forced oral sex)
	Palatal lesions and scars
Neglect	Poor hygiene
	Rampant caries, early childhood caries
	Unmet medical or dental needs
	Lack of regularity of dental hygiene appointments
	Poor or no parental supervision
Sexual abuse	Petechiae on soft palate (may be a sign of forced oral sex)
	Venereal warts (condyloma acuminatum) on lips, tongue, palate, or gingivae
	Venereal disease (in prepuberty)
	Itching of genitalia
	Difficulty in walking or sitting
Emotional maltreatment	Withdrawn or fatigued
	Record of suicide attempts
	Parent or caregiver:
	Constantly blames or berates child
	Is unconcerned about child
	Overtly rejects child

*Normal childhood injuries tend to occur on bony protrusions, e.g., knees and elbows. Bruises caused by abuse are often found on nonbony areas, e.g., arms, legs, and neck.

Copyright © 2010 by Saunders, an imprint of Elsevier Inc. All rights reserved.